Diseases in the cranio-cervical junction

Diseases in the cranio-cervical junction

Anatomical and pathological aspects and detailed clinical accounts

Edited by
D. Voth and P. Glees

In collaboration with
K. Schürmann and F. Schilling

Walter de Gruyter
Berlin · New York 1987

Prof. Dr. med. Dieter Voth
Klinikum der Johannes-Gutenberg-Universität
Neurochirurgische Klinik und Poliklinik
Langenbeckstr. 1 · D-6500 Mainz

Prof. Dr. med. Paul Glees
University of Cambridge · Department of Anatomy
Downing Street
Cambridge CB2 3DY · Great Britain

This book contains 254 illustrations and 57 tables.

CIP-Kurztitelaufnahme der Deutschen Bibliothek

Diseases in the cranio-cervical junction:
anatomic. and patholog. aspects and detailed clin. accounts / ed. by D. Voth and P. Glees. In collab. with K. Schürmann and F. Schilling. – Berlin ; New York : de Gruyter, 1987.
ISBN 3-11-011122-5 (Berlin)
ISBN 0-89925-265-6 (New York)
NE: Voth, Dieter [Hrsg.]

Library of Congress Cataloging in Publication Data

Diseases in the cranio-cervical junction.

Proceedings of a conference held at Mainz University.
Dedicated to the memory of Johann Wolfgang Goethe.
Includes bibliographies and indexes.
1. Vertebrae, Cervical– –Diseases– –Congresses. 2. Skull– –Diseases– –Congresses. 3. Vertebrae, Cervical– –Wounds and injuries– –Congresses. 4. Vertebrae, Cervical– –Surgery– –Congresses. I. Voth, D. (Dieter), 1935– II. Glees, Paul. [DNLM: 1. Brain Diseases– –congresses. 2. Cervical Vertebrae– –congresses. 3. Skull– –congresses. 4. Spinal Diseases – –congresses. WE 725 D611]
RD763.D54 1987 617'.53 86-29210

ISBN 0-89925-265-6 (U.S.)

 Typesetting and Printing: Arthur Collignon GmbH, Berlin. – Binding: Dieter Mikolai, Berlin. – Cover design: Rudolf Hübler, Berlin. – Printed in Germany.

This book is dedicated to the memory of the great natural philosopher and celebrated poet Johann Wolfgang von Goethe (born 1749 in Frankfurt (Main), died 1832 in Weimar).

Goethe devoted much of his time studying comparative morphology in particular the skull and we quote:

Ebenso war der Aufbau des Schädels aus Wirbelknochen, einmal zugegeben, von wichtigen Folgen, denn die Identität aller noch so entschieden geformten Einzelheiten des Typus war hierdurch gleichfalls gesichert.

(J. W. Goethe, Zur Morphologie, Zweiten Bandes zweites Heft, 1828)

Daß die drei hintersten Knochen des Schädels aus Wirbelknochen abzuleiten seien, läßt sich mit den Augen des Leibes gar wohl erkennen. Es sind nicht nur drei, es sind sechs Wirbelknochen, aus denen der Kopf zusammengesetzt ist.

(J. W. Goethe, Paralipomena 21, 1817 – 1824)

Die Pflanze geht von Knoten zu Knoten und schließt zuletzt ab mit der Blüte und dem Samen. In der Tierwelt ist es nicht anders. Die Raupe, der Bandwurm geht von Knoten zu Knoten und bildet zuletzt einen Kopf, bei den höher stehenden Tieren und dem Menschen sind es die Wirbelknochen, die sich anfügen und anfügen und mit dem Kopf abschließen, in welchem sich die Kräfte konzentrieren.

(J. W. Goethe, Gespräche mit Eckermann, 13. 2. 1829)

Preface

The transitional area between cranium and cervical vertebrae has many specific anatomical and clinical particularities. No other body region is threatened to such a degree by critical diseases and traumatic dislocations. In recent years, modern methods of investigation have made it possible to foresee threats to health and have opened the way to new approaches to dealing with states of emergencies and to modes of treatment.

Traditionally, the Symposia at Mayence University aim to gather a wide spectrum of contributions from neurosurgery, orthopaedy, accident surgery, neurology and clinical medicine. Furthermore functional anatomy and embryology, general and special pathology have fully been considered.

We sincerely hope that these contributions convey the rapid diagnostic and therapeutic advances to the medical profession to direct their patients into the right channels for specialised treatment.

Mainz/Cambridge, Spring 1987 D. Voth and P. Glees

Contents

III Traumatic lesions

IV Malformations, system diseases and functional disturbances

V Inflammatory and degenerative lesions

I Introduction

The cranio-cervical junction in the light of a socio-logical cultural analysis (an introductory address)

D. Voth

When going through Western cultural history one interesting fact emerges related to our theme of this meeting namely that the head detached at the cranio-cervical junction (becoming essentially a skull) takes on a *'pars pro toto'* function and represent man. The head or skull acts as a human symbol, both in fairy tales and myths and is endowed with the spirit of man be it enemy or friend.

When Hamlet addresses the skull of Yorick at the beginning of the 5th act, "Where be your gibes now? Your gambols? Your songs? Your flashes of merriment, that were wont be set the table on a roar? Not one now, to mock your own grinning? Quite chap-fallen? Now get you to my lady's chamber and tell her, let her paint an inch thick, to this favour she must come; make her laugh at that."

The numerous 'talking' heads and skulls in the literature of black romantic need only to be mentioned, but even in more recent literature we find the motive of

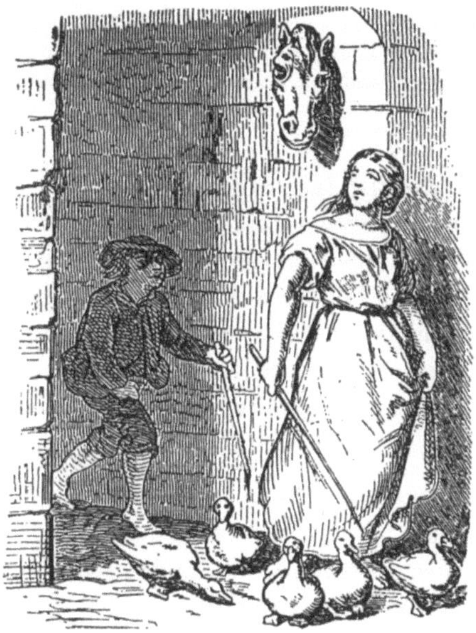

Fig. 1 The king's daughter as goose maid and the talking head of the horse Falada. Illustration by Oswald Sickert (born 1828).

'pars pro toto' like in the novel by Thomas Mann 'Die vertauschten Köpfe' (The exchanged heads). In this tale the head is the real person and when transplanted onto the body of another person gives the whole of this other body the identity of the head. Fairy tales confirm the believe that the head is the essential part, for one of Grimm's story 'The goose maid' gives a vivid account of the speaking horse Falada, still faithful to the maid after its death. The head of horse, nailed to the arch of the gate (fig. 1) still keeps its ability to talk to its mistress, instrumental in her final return as the king's daughter.

Following a short expedition into the realm of myths and legends, as for example the "head of Gorgo" – Perseus beheaded Gorgon Medusa – Athena wore the painted head on her shield as a petrifying fright. It is somewhat typical for the variability of these early pictures and archetypes, that the bugbear with boar teeth and put out tongue later changed to the head of a beautiful woman with hair interlaced with snakes (fig. 2).

a b

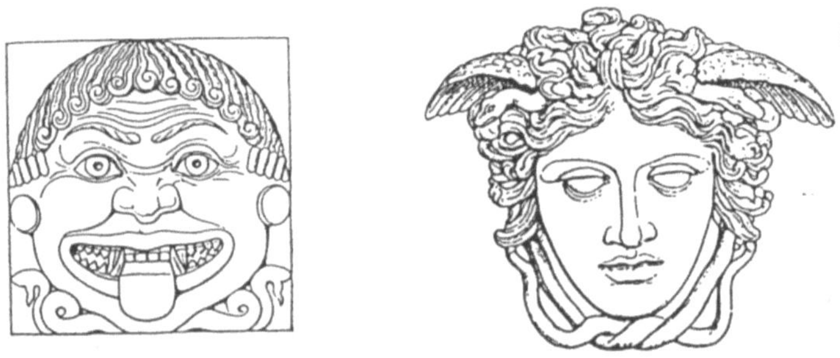

Fig. 2 Presentation of the Gorgoneion, the head which Perseus cut off the Gorgon Medusa. In early presentations (a) it decorated weapons, amulets and architecture objects as a fright which should scare away harm (Apotropaion). In the later art this fright changed to the presentation of a beautiful, in a death-struggle stiffened head of a woman, like the Rondaninic Medusa (b).

Salome's dance around the head of John the Baptist (fig. 3) was thought of in earlier times to be the expression of vengeance but was modified in the 19th Century to symbolise the possession of a lover's head – as *pars pro toto* – when the whole person was for ever unobtainable. This version was extensively used by numerous writers (Oscar Wilde, Gustave Flaubert, Jules Laforgue, Antoine Sabatier) and painters (Gustave Moreau, Aubrey Beardsley, Henri Ragnault, Jean Lorrain, Max Klinger) and set into music by Richard Strauss (1864 – 1949).

Looking back once more on ancient rites, preserved even in modern times we can refer to the customs of farmhouses in Lower Saxony of having horses skulls made of wood fixed to their roof. They symbolise protective and magic properties of the farmer's most favoured animal since heathen times (fig. 4).

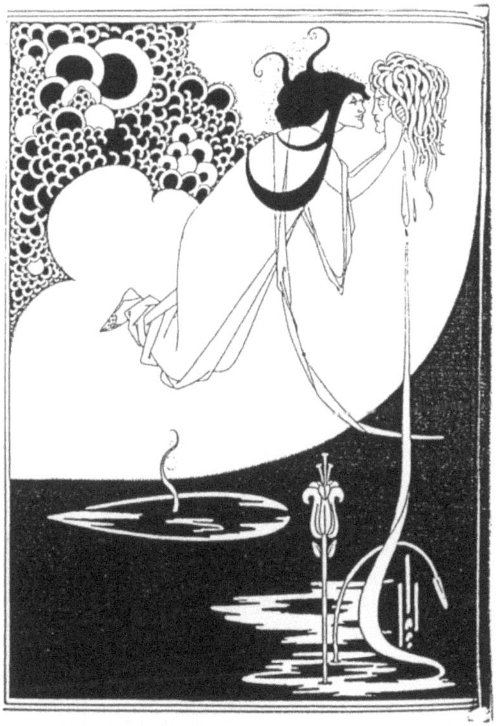

Fig. 3 Aubrey Beardsley – Illustration for Oscar Wilde "Salome".

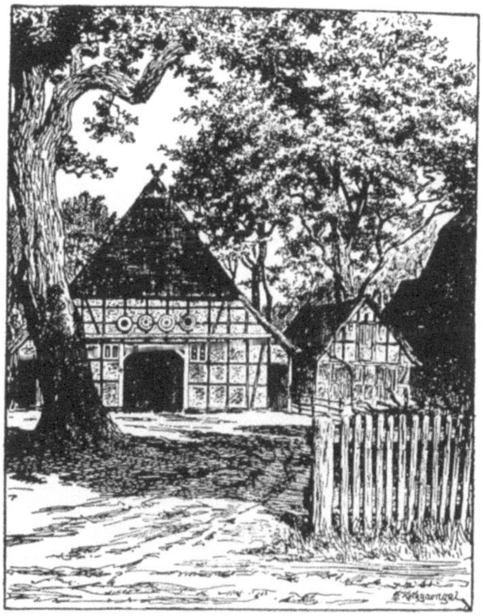

Fig. 4 Horses skulls made of wood on the roof of the farmhouses in Lower Saxony (Illustration for Hermann Löns "Die Häuser von Ohlenhof", with permission of the Adolf Sponholtz Verlag, Hameln).

The practise of the German hunter nailing the skulls of animals on his wall (fig. 5) seems an atavistic trend at first sight, but it is certainly more and the hunter not only demonstrates his skill in hunting but believes that the strength and vigour of the animals, represented by their heads on his wall might permeate to him.

After this historical and psycho-analytical discourse we came to the most relevant and early scientific explorer and genius of the late 18th and 19th Century Johann Wolfgang von Goethe to whom the German culture owes so much, in the field of literature, education and in natural sciences.

Goethe's scientific interest finds expression in the fact that 14 volumes of the Weimar edition of his works are concerned with scientific facts. Characteristic for Goethe's work as well as his poetry is his intensive endeavour after natural sciences. It is part of his life and began during his years of study in Straßburg where he heard lectures on chemistry and anatomy of Spielmann and Lobstein, clinical lectures of Ehrmann sen. and of his son on gynecology. Shortly before he died, in the year 1832 he cooperated in the differences between Cuvier and

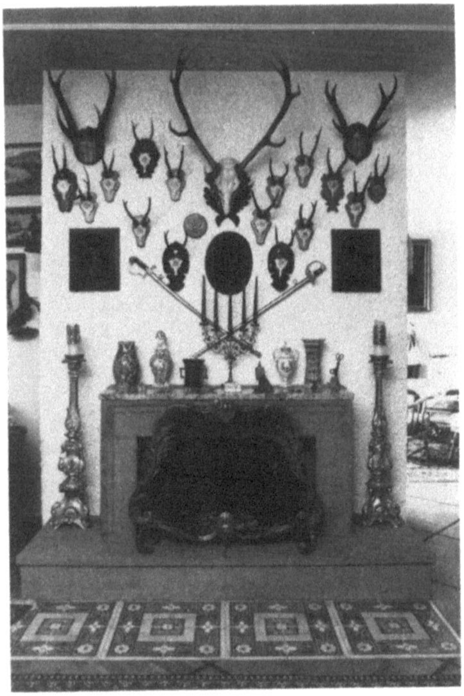

Fig. 5 Arrangement of hunting trophies, typical for the German state of civilization. This custom originates from magic or mystic imaginations, even though these sources are not alive anymore to modern human beings.

St. Hilaire, wrote an essay on osteologic objects and synthetic and analytic methods in natural sciences in general.

In the scientific field [6 – 13] Goethe's name is closely associated with his work on the metamorphosis of plants [17] but to us his researches into the development of the human skull are of fundamental importance [21, 22] and directly relevant and still stimulating for the discussions on the topics of our meeting. Goethe always has advocated the application of evolutionary principles in research [3, 4, 5, 14]. This is clearly seen in studies of fossil remains in search for a "Urpflanze" (fig. 6) or archetype of plants [12, 15]. Relevant to our meeting when refering to skull development Goethe's evidence for man's intermaxillary bone being a separate bone and in line with primate evolution is of importance. This independent origin of the incisive portion of the human maxilla (fig. 7) the naso-medial processes shows it to be homologous to the pre- or intermaxillary bone of lower vertebrates.

Furthermore Goethe [16] suggested that the skull could have developed from a complex fusion of six upper vertebrae [3, 10, 14, 18, 19, 23]. The abrupt change from the metamerely structured spine to the obviously completely different structural principles of the skull was for Goethe and his contemporaries an important challenge to seek in detail the ruling principles. And so the structure

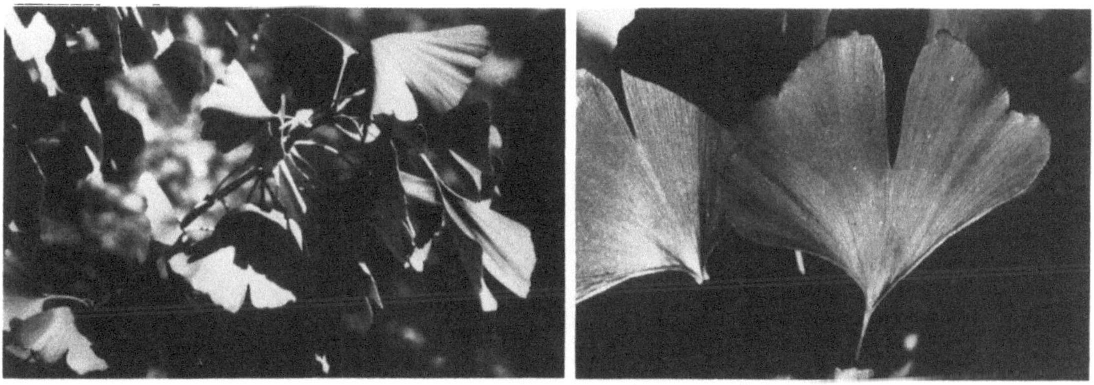

a b

Fig. 6 Branch (a) and leafs (b) of the Gingko biloba, which provided Goethe the essential impulses for the development of his imaginations of the primary plant ("Urpflanze"). This climatically very adaptable tree is quite frequently found in Europa today.

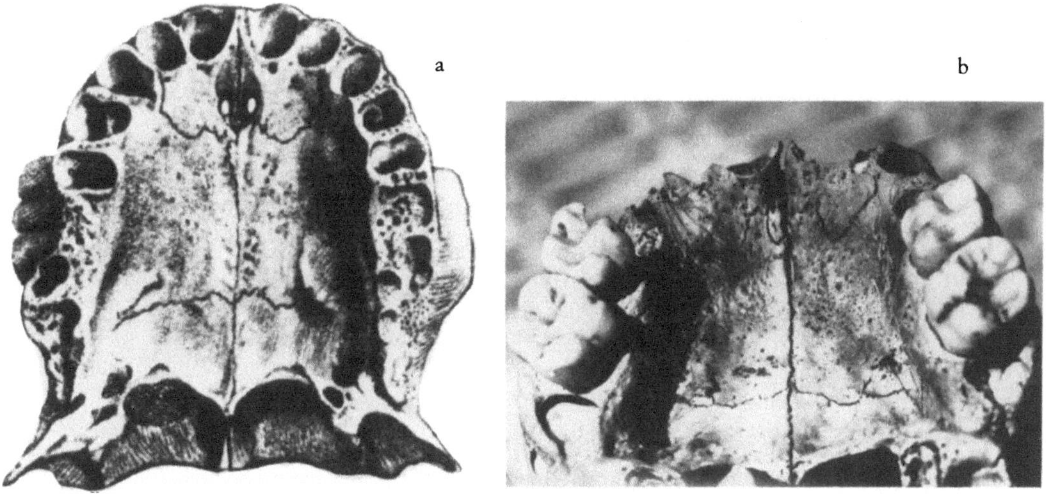

a b

Fig. 7 Illustration of Os intermaxillare of a human maxilla by Goethe (a) and in an infant's maxilla from a grave of the 30 years war (b) [Author's collection].

of the skull into six vertebrae seemed to Goethe, at the inspiration of the moment, clear and proved. He sketched his conceptions (fig. 8) the same day, happy, glad; he gave his idea around a gay circle at night and had to experience that one of the interlocutors, i. e. the certainly well-known Lorenz Oken, included this idea in an own essay which was just in print and so one can say that he has stolen

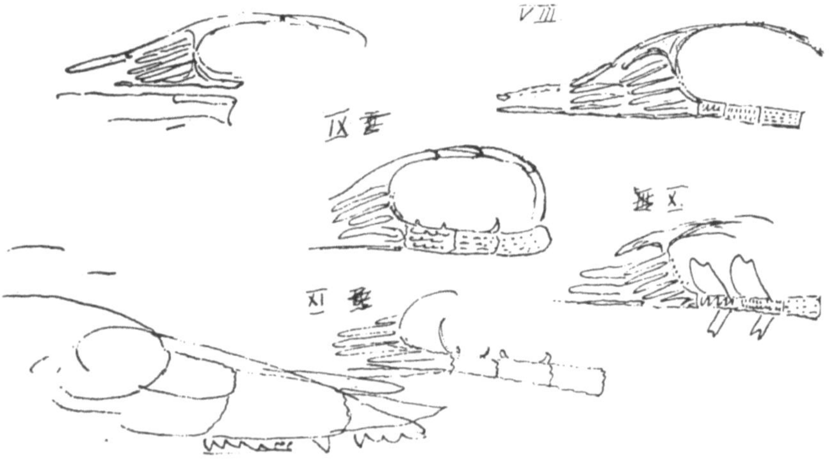

Fig. 8 Sketches made by Goethe illustrating his theory of skull formation, which he assumed developing from six vertebrae, three of which for the occipital bone, the posterior and anterior sphenoid, while the other three form the palate, maxilla and outermaxillary bones.

Goethe's inspiration! So Boisserée [2] said in 1815: "The head, nothing but a vertebra. Oken has stolen this idea from Goethe!".

In any case developmental anatomical studies, cases of malformations and clinical observations by contributors to this meeting will prove to the audience the significance of Goethe's early observations on skull development and of his work in general as clearly illuminated by Rudolf Virchow in 1861 [20] and Gottfried Benn [1] in 1949.

References

[1] Benn, G.: Goethe und die Naturwissenschaften. In: Goethes naturwissenschaftliche Schriften, pp. 7–41. Droemer, Berlin – Zürich 1962.

[2] Boissserée, J. S.: Briefe. (Mathilde Boisserée, ed.) 2 vols. Stuttgart 1862.

[3] Bratranek, F. Th.: Goethes naturwissenschaftliche Correspondenz. Leipzig 1874.

[4] Carus, C. G.: Goethe: Leipzig 1843. Benutzte Ausgabe: Rotapfel Verlag, Zürich 1948.

[5] Fischer, H.: Goethes Naturwissenschaft. Zürich 1950.

[6] Goethe, J. W. von: Goethes Werke. Großherzogin Sophie von Sachsen (ed.) 2. Abteilung "Naturwissenschaftliche Schriften", Bd. 1 – 13, Weimar 1887 – 1919.

[7] –, –: Versuch die Metamorphose der Pflanzen zu erklären. Gotha, Carl Wilhelm Ettingen 1790.

[8] –, –: Der Kammerberg bei Eger. Leonhards Taschenbuch für die gesamte Mineralogie. Frankfurt 1809.

[9] –, –: Sammlung zur Kenntnis der Gebirge von und um Karlsbad angezeigt und erläutert von Goethe. Leonhards Taschenbuch für die gesamte Mineralogie. Frankfurt 1809.

[10] –, –: Das Schädelgerüst aus sechs Wirbelknochen aufgebaut. Zur Morphologie. Zweiten Bandes zweites Heft 1824.

[11] –, –: Principes de Philosophie Zoologique, Discutés en Mars 1830 au sein de l'académie royale des sciences par Mr. Geoffroy de Saint-Hilaire. Paris 1830. Jahrb. für wiss. Kritik, Berlin 1830, 1832.

[12] –, –: Versuch über die Metamorphose der Pflanzen. Übersetzt von Friedrich Soret, nebst geschichtlichen Nachträgen. Cotta, Stuttgart 1831.

[13] –, –: Über den Zwischenkiefer des Menschen und der Tiere. Jena 1786. Verhandlungen der Kaiserlichen Leopoldinisch-Karolinischen Akademie der Naturforscher. 1. Abtl., Bd. 15, Bonn 1831.

[14] Haecker, V.: Goethes morphologische Arbeiten und die neue Forschung. Jena 1927.

[15] Hein, W.-H., D. Andernacht: Der Garten des Apothekers Peter Saltzwedel und Goethes Gingko biloba. In: Festschrift P. W. Meister, Hamburg 1974.

[16] Matthaei, R., D. Kuhn, O. Wagenbreth, et al. (eds.): Corpus der Goethezeichnungen. In: Bd. V, A und B. Naturwissenschaftliche Zeichnungen. Leipzig 1963, 1967.

[17] Meyer-Abich, A.: Biologie der Goethezeit. Stuttgart 1949.

[18] Peyer, B.: Goethes Wirbeltheorie des Schädels. Zürich 1950.

[19] Veit, O.: Über das Problem Wirbeltierkopf. Kempen 1947.

[20] Virchow, R.: Göthe als Naturforscher und in besonderer Beziehung auf Schiller. August Hirschfeld, Berlin 1861.

[21] Vogel, C.: Die letzte Krankheit Goethe's beschrieben und nebst einigen andern Bemerkungen über denselben mitgetheilt von Dr. Carl Vogel. Journal der praktischen Heilkunde 1833.

[22] Wagner, R.: Samuel Thomas Sömmerings Leben und Verkehr mit seinen Zeitgenossen. 1. Abt., 1. Bd., Leipzig 1844.

[23] Wohlbold, H.: Die Wirbelmetamorphose des Schädels von Goethe und Oken. München 1924.

II Basic research and diagnostic methods

Embryological and neuro-anatomical aspects of the cranio-cervical region

P. Glees

Introduction

Before focusing on the development of the cranio-cervical juntion a general description of skull and brain development will be necessary for only this will explain the obvious abrupt anatomical nature of this junction. For this understanding it is helpful to divide the components into neural and visceral portions. Probably the most ancient portion is the visceral one and centered around the oral opening, the beginning of the digestive tube. This concept will bring the gill arches as foremost parts in particular the first and second arches. The first arch is primarly guarding the oral opening by division of the 1st arch into a maxillary and mandibular component. While the first arch is concerned with food intake, the second is already a part of the respiratory system but partically becomes drawn into the making of the skull. But not only the brain has to be housed separately also the sense organs have to be fitted into the neural portion of the skull and encasing the brain and the long distance sense organs

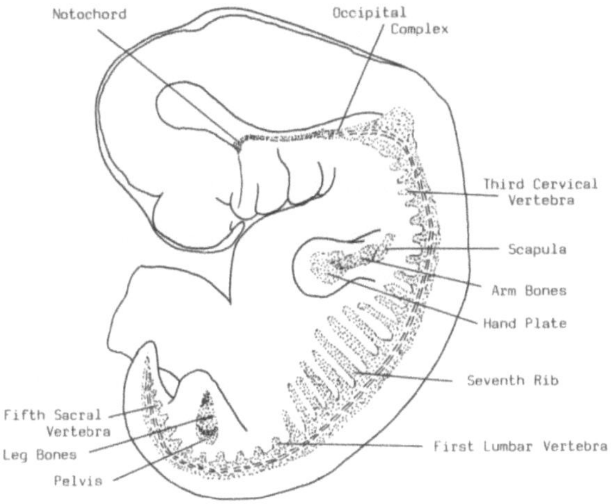

Fig. 1 The forerunner of the axial skeleton is the notochord, which reaches cranially to the pituitary fossa. Around the notochord mesenchym is formed supplying the material for the subsequent stages (Diagram represents a 10 mm stage).

for olfaction, vision and hearing. For this task not only the evolutionary old cranial floor has to be used but also a new portion, the vault for the brain. While the old portions stemming from arch material have a cartilagenous or endochondrial origin the newly added parts such as vault are membranous and do not pass through a cartilagenous stage. To achieve the formation of the mammalian skull an intense moulding process by fusion of the different parts occurs, making precise identification of all these parts almost impossible.

The embryological stages of skull formation

The earliest signs of skull formation is a mesenchymal thickening around the notochord (fig. 1) and extends frontally. This mesenchymal plate become the cartilagenous basis for the brain and has been termed chondro-cranium (figs. 2 a, b). Phylogenetically speaking this is the oldest portion of the brain envelope and reminds the comparative anatomist of the brain encasing in primitive cartilagenous fishes such as the elasmobranches whose supporting skeleton does not use osseous materials but cartilage.

In the human embryo the cranial floor to start with is cartilagenous, including the capsules for the inner ear and the nasal cavities (fig. 26 b). Furthermore the cartilages of the gill arches I – V are either used in the ‚construction‘ of the skull (chondro-cranium) or for the cartilages of the larynx. While the chondro-cranium

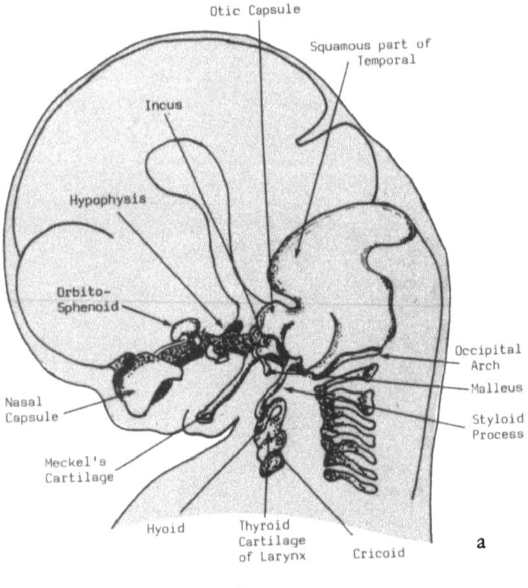

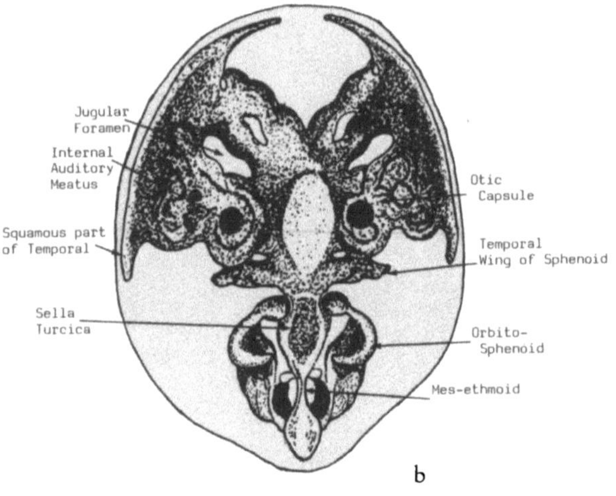

Fig. 2 a, b The chondro-cranium of a human embryo about the 8. – 9. week. A lateral view, B cranial cavity seen from above (modified from Patten [3]).

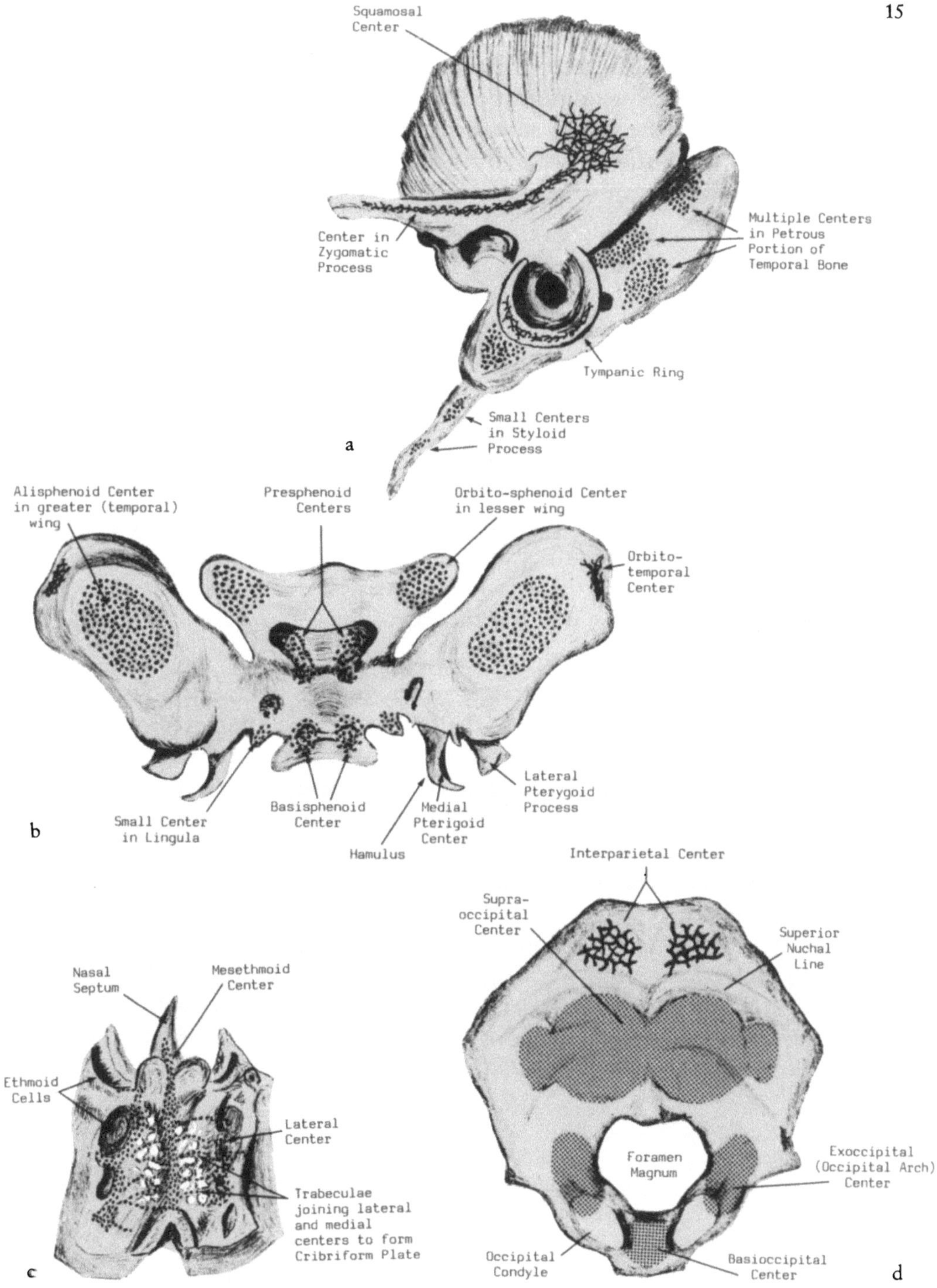

Fig. 3 a – d Diagrams illustrating ossification centers in four of the principle bones of the skull. Intramembranous centers stippled black and enchondral centers in large block dots against shaded background outlining the definite chape of the bone (modified from Patten [3]).

arises from a mesenchymal area of fusion, without distinct boundaries related to the early embryology, the different portions become clearer when ossification centres appear. But as the skull is such a composite arrangement of many centres, not every bone can be traced easily to its ancestral origin, but to some extent it seems that multiple centres of ossification in a bone indicate also multiple evolutionary origins.

As the main theme of our meeting is the cranio-vertebral junction, we first present the features of the base of the skull. This base is composed of the occipital bone framing the foramen magnum, the sphenoid caudal to pituitary fossa and the ethmoid harbouring the front of the forebrain reaching into the nasal area to provide cover for the olfactory bulb.

We find in the occipital bone a number of ossification centres (fig. 3 a). They arise in the endochondral matrix and in the intra-membranous paired centers, giving origin to the inter-parietal ossification centres above the superior nuchal line (fig. 3 a). The intra-membranous, inter-parietal centres show loosely arranged bony trabeculae while the supra-occipital centre is of firmer structure and appears in the 9th or 10th week. The other centres are visible somewhat later. All these centres fuse between the first and fourth year of life.

The sphenoid bone has five pairs of enchondral centres for the lesser wings, orbito-sphenoid, the temporal or greater wings, for the rostral part of the body of the sphenoid, for the caudal part of the body and small centres for the tongue like processes, the lingulae. In addition intra-membranous centres make up the sphenoid bone, contributing to the orbio-temporal wings, the medial lamina of the pterygoid processes (fig. 3 b). At the birth the whole complex is as yet not fused and 3 parts of the sphenoid or pterygoid bone are visible. The ethmoid is a part of the chondro-cranium and has medial and lateral portions. The details can be seen in figure 3 c. The temporal bone stems from the capsule of the inner ear, a part of the cartilagenous cranium and secondary additions of membranous bone, the squama temporalis (fig. 3 d), while the styloid process is a part of the second gill arch (fig. 3 d). The tympanic ring (fig. 3 d) begins to ossify in the 10th week. One of the two endochondral ossification centres can be seen at birth, the second two years later.

Membranous contributions to the cartilagenous portions of the skull

Substantial contributions are made by mesenchyme and refered to as membranous bones, without passing through a chondrogenous stage. In this way the sides and the entire roof capsule of the skull are membranous in origin (fig. 4). The parietal

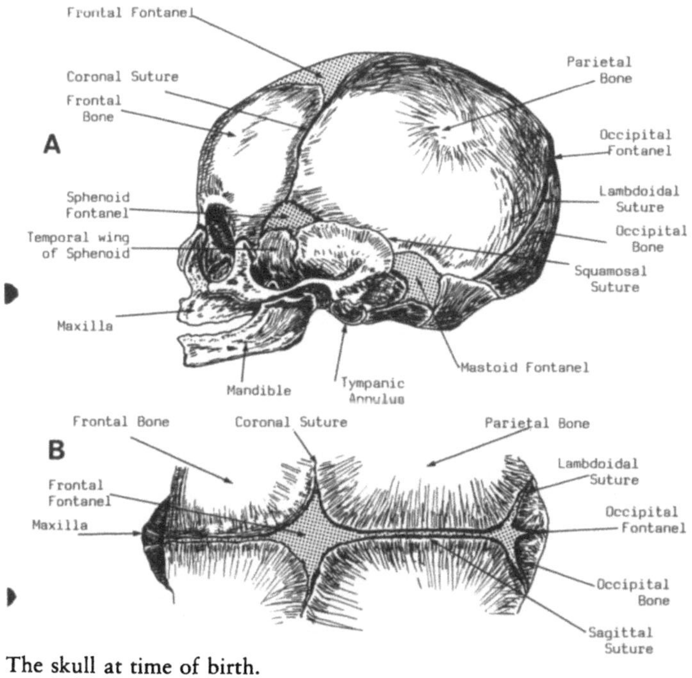

Fig. 4 The skull at time of birth.

bones develop from a single centre and the frontal bones from paired centres. The fusion between the parietal and adjacent bones is delayed and the areas called the fontanelles. These fontanelles allow for 'evasive' action of the skull at birth and for growth afterwards (fig. 4). The nasal, lacrimal and zygomatic bones all derive from a membranous origin.

The branchial arches contributions: The first arch material supplies the maxillary and mandibular process, but this cartilagenous contribution is more ancestral, for the bone formation itself is entirely membranous although Meckel's cartilage is clearly to be seen inside the mandibular process and may serve as a guiding structure for the inferior dental nerve and artery and to provide their entrance into the mandibular foramen.

But Meckel's cartilage contributes to the ossicles of the middle ear, the malleus, incus and the spheno-mandibular ligament. The second branchial arch cartilage provides the stapes and the styloid process which fuses with temporal bone while the distal part of the arch is transformed into the stylo-hyoid ligament. The lesser wing of the hyoid is developmentally a part of the second branchial cartilage.

The cartilage of the third arch is used for the greater horn and the fused plates of the arch the body of the hyoid.

The other two remaining arches deliver the material for the thyroid cartilage and the smaller cartilages of cuneiform, corniculate and cricoid.

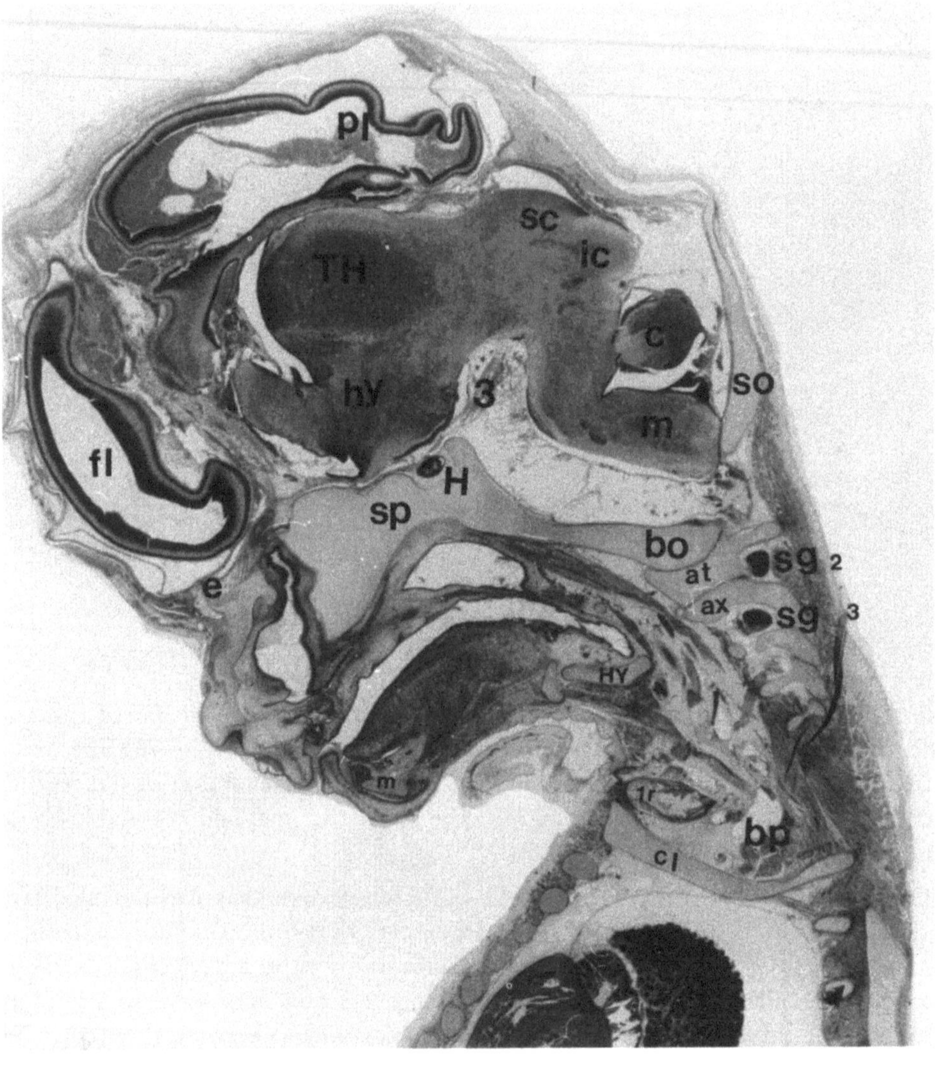

Fig. 5 Sagittal and lateral section through the head of an embryo of 11–12 weeks (Author's collection).
Read from left to right: pl = future parietal lobe; Th = thalamus; hy = hypothalamus; sc = superior colliculus; ic = inferior colliculus; c = cerebellum; m = lower medulla; SO = supra-occipital part of occipital bone; bo = basi-occipital part of occipital bone; at = atlas; ax = axis; e = cribriform plate of ethmoid; SG_2 = Spinal ganglion of C_2; SG_3 = spinal ganglion of C_3; bp = brachial plexus and subclavian artery between 1st rip (1r) and clavicle (cl); HY = hyoid bone; m = mandible; sp = sphenoid; H = hypophysis; 3 = third nerve; fl = frontal lobe.

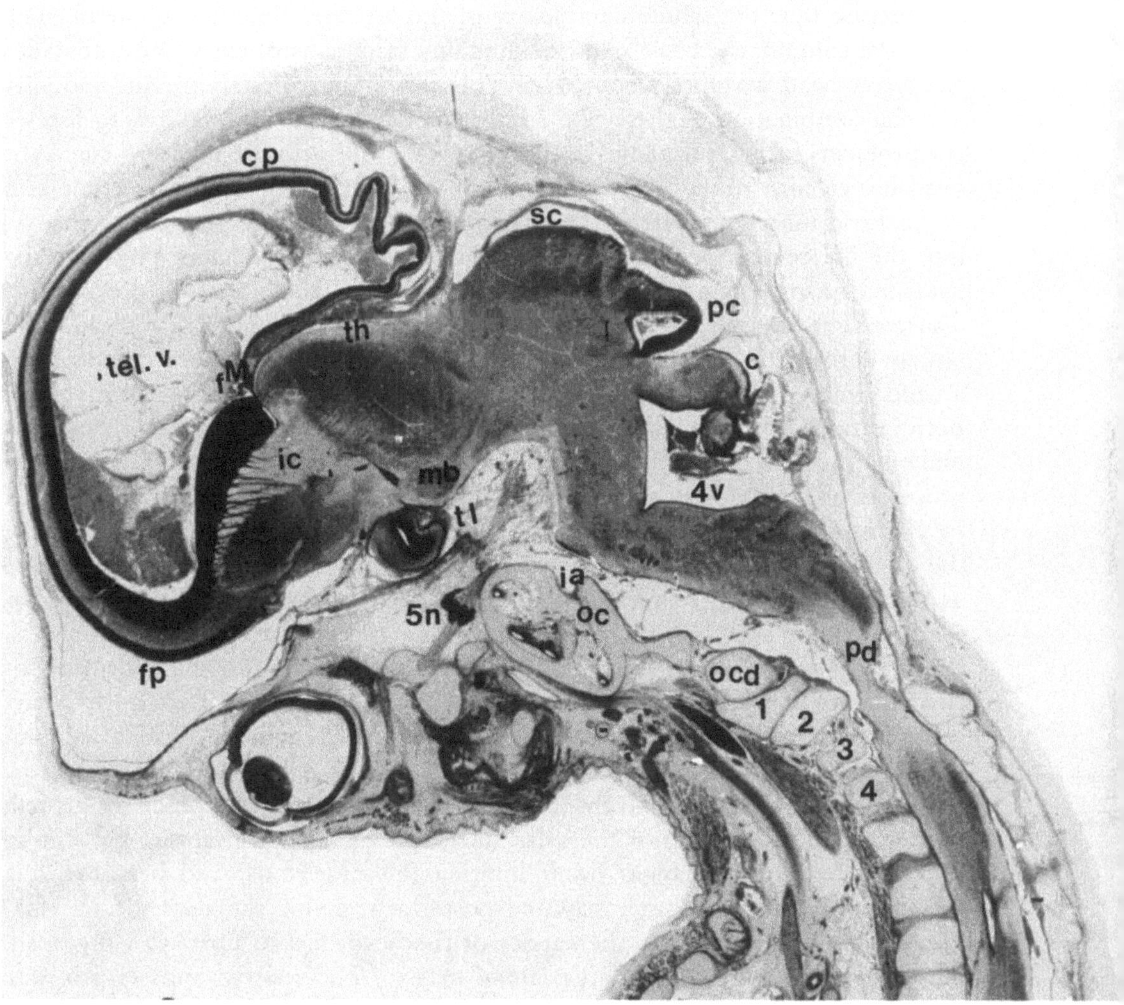

Fig. 6 Sagittal section illustrating cranio-cervical transition through a foetal head (about 11 weeks). Note the large size of medulla and midbrain when compared to thalamus and in particular to the telencephalon. The plexuses of the brain stem eventually will disappear when the base of the skull provides more space, if not malformations and dislocation of brain stem and cerebellum will occur (Author's collection).

cp = cortical plate (neo-cortex); th = thalamus; sc = superior colliculus; pc = posterior colliculus; c = cerebellum; 4v = 4th ventricle; pd = pyramidal decussation area; ocd = occipital condyle; 1–4 = cervical vertebrae; oc = otic capsule, containing inner ear formations; ia = internal auditory meatus; 5n = trigeminal nerve and ganglion; tb = temporal lobe (uncus); mb = mamillary body; ic = internal capsule; fM = foramen of Monroe; tel. v. = telencephalic ventricle; fp = frontal pole.

After this brief survey of the skull's development we must turn our attention to the cervical component of the junction, the upper part of the vertebral column, considering this, the whole complexity of the junction becomes apparent. The vertebral column, the basic pillar of the bony frame has to carry and to balance the heavy head weighing about 6 kg. This task is one of stability and mobility and the combination of these two conflicting demands already allows to foresee the problems facing our clinical colleagues. The problems are made worse as the head has to turn round a pivot the odontoid process, whose construction as a vertical rod inherently carries the possibility of breaking by accident or disease into the life centers of the lower medulla. To prevent this happening specially firm and secure ligaments have to anchor the dens and normally prevent this disaster. The design of the dens in phylogeny and ontogeny is complex and largely derives from the body of the atlas. The body of a vertebra derives from a caudal more compact part of embryonic sclerotome and a looser cranial half. Both portions form the definite vertebrae. From the dense half dorsal extensions make up the vertebral arch and paired ventro-lateral processes, the future costal processes or ribs. Mesenchymal tissue fills in the new intervertebral space caused by the fusion of two different slerotomal portions and lays the foundation for the intervertebral discs, which harbour the remnants of the notochord refered to as nucleus pulposus. Centers of chondrofication appear in the 7th week, 2 for the body, 1 for each half of the arch and a separate one for the costal process. In the tenth week ossification starts, usually a single centre for the body, one for each half of the arch and uniting several years after birth. Late at 17 years secondary centres arise in the cartilage covering the cranial and caudal ends of the vertebral body forming discs and like an osseous epiphysis joining with the body of the vertebrae around the 20th year of life. These discs provide for growth in length. The formation of the atlas starts like all other vertebrae, but due to odontoid formation changes occur limiting this uppermost and head-carrying vertebra to two arches anteriorly and posteriorly, giving the atlas a final ring-like shape. The atlas being the carrier of the head, has to turn with the head. This is possible only by the large lateral masses. These lateral masses protrude and can be felt between mastoid process and angle of the jaw. Each lateral mass has a large superior joint surface with the condyle of the occipital bone above and an inferior joint surface with the second vertebra, the axis or epistropheus. Both rotary joints are divided in 6 separate chambers, two between atlas and skull and 4 between atlas and axis. The odontoid process of the axis can be divided in an apical portion, giving rise to the apical ligament, probabely a remnant of the notochord and a caput and a collum. The upper joint surfaces of the dens are flat roller joints providing seats for the convex lower articular processes of the atlas.

Functional considerations

In horizontal rotation one tubercle of the atlas glides alternately from the upper axis tubercle foreward, and the other posteriorly and downwards about 2 mm. This shortening is a compensation for the lateral movement of posterior arch of the atlas preventing a shearing of the spinal cord. The nodding movement of the head occurs in the atlanto-occipital joint using as an axis a line running closely behind the external meatus across both mastoid processes and moved, delicately balanced, by the muscles of the neck. A more detailed anatomical description of the region will be given in the next communication by Lang.

When we are tired having a reduced tone in the activating reticular formation these muscles loose tone and our head falls forward indicating our sleepy condition. The head of the baby falls back having a relatively heavier back of the skull and weaker ligaments, esp. the tectorial membrane and anterior and posterior longitudinal ligaments normally limiting the bending backward. The short muscles, acting between vertebrae and the basilary portion of the occipital bone have the same significance for head movements as the small muscles of hand for delicate finger movements namely, executing delicate head movements in support of visual eye movements. Their proprioceptive innervation including all the many joint receptors is of the greatest importance for maintaining posture in upright position in relation to the skull. The headjoints when acting together can be considered as a large ball and socket joint, where the skull represents the ball and the upper two vertebrae the sockets.

The central nervous system responds to the important role of the upright position of the human head by forming a special proprioceptive medullary relay nucleus, the lateral cuneate nucleus. The great number of proprioceptive sense organs located in the head muscles and joints demand the distribution of their signals to the cerebellum and the reticular formation.

Neuro-embryologico-neurological aspects of the cranio-cervical region (some aspects of development have also been discussed in a previous contribution, c. f. Mainz Proceedings, Glees, [1]). The complexity of the neural structures above the foramen magnum when compared to the organisational simplicity of the spinal cord is enormous (figs. 5 – 8). It is not only the opening of the central canal into a IV ventricle (fig. 8) or the greater mass of nervous tissue, the complexity lies in the new elements of the medullary switchboard. These new elements are those of the reticular formation, the neurons serving special senses and the provision for centers of cardiac and pulmonary activity, such as the vagal nerve with its para-sympathetic component (fig. 9). These additional neurons are superimposed on a basic spinal cord organisation and their destruction is so disastrous by a fracture of the odontoid process.

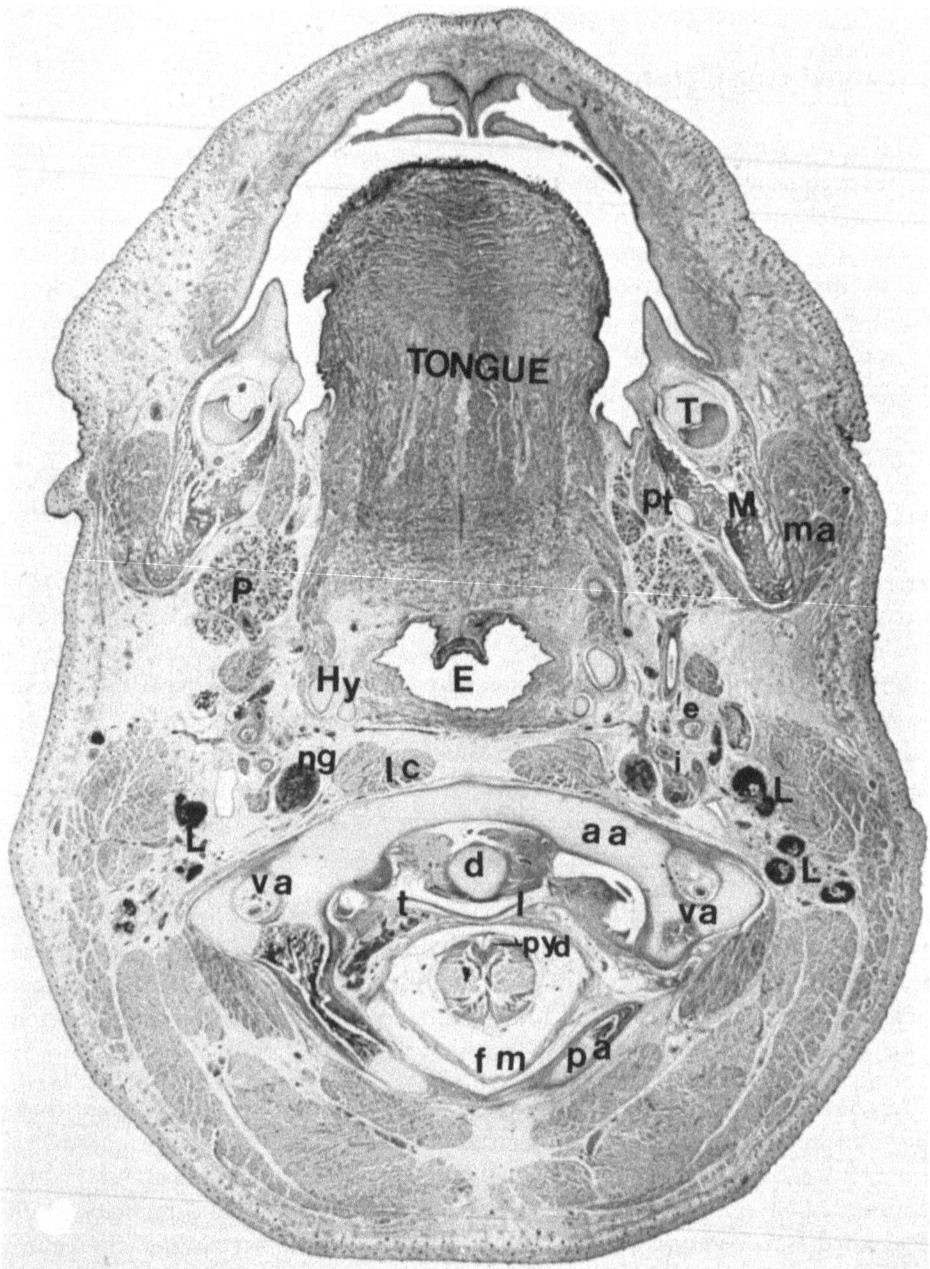

Fig. 7 Horizontal section through a foetal head illustrating the relation of the dens or ondontoid process in the foramen magnum towards transitional area of medulla and spinal cord (Author's collection).

T = tooth development; M = mandible; ma = masseter; pt = medial or internal pterygoid muscle; e = external carotid artery; i = internal carotid artery; L = mastoid (deep) lymphnodes; va = vertebral artery; d = dens or odontoid process; cl = transvers ligament; aa = anterior arch of atlas; pyd = pyramidal tract decussation; pa = posterior arch of atlas; fm = foramen magnum; ng = nodose ganglion of X; Hy = hyoid cartilage; E = epiglottis; P = retro-mandibular part of parotic gland.

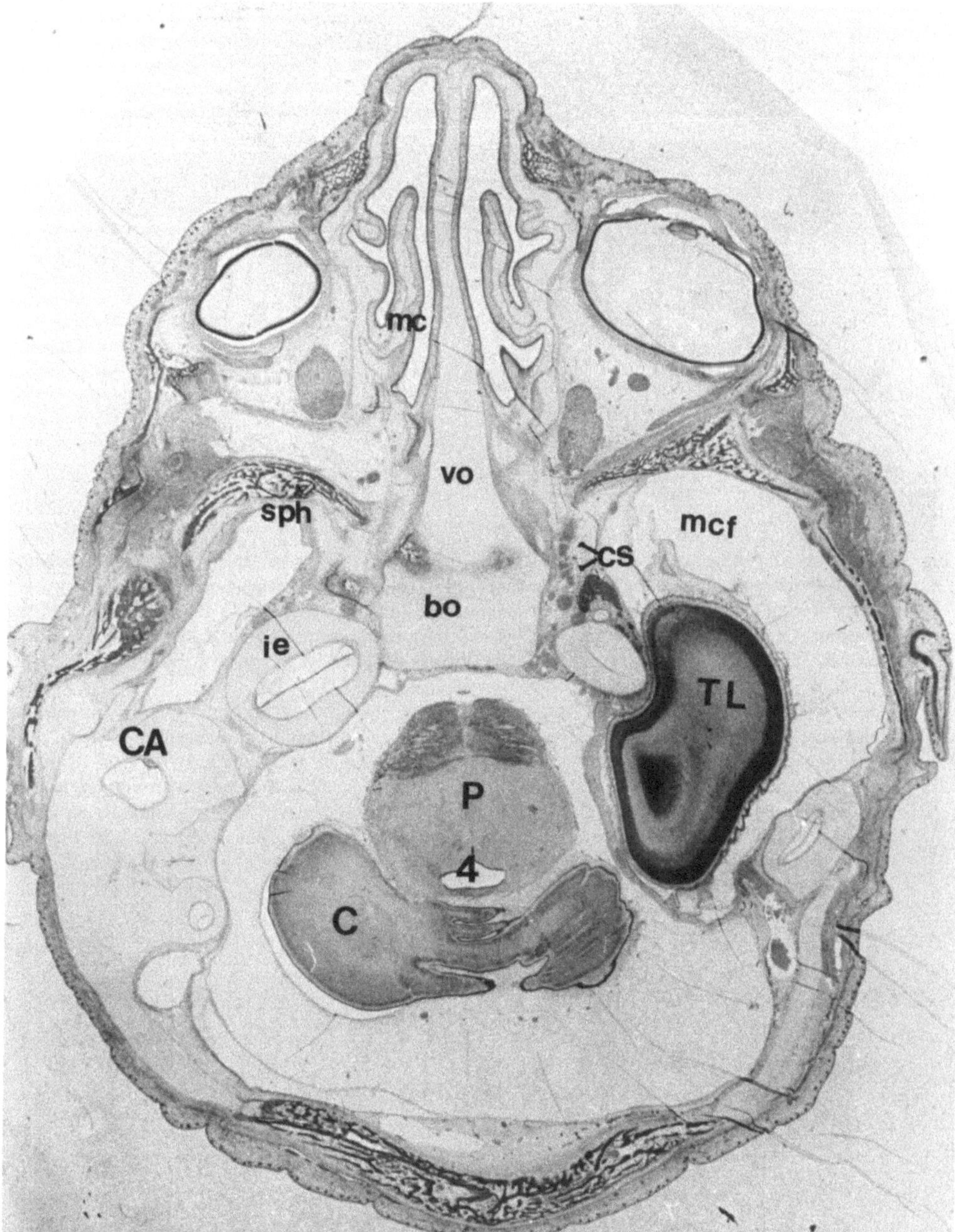

Fig. 8 Horizontal section through a foetal head, showing the posterior cranial fossa and the relation to pons and cerebellum (author's collection).
mc = middle concha; vo = vomer; bo = basi-occipital cartilage; cs = cavernosus sinus with contents III, IV, V, VI nerves and carotid artery; mcf = middle cranial fossa; TL = temporal lobe; P = pons; C = cerebellum; 4 = 4th ventricle; CA = crista ampullaris of semicircular canal; ie = internal ear; sph = sphenoidal bone ossification.

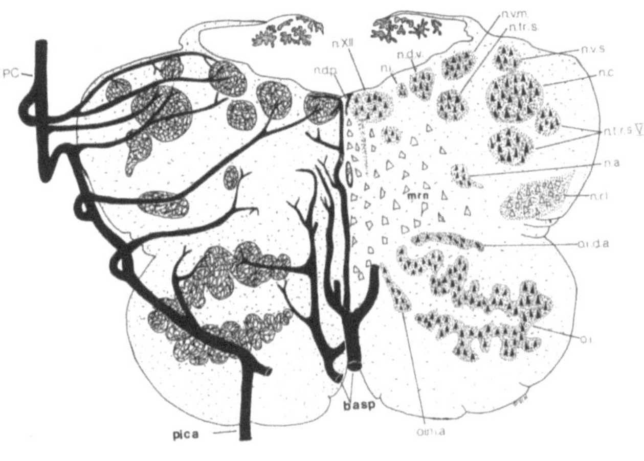

Fig. 9 A composite diagram of the medulla showing blood supply on the left half and neuronal nuclear groups on the right. Note that blood supply areas and neuronal groupings are coexistential. The blood vessels can be divided into a medial group from branches of the vertebral arteries, which eventually by fusion form the anterior spinal artery, a descending vessel. The dorso-lateral position of the medulla is supplied by the posterior inferior cerebellar artery.
n. d. p. = para median dorsal nucleus; n. XII = hypoglossal nucleus; n. i. = intercalate nucleus; n. d. v. = dorsal nucleus of vagus; n. v. m. = medial vestibular nucleus; n. tr. s. = nucleus of tractus solitarius; n. v. s. = nucleus vestibularis, spinal part; n. c. = cuneate nucleus; n. t. r. s. V = descending or spinal nucleus of V; n. a. = nucleus ambiguus; m. r. n. = medial reticular nucleus; n. r. l. = lateral reticular nucleus; o. i. d. a. = dorsal accessory olive; o. i. = inferior olivary nucleus; o. i. m. a. = accessory medio inferior olive; basp = branches of anterior spinal artery; pica = posterior inferior cerebellar artery; PC = branch of pica to cerebellum.

Fig. 10 Myelin stained section of lower medulla at the level of posterior column relay nuclei (author's collection).
dt = descending trigeminal fibres, mainly from ophthalmic division; 5n = descending or spinal nucleus of V; co-sp = cortico-spinal tract before decussation; sp-th = spino-thalamic tract but mixed with spino-tectal, spino-reticular and spino-cerebellar fibres; pcnm = medial post. col. nucleus for leg fibres; L = lateral post. col. nucleus for arm fibres; cml = crossing medial lemniscus fibres from pcnm.

Important too is to consider the delicate blood supply of the medulla so easily interfered with, when a neurosurgical severence of the pain tract is carried out (fig. 10). The neurosurgeon can interrupt at medullary level both the pain fibres from the ophthalmic division of the trigeminal nerve, e.g. those fibres from the cornea in case of an extremely painful ulcer and the spino-thalamic tract which is easily accessible above the inferior olive at lower medullary level (fig. 11). But each small blood vessel cauterised may abolish the blood supply to an important medullary group of neurons. The clinical and experimental findings on pain pathways have been summarised by Glees, [2].
This brief discussion of the transitional region between spinal cord and medulla together with the illustrations of the developmental aspects should provide a background knowledge for the neurological and neurosurgical problems of the cranio-cervical junction.

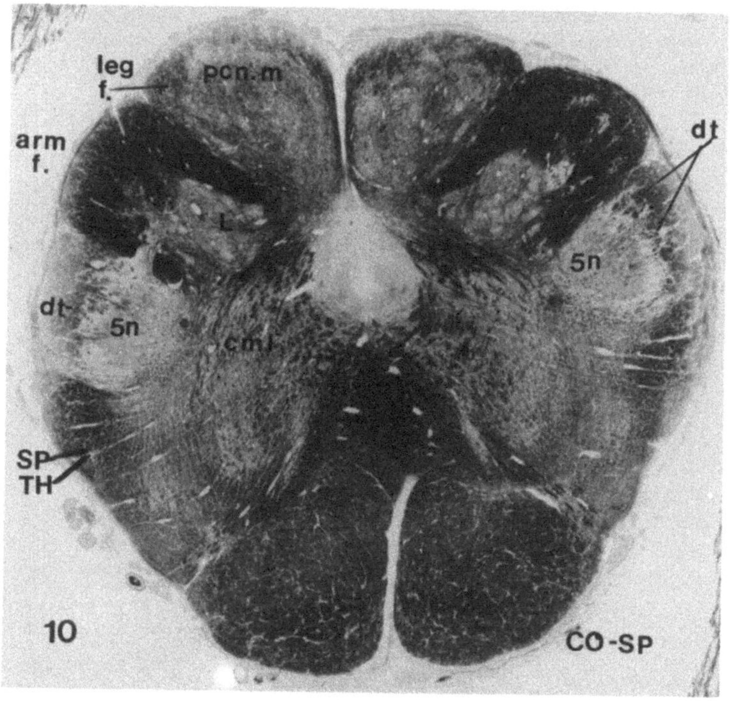

Fig. 10

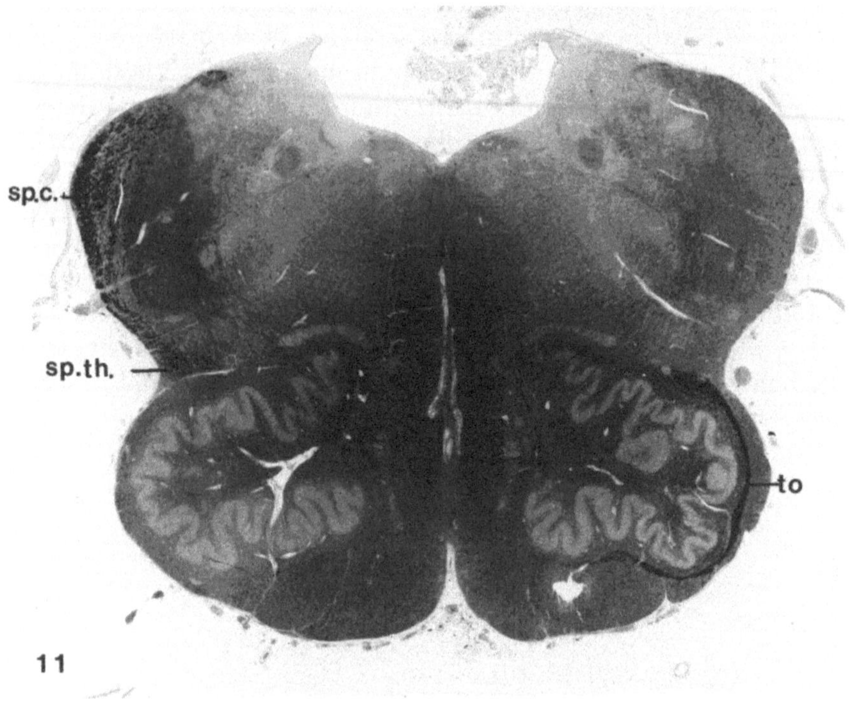

Fig. 11 Marchi section of human medulla illustrating on the left the position of the spino-thalamic tract (sp. th.). The tract is degenerated after surgical intervention of Th 4. Dorsal and ventral spino-cerebellar fibres (sp. c.) have been severed as well. On the right half of the section the tegmento-olivary fibres are shown (to).

Acknowledgement

The author wishes to thank Mr. D. A. McBrearty, M. A. and Mr. S. F. Crane for their excellent art work.

References

[1] Glees, P.: Evolutional, developmental and clinical aspects of brain stem organisation. In: D. Voth, P. Gutjahr, C. Langmaid (eds.): Tumours of the central nervous system in infancy and childhood, pp. 190 – 198. Springer, Berlin – Heidelberg – New York 1982.

[2] Glees, P.: The central pain tract. Acta neuroveg. 7 (1955) 160 – 174.

[3] Patten, B. M.: Human embryology. Churchill Ltd., London 1947.

The cranio-cervical junction – Anatomy

J. Lang

Introduction

Without a detailed knowledge of the anatomy of a region it is not possible to give an adequate explanation of its functions. Anatomical knowledge is a prerequisite if radiographs, angiograms, CT scans or NMR pictures are to be correctly interpreted. For surgical procedures and hence, the well-being of the patients, knowledge of the anatomical structures and their functions are essential [1, 12, 44, 61, 82, 103, 106]. The cranio-cervical junction can be approached from behind (dorsally), dorso-laterally and from the front, as well as from below and anteriorly. In its strict sense the cranio-cervical junction includes only the foramen magnum, the occipital condyles and the upper two cervical vertebrae, which apart from their function as joints, surround and protect the nervous structure inside. On account of the various approaches, the surgeon has to deal with the adjoining vessels and nerves which run through the region, as well as the surrounding muscles.

Clinical significance of evolutionarily old structures

So-called chordomas [84, 85, 91] can develop from the notochord around the cranio-cervical junction [94], the nasal and pharyngeal cavity, in the sphenoidal sinus and within the skull. These have been recognised since 1858 (fig. 1). The cartilaginous shell of the posterior cranial fossa can be subdivided into a central portion, the subsequent basi-occiput and the part derived from the body of the sphenoid, a lateral portion formed from the lateral occipital bone and also a dorsal part. Apart from this, the central portion of the otic capsule for the stato-acoustico-kinetic sensory organ is formed laterally, and so are the initially wide openings or grooves for the vessels and nerves. In a 52 mm embryo a part of the basi-occiput is already calcified, as well the posterior sections of the lateral occipital bone [11]. Also the dorsal rim, which still has a posterior notch (incisura posterior) in a 93 mm fetus, is still cartilaginous (with the exception of a small ossicle in the posterior midline portion).

* This work is dedicated to Professor Dr. Jochen Staubesand, head of Department of Anatomy, University of Freiburg/Br., to his 65th birthday.

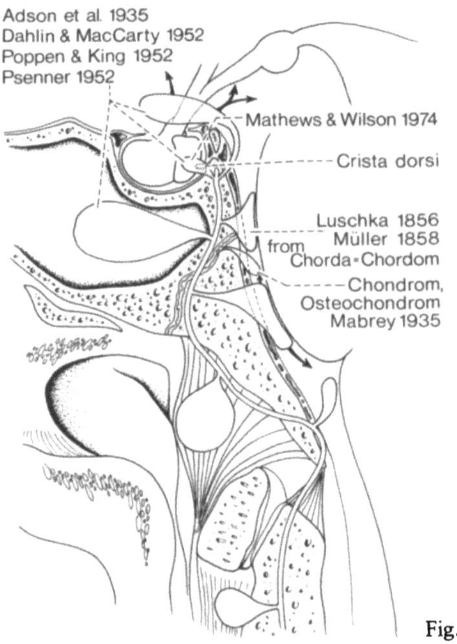

Fig. 1

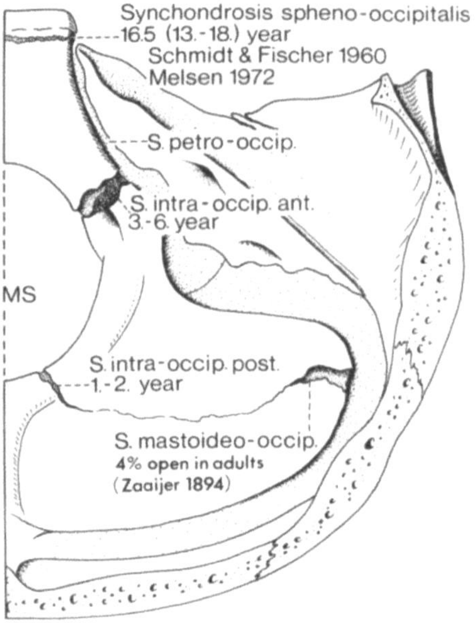

Fig. 2

Fig. 1 Clivus area, viewed on a median sagittal section, course of the notochord and occurrence of chordomas and chondromas in the area of the cervicocranial junction.

Fig. 2 Synchondroses in the posterior fossa area and the time of its synostoses.

The greater part of the posterior part of the floor of the posterior fossa is preformed in cartilage from the so-called tectum posterius. This part belongs to the *pars nuchalis* of the occipital squama. The pars occipitalis, above this, arises from membranous bone. In the lateral border region there is always in the new born, but rarely in adults, a cleft or else a suture, the *sutura Mendosa*, which is not only of forensic but also of practical interest (confusion with fractures). At the end of the second month ossification centres arise in the basi-sphenoid, in the third month also in the presphenoid [107]. Around the perinatal period these two bony sections fuse from the inner aspect of the skull towards the outside. The dorsum sellae only ossifies post-natally as a part of the basi-sphenoid.

The cartilaginous joint between the basi-sphenoid and the pre-sphenoid is at the anterior border of the pituitary fossa. Behind the dorsum sellae [25] the clivus is divided by the spheno-occipital synchondrosis, which is responsible particularly for the lengthwise growth of the skull, and which as a rule persists until the 12th – 18th year. Afterwards, the syn*ostosis* develops from the inner aspect of the skull, outwards towards the under side of the clivus (fig. 2).

Development of the skull – Comparative anatomy

The significance of malformations of the cranio-cervical junction has been dealt with particularly by Albrecht [4] and many others [32–35, 48, 62, 112]. According to this, the basilar portion of the occipital bone or a portion of this section of the clivus arises from 3–4 (or 5) vertebral body rudiments (anlage) rostral to the atlas, which have become incorporated in the skull. Immediately in front of the atlas there was originally a so-called pro-atlas, which consisted of an anterior and posterior arch [38, 39]. The anterior portion of this arch may be incorporated in the basilar portion of the occipital bone, particularly in the region of the condyles. The dorsal section is said to become the upper joint surface of the atlas and its posterior arch.

Medical significance

a) Occasionally the superior articular facet of the atlas is separated into an anterior and a posterior portion. The posterior portion is said to originate from *pro-atlas material*. Von Schuhmacher [105] found within the anterior and posterior atlanto-occipital membranes various *bony bars* not connected with the occiput, which he likewise interpreted as remnants of the *pro-atlas*.

b) Occasionally an arcus *prebasio-occipitalis* can be found, which resembles a portion of the anterior arch of the atlas having partly fused with the anterior rim of the foramen magnum.

c) At the anterior rim of the occipital condyle there may be smaller or larger bony projections which are described as *basilar processes*.

d) *The condylus tertius* (third condyle) placed median or paramedian is said to be part of the pro-atlas fused with the occipital bone. This can articulate with the tip of the dens of the axis, with the anterior arch of the atlas, or with both.

e) Possibly the *ponticuli*, which bridge over the vertebral artery in the arterial sulcus also represent remnants of the pro-atlas.

f) The atlanto-occipital membrane might also be a vestige of the pro-atlas.

g) Possibly the *ossicula terminalia* [10] are remains of the anterior portion of the pro-atlas [47, 48]. Von Torklus and Gehle [119] illustrate specimens from Geipel [40] which show in the tip of the dens a separate centre of ossification from which the *ossiculum terminale* develops. This can become incorporated in the tip of the dens as a result of a vacuole formation. In our material, not uncommonly a bony process juts out from the tip of the dens upwards, upwards and forwards, or upwards and backwards.

h) Also in various cases of atlas assimilation the pro-atlas appears to have developed as a union *between the posterior arch of the atlas and the occiput* (fig. 3).

i) Kollmann [62] described *'labia'* of the foramen magnum on the underside of the skull, *paracondylar processes* (= *paramastoid*) and also duplications of the hypoglossal canal, which are also regarded as parts of the pro-atlas incorporated into the skull.

j) Froriep [31 – 35] described the basilar tubercles (basilar processes, papillary processes) more accurately and also found unpaired protuberances in the midline, which enclosed a short canal: *Arcus prebasio-occipitalis*. He emphasised that the canal did not represent a *canaliculus of the notochord*, as this can exist simultaneously and penetrate the occipital bone above the former. When markedly developed this variation gives rise to a Condylus tertius (third condyle) which articulates with the dens of the axis.

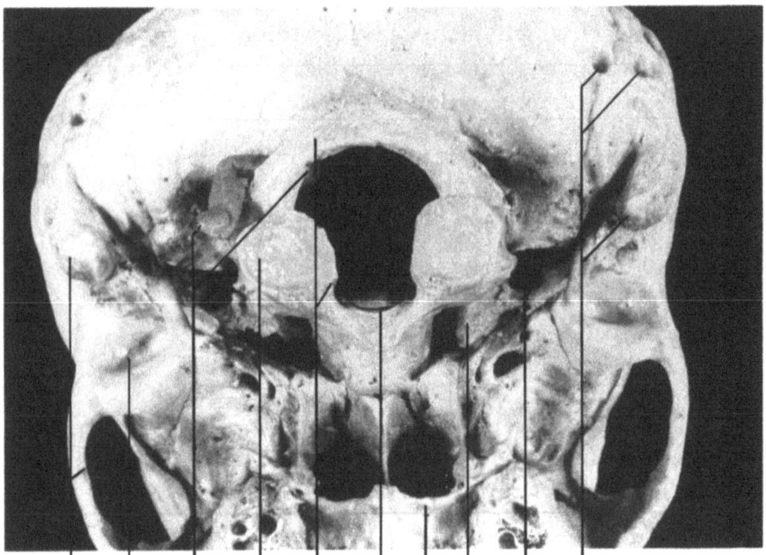

Fig. 3 Atlas-assimilation (complete), viewed from below.
1. Mastoid process and zygomatic arch; 2. Mandibular fossa; 3. Vertebral artery, course; 4. Facies articul. inf. atlantis; 5. Dorsal and ventral arch of atlas; 6. Facies articularis dentis; 7. Hard palate; 8. Petrous part of temporal bone; 9. Canalis caroticus and foramen jugulare; 10. Foramina mastoidea and mastoid process.

Sphenoid-clivus angle

In our material the angle between the planum sphenoidale and the clivus tangent on the inner aspect of the skull was measured [100]. It showed an average angle of 117.68 (96 – 143)°. Most values lay between 115 and 127°. Bergerhoff and Stilz [9] found an average value of 117.5°. It was stressed that with assimilation of the atlas a flattening of the skull base angle [67] was found. Lang and Brückner [73] examined the sphenoid-clivus angle in 67 children's skulls and found in the new-born there was an average angle of 133.25°, in one-year-olds one of 127.66°, in five-year-olds one of 115.16° and in 16 – 17 year-olds one of 112°. According to Landzert an abnormal development of the skull-base angle was assumed. Becker [7] arrived at similar findings after measurements from X-ray plates. A very large angle corresponds with a platybasia. According to McGregor [87] platybasia was first described by Ackerman [2] and then by Boogaard [16].

Basilar impression (fig. 4)

After Ackermann [2] and Virchow [111] McGregor [87] in particular studied the basilar impression. As with earlier workers (Virchow) he classified it into a primary form, as a congenital anomaly, and a secondary in osteoporotic illnesses (osteomalacia, Paget's disease, hyperparathyroidism, osteogenesis imperfecta, chondro-osteo-dystrophy etc). In addition local bone changes associated with tumours or infections, thinning of the skull bones as a result of hydrocephalus or injuries (with "ring-fractures") can also be followed by basilar impression.

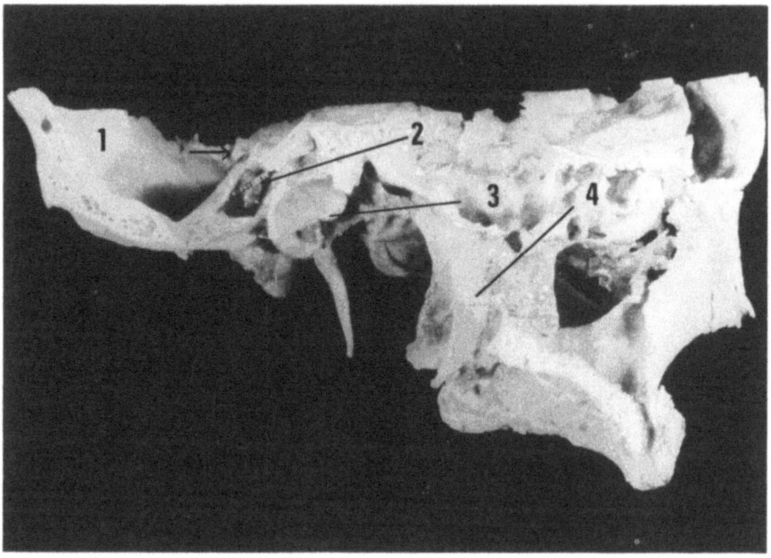

Fig. 4 Basilar Impression.
1. Basilar impression; 2. A. vertebr., course; 3. Atlas, synostosed; 4. Proc. pterygoideus.

Some angles and reference-lines

Boogaard's foramen magnum-clivus angle. Boogaard [16] measured the angle between the anterior and posterior margins of the foramen magnum and the plane of the clivus. In his material this came to 119.5 – 136°. In our material the angle between the anterior and posterior borders of the foramen magnum and the Frankfurt horizontal plane was determined. This amounted to –13.7° (–2.1 – –27.0°) [100]. With basilar impression the upper cervical vertebra and the dens of the axis [14], possibly with atlas assimilation – see figure 4 – together with the foramen magnum and its surroundings is invaginated into the skull. Von Torklus and Gehle [114] stress that it is not a question of an impression, but that we are dealing with an occipital hypoplasia with a reduced descent of the base of the skull. The term impression is really applicable only to secondary, that is to say acquired, basilar invagination. Primary basilar impression associated with an occipital dysplasia occurs in about 1% [102]. In addition shortenings of the clivus are distinguished (median from paramedian basilar impressions). A series of reference lines for the assessment of platybasia, basilar impression and other malformations in the cranio-cervical region will be described.

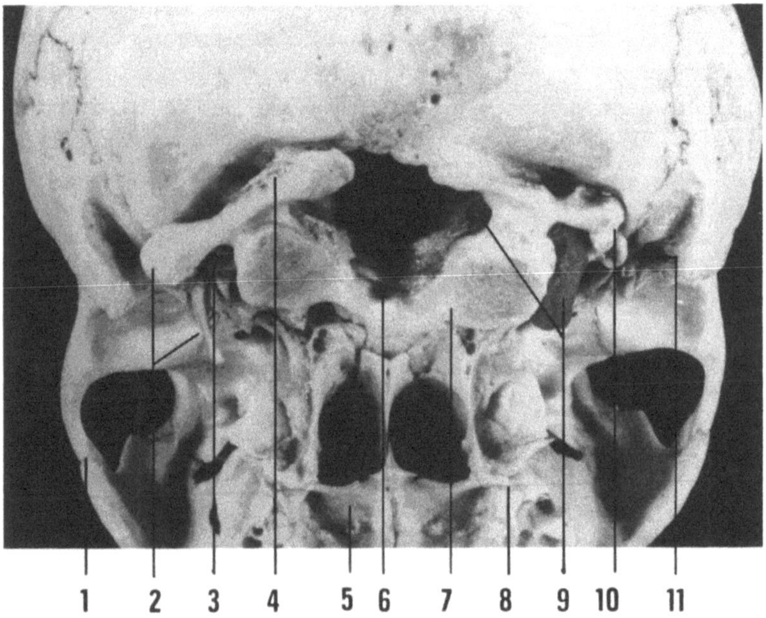

Fig. 5 Atlas-assimilation, viewed from behind.
1. Zygomatic arch; 2. Massa lateralis atlantis united with occiput and styloid process; 3. Foramen transversum; 4. Bony bridge between dorsal arch and occipital bone; 5. Hard palate; 6. Facies articularis dentis of anterior arch; 7. Facies articularis inferior atlantis; 8. Hamulus pterygoideus; 9. Course of the right vertebral arteries; 10. Massa lateralis atlantis, not completedly united with occipital bone; 11. Mastoid process.

McGregor's line [87], Weisbach's facial angle, Chamberlain's [21] line (between foramen magnum and posterior edge of the hard palate), McGregor's basal angle (Nasion – centre of the pituitary fossa, and centre of the pituitary fossa to the anterior margin of the foramen magnum) = 134 (124 – 147)°, mastoid line, etc.

Craniovertebral anomalies [113]. Clinical significance (fig. 5)

Bharucha and Dastur [13] examined 40 patients with craniovertebral anomalies (23 atlas assimilations, six basilar impressions, and others). They stress that with atlas assimilations (19 cases) there is, as a rule a short neck and a low hair line and in 16 of the patients the neck movements were restricted. In four of the patients there were lesions of the lower cranial nerves (dysphagia, disturbances of swallowing, and also impairment of the trigeminal nerve etc). Pyramidal signs [57) were frequent, and ataxia not only in atlas assimilation but also in basilar impressions. Occasionally in cases of basilar impression, disturbances of continence and respiration were observed, as well as more rarely, vertigo, vomiting, ataxia, loss of sensation in the upper limbs and chest. Wackenheim and Wackenheim et al. [122 – 126], as well as von Torklus [113] and von Torklus and Gehle [114] demonstrated radiologically a whole series of malformations of the cranio-cervical junction.

The cranial part of the cranio-cervical junction

a) Inner aspect of the clivus of the skull

The upper part of the clivus, including the dorsum sellae belongs to the body of the sphenoid bone, the lower part to the basilar portion of the occipital bone. As a rule the two portions are separated from each other by the spheno-occipital synchondrosis until the age of 16.5 (13 – 18) in males, and 14.4 (12 to 15) in females [102]. The ossification [68] normally proceeds from within outwards. In our material the length of the clivus in adults, measured between klition (a point on the highest edge of the dorsum sellae in the midline) and the basion (anterior border of the foraman magnum in the median sagittal plane) is 45 (37 – 52) mm [63]. In addition the lengths of the upper and lower parts of the clivus were determined in children from 0 – 6 years (fig. 6). According to Schmidt and Fischer [102] the length of the basilar portion of the occipital bone is 3.1 – 0.3 cm, in occipital hypoplasia 2.4 (± 0.3) cm, occasionally however it is only 1.7 cm. The thicker part of the clivus is in the anterior and superior part, and the thinner portion in the lower and posterior part. The upper and lower aspects consist of compact bone between which there is cancellous bone. As a rule the basal (outer) compact layer is thicker than the dorsal (inner) layer.

Basilar canals (Canales basilares)

It is rare, that a diploic vein traverses the clivus – the canalis basilaris. Gruber [43] examined 5000 skulls and distinguished superior, inferior and bifurcated basilar canals from each other. Hori [50] found altogether in 400 skulls from Japan, nine median basilar canals, among which were five superior median basilar canals, which drained upwards, two bifurcated median basilar canals which penetrated the clivus and likewise two median uniperforate basilar canals. Oehmke [93] described further sub-types of these diploic veins.

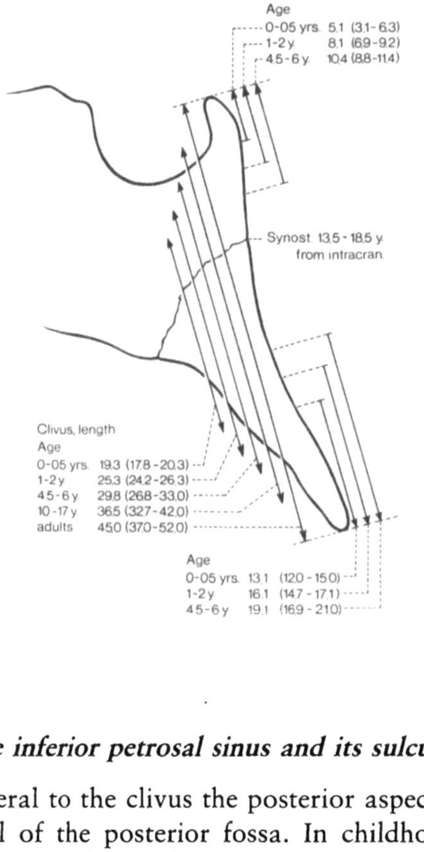

Fig. 6 Measurements of the length of the clivus and clivus parts in the median sagittal plane. Given are also some values of the sphenoidal and occipital clivus part in the postnatal time.

The inferior petrosal sinus and its sulcus [17]

Lateral to the clivus the posterior aspect of the petrous bone forms the anterior wall of the posterior fossa. In childhood and adolescence the sphenopetrosal (above) and the spheno-occipital (below) synchondroses are found between these two bones. In the region of this synchondrosis runs the inferior petrosal sinus. As the lower part of the clivus is wider than the upper, anatomists have for many years made a distinction between a longitudinal and a transverse portion of the inferior petrosal sinus. The pars longitudinalis is 7 – 10 mm, and the pars transversal is 2.85 (0.5 – 5.0) mm wide. The abducens nerve is enclosed in the upper part of the sinus, surrounded by a sheath of dura and arachnoid. Most frequently the inferior petrosal sinus drains, after penetrating the dural/pericranial layer, into the jugular foramen between the ninth and tenth cranial nerves (48%). In 30% it gets to the jugular foramen anterior to the ninth nerve, in 16% between the ninth and tenth and in 5% between the tenth and eleventh. It may be stressed, that duplication of the passage of the sinus through the jugular foramen is possible. The inferior petrosal sinus can enter the jugular foramen at varying levels, to join the internal jugular vein, sometimes even far below the base of the skull. Duplications of the internal jugular vein were also demonstrated in our material (with the development of several jugular foramina). Veins which pass through the pars petrosa of the internal carotid venous plexus, flow into the inferior petrosal sinus. We have designated these veins which we were able to find in 46% as medial intrapetrosal, and the lateral petrosal veins which were found in 50%.

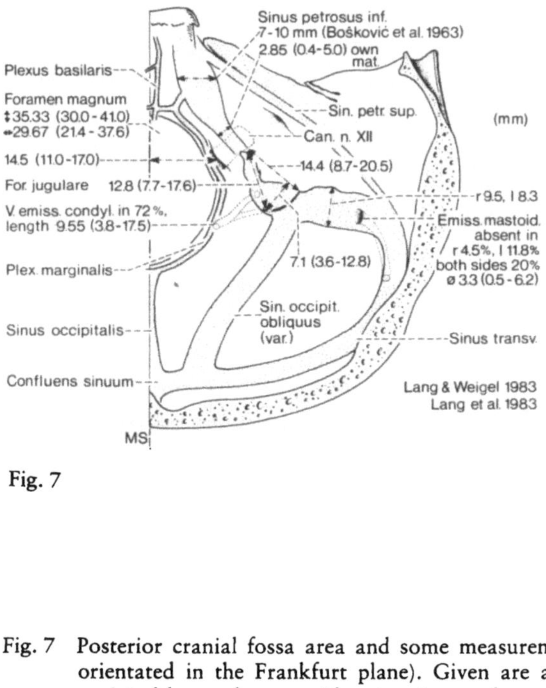

Fig. 7

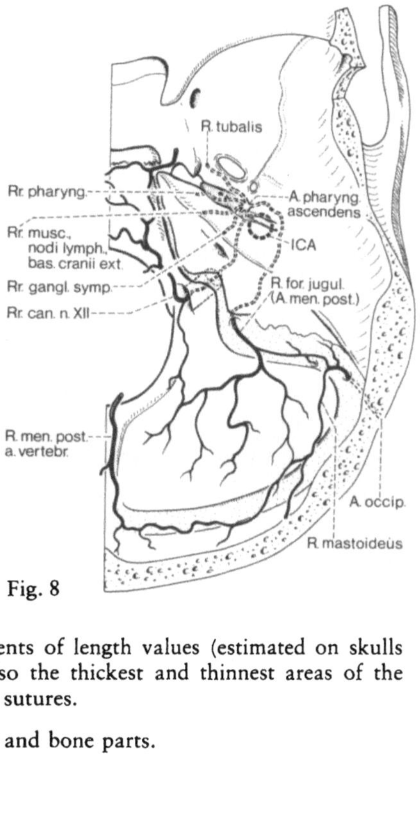

Fig. 8

Fig. 7 Posterior cranial fossa area and some measurements of length values (estimated on skulls orientated in the Frankfurt plane). Given are also the thickest and thinnest areas of the occipital bone, the mastoid emissarium and some sutures.

Fig. 8 Posterior cranial fossa, arteries of the dura mater and bone parts.

Jugular foramen

Repeated osteological investigations of the jugular foramen have been carried out on our material [8, 15, 78]. Single and multiple openings of various types were demonstrated. In the medial part of the jugular foramen a bony canal can be found, through which passes the inferior petrosal sinus with the glossopharyngeal nerve, or either structure on its own [78]. Medially the inferior petrosal sinus is connected with the basilar plexus. This takes various forms and runs between the dorsum sellae and the basion. In this region the clivus shows a depression not only in the longitudinal but also in the transverse axis. Twigs of the meningeal arteries run within the basilar plexus (and in the dural sinuses in general) and anastomose with each other. As a rule a branch of the ascending pharyngeal artery enters the skull through the jugular foramen [75]. The average diameter of this vessel is 0.63 (0.2 – 1.1) mm. From above, dorsal rami of the carotico-cavernous branches run into the basilar plexus and onto the posterior aspect of the petrous temporal bone, while from below twigs reach the vascular network from the meningeal branches of the vertebral artery [76]. Figure 7 gives details about the openings in the posterior cranial fossa, including the condylar and the mastoid emissary veins. Meningeal rami from the occipital artery run into the skull through the mastoid emissary (frequently double, rarely triple, occasionally very wider) (fig. 8). Occasionally we found meningeal branches to the floor of the posterior fossa from the posterior inferior cerebellar artery (fig. 277, in [71]). At both sides of the foramen magnum the oblique occipital sinus runs from the straight sinus obliquely forwards and laterally to the jugular foramen. These are developed more frequently in fetuses and small children than in adults (fig. 89 in [69]). A venous network of variable density surrounds the foramen magnum itself. This is connected with the basilar plexus, with the venous plexus in the hypoglossal canal and with the suboccipital venous network. The illustration shows its position, course and angulation. It may be stressed that not uncommonly the foramen for the hypoglossal nerve is duplicated and the nerve may run through two bony canals. The nerve fibre bundles are likewise surrounded by sheaths of dura and arachnoid and are usually accompanied by a meningeal branch from the ascending pharyngeal artery. The nerve bundles usually come together before the external, inferior opening of the hypoglossal canal. The venous plexus of the hypoglossal canal communicates with the condylar emissary vein, those in the jugular foramen as well as with the large diploic veins of the jugular tubercle.

b) External aspect of the skull in the region of the clivus

For the transorsal (transnasal) approach to the clivus it is important for the surgeon to know its dimensions and the position of the adjoining structures. As on the inner aspect of the skull, there is also on the outside a smaller, anterior portion of the clivus, whose width is 25.5 (13 – 28) mm. This section is about 11 mm long. Below and posteriorly the clivus widens up to 42.7 (33 – 52) mm, at the medial border of the jugular foramen. This part measures 14.3 (8 – 20) mm. It must be stressed that the external openings of the two hypoglossal canals at their anterior limit are 28 mm, and at their posterior border something over 42 mm separated from each other. In the skulls of newborns and children the external opening is usually visible from below. Later, this becomes for the most part overgrown by the occipital condyle (fig. 9). The amount of room available between the openings for the great vessels and the nerves of the base of the skull can be seen in figure 9. It may be stressed that lateral to the occipital condyle there are usually longer or shorter canals on the outer aspect of the skull base, which transmit veins e.g. inferior condylar canal (fig. 327, in [71]).

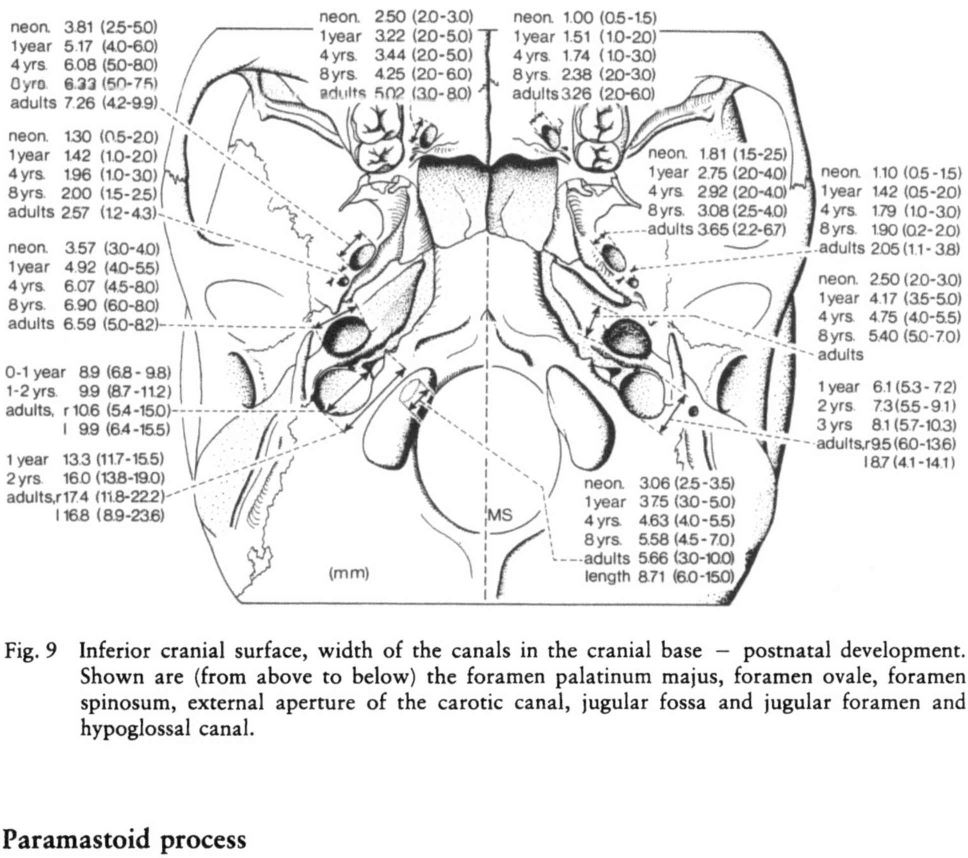

Fig. 9 Inferior cranial surface, width of the canals in the cranial base – postnatal development. Shown are (from above to below) the foramen palatinum majus, foramen ovale, foramen spinosum, external aperture of the carotic canal, jugular fossa and jugular foramen and hypoglossal canal.

Paramastoid process

Gruber [41] found a process with an articular facet, on the outer surface of the jugular process of the occipital bone, which articulated with the transverse process of the atlas. The articular process measured up to 24 mm on its dorsal aspect. Such paramastoid processes were also seen in our material (fig. 122, in [69]). These processes were also considered to be parts of the pro-atlas fused with the occiput. For further details see also Wackenheim [125] and von Torklus and Gehle [114] who observed these processes both with and without articulations with the atlas.

Occipital condyle

Both condyles are usually long and oval in shape, sometimes even reniform shaped. Between the third and sixth years their more anterior, smaller and medial portion is separated from the posterior, larger and lateral part by the anterior intra-occipital synchrondrosis. This synchondrosis also ossifies from within outwards. As a rule the condyle is twice as long as it is wide. Strecker [110] has described a whole series of different shapes (very short and wide, flat and long, narrow and markedly convex!). Slight asymmetries occur quite frequently, more marked ones less frequently. According to Ingelmark [51] in newborns the long axis of the occipital condyle makes an angle with the midline on average of 35.5°, in adults one of 28°. Apparently during the post-natal widening and lengthening of the foramen magnum the anterior segments of the two condyles become more separated from each other than the posterior. In our material the distances between the anterior and posterior ends of the occipital condyles as well as their angulation were determined afresh (fig. 10).

The lateral surface of the condyle lies higher than the medial. If one draws tangents in the frontal plane, the so-called frontal joint axial angle amounts to an average of 124° in men and 127° in women [60] (fig. 11). There are high and low occipital condyles, as McRae [88] has also pointed out. With hypoplasia of

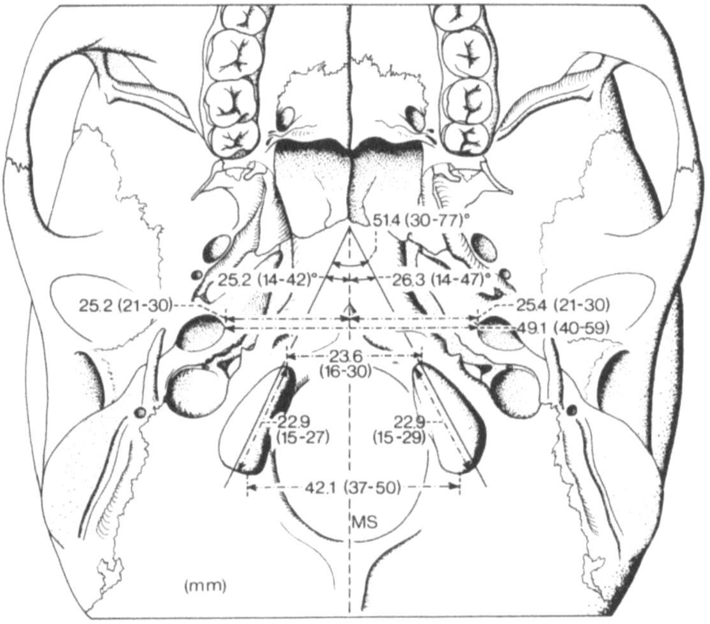

Fig. 10 Inferior surface of the skull, axis of the occipital condyles, its anterior and posterior distances from the median sagittal plane and its length. Given are also distances of the medial border of the canalis caroticus.

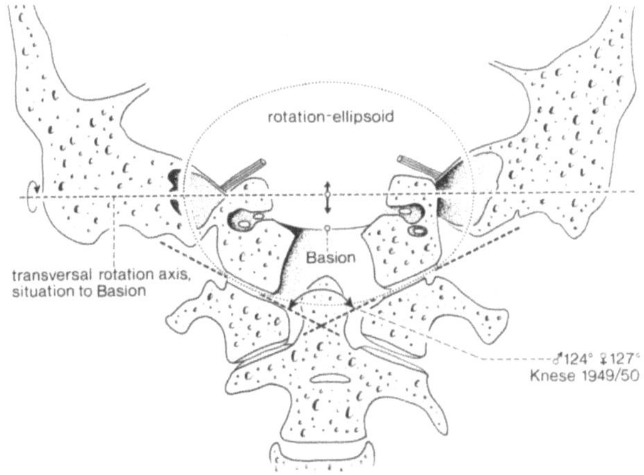

Fig. 11 Coronal axis of the atlanto-occipital joint and transversal rotation axis – its situation to basion.

the condyles the frontal joint axis angle increases up to 152° [60] or even to 160° [109]. Above the occipital condyle the hypoglossal nerve traverses the bone and above this the jugular tubercle is found on the inside of the skull. In our material the distance between tuberculum and condyle was 19.6 (12.4–25.1) mm.

Atlanto-occipital joint – axis of rotation (fig. 12)

In our material, in each case both occipital condyles from 42 skulls and 35 heads were modelled with Optosil [36], as only the two occipital condyles are able jointly to articulate with the upper articular facets of the atlas. With the computer T50 of the computer centre Wurzburg an attempt was then made to adapt the joint surfaces, which was possible with the help of a rotation ellipsoid. By calculating in this way, the interval from the transverse axis of the atlanto-occipital joint to the basion measured 20.53 (± 1.18) mm and a distance from the Frankfurter horizontal of 9.57 (± 0.45) mm.

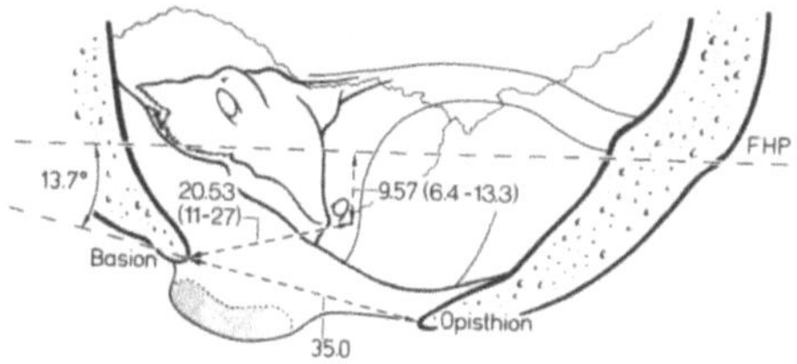

Fig. 12 Position of the transverse axis of the atlanto-occipital joint, reconstructed by Fuchs [36]. The transverse axis is situated 20.53 mm behind the basion and 9.57 mm below the Frankfurt horizontal plane (mean values). Given is also the angle between the anterior and posterior borders of the foramen magnum and the Frankfurt horizontal plane [100] and the length of the foramen magnum is also estimated on our material. All values in mm (extremals).

Basal process

Anterior and medial to the occipital condyle there may be small or larger tuberosities on the outer side of the skull, which according to Bolk (1921) may represent incompletely involuted rostral portions of the condyle, or else remnants of the pro-atlas which have fused with the occipital. These processes were found by Kalenscher [53] in 14% and by Bystrow [19] in 9% of cases.

The atlas in adults

a) The atlas from above (fig. 13)

The atlas consists of the anterior arch with the anterior tubercle (tuberculum anterius) anteriorly (figs. 15, 16) and the facet for the odontoid process (fovea dentis) behind [55], the posterior arch with a groove for the vertebral artery and the posterior tubercle. At the side, the lateral mass juts out further laterally than in the lower cervical spine. It is perforated by the foramen transversarium, which gives passage to the vertebral artery and its accompanying venous plexus, as well as the vertebral nerve(s). Their medial margins are 52.3 (44 – 59) mm apart, the lateral ones 64 (56 – 70) mm. The medial parts of the margin may be overlapped by the superior articular facet of the atlas. The dens (figs. 15, 16) articulates with a facet on the posterior aspect of the anterior arch. The posterior arch forms about two-fifths of the total circumference of the atlas (fig. 14).

The greatest length of the vertebral foramen on the upper aspect of the atlas is 34.5 (28 – 38) mm, the greatest width 30.2 (25 – 40) mm. According to Tsusaki

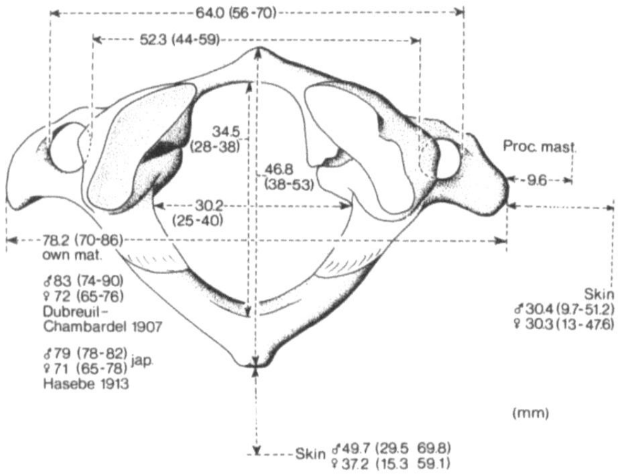

Fig. 13 Atlas from above, measurements.

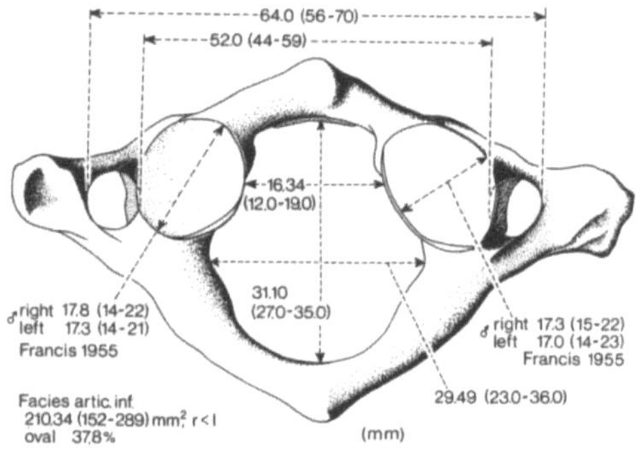

Fig. 14 Atlas from below. Measurements in mm (extremals).

[115] the sagittal measurement between the anterior and posterior tubercles is 39.8 – 48.0 mm, but most frequently it measures between 42 and 46 mm. In our material it was 46.8 (28 – 53) mm. In European males the average figure was 46.5 and in females 43.2 mm. In the Japanese the figures are somewhat smaller. The greatest transverse diameter in European males is 83 (74 – 90) mm and in females 72 (65 – 76) mm [26]. In our material the greatest width was 78.2 (70 – 86) mm. The vertical diameter of the anterior arch of the atlas was found by Hasebe [46] to be 10.1 (9 – 11) mm, that of the posterior arch 9.9 (4.0 – 13.0) mm. The foramen transversarium is often not closed, laterally or antero-laterally (see Fig. 119 and 120 in [69]). In about 3% there is a posterior cleft in the atlas, and occasionally even a completely cleft atlas is found (figs. 120 and 121, in [69]).

The bridge over the vertebral artery in the sulcus for the artery is called ponticulus. Ponticuli posteriores bridge over the artery (and accompanying veins), as well as the suboccipital nerves, from behind, ponticuli laterales from laterally and anteriorly. Ponticuli dorsales occur in ca. 10% [6], ponticuli laterales in 2.3% (Barge) or else 2.9% [48]. According to Lamberty and Živanović [66] it is completely bridged over in about 7.6%.

In the lateral part of the arch of the atlas is situated the superior articular facet (fovea articularis superior). Not uncommonly this articular facet shows a division into two, which can be explained developmentally (v. s.). In shape the articular facet corresponds to the respective occipital condyle. In the "Nomina anatomica" (1983), these fluted surfaces are called the superior articular facets (Facies articularis superior). According to Tsusaki [115] the length of the superior articular facet on the right is on average 22.3 mm, on the left 22.8 mm. The limits are between 19.8 and 25.9 mm. The greatest width, measured vertical to the length in our material was 10.3 mm right and 10.0 mm left. The limits were 8.2 and 13.3 mm. Other investigators found, as a rule, the joint surface bigger on the right than on the left.

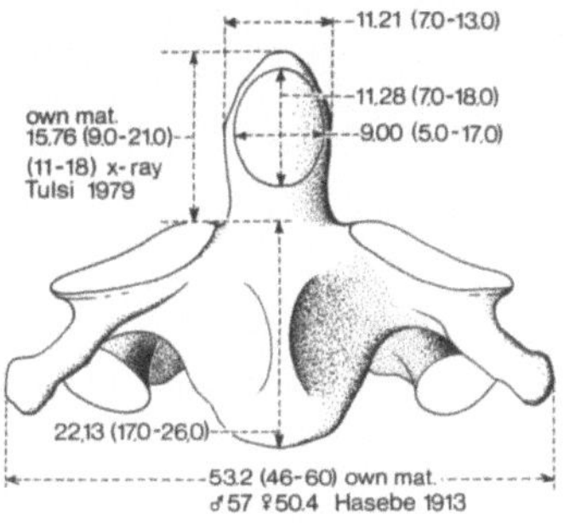

Fig. 15 Axis, measurements in mm (extremals).

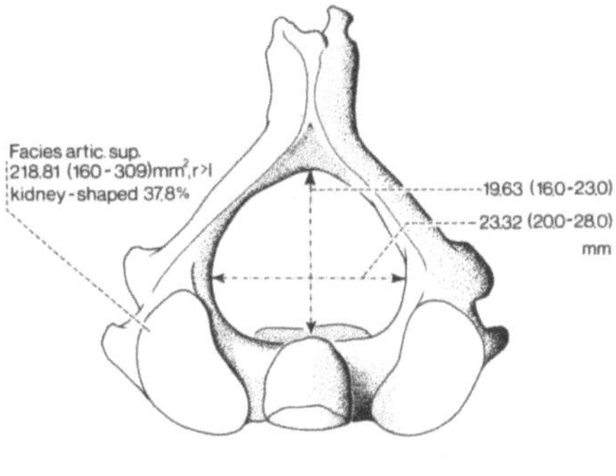

Fig. 16 Axis from above.

Medially and below the superior articular facet there are small tubercles and areas for the entry of blood vessels near the area of attachment of the transverse ligament of the atlas: the tuberculum ligamenti transversi atlantis. Slightly dorsally a smaller accessory tuberculum is found from which the accessory atlanto-axial ligament may arise. Around the kidney-shaped superior articular facets, described by Cave [20] there are in 50% grooves for the recesses of the joint cavity (medial recesses).

Atlas assimilation [127]

a) Varieties

Ingelmark [51] distinguished genuine atlas assimilation, pathological fusions between the atlas and the occiput (tuberculosis, non-specific infections, spondylo-arthritis ankylopoietica), assimilations as a result of lesions in the occiput and assimilations after dislocations. According to X-ray findings assimilations of the atlas were shown in 0.4% [114]. In our material also, as with earlier investigations of atlas assimilation, they are usually associated with other malformations [90]. Complete, and thick bony ridges between the posterior border of the foramen magnum and the posterior arch of the atlas may well be interpreted as remnants of the pro-atlas, fused with the occiput and the atlas (fig. 3). These can attain a height of 17 mm. Not uncommonly unilateral fusions of the atlas with the occiput are found e. g. the lateral mass and the posterior arch completely fused with the occiput on one side, and incomplete fusion on the other side (fig. 5). Frequently with assimilations of this sort between basion and the anterior arch of the atlas a hole can be identified. Occasionally there is no foramen for the passage of the vertebral artery. Not uncommonly atlas assimilation is associated with a platybasia. In one of our specimens with basilar impression there is also a small "third condyle" (condylus tertius) and on the inferior aspect of the completely assimilated atlas a large articular facet concave downwards.

Craniocervical junction, joint capsules and ligaments

Atlanto-occipital joint (fig. 17)

The fibrous capsule of the atlanto-occipital joint is attached around the occipital condyles as well as in the region of the upper articular facet of the atlas. It is thinner anteriorly and medially than behind and laterally. On the medial side of the joint there are occasionally defects which can exist in the attachments with the joint cavity between the dens and the transverse ligament of the atlas [20, 56].

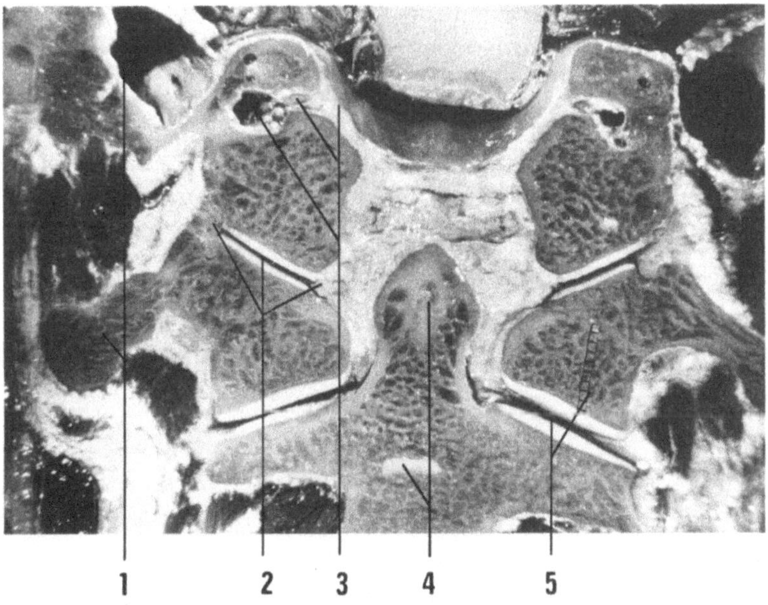

Fig. 17 Coronal section through cervicocranial junction, viewed from behind.
1. Fossa jugularis and transverse process of atlas; 2. Articulatio atlanto-occipitalis, capsule and synovial pads; 3. Hypoglossal nerve bundles, hypoglossal canal and dura mater; 4. Dens axis and subdental synchondrosis; 5. Articul. atlanto-axialis lateralis and mm-graph.

Recesses and depth

At the anterior margin of the occipital condyle there was, in our material, a recess, on average 4.6 mm deep, laterally the recess was 3.8 mm and medially 2.6 mm deep; dorsally there was an average depth of 2.8 mm [36]. The deepest part of the recess was in the region of the upper surface of the atlas, on its lateral surface (5.2 mm). Anteriorly the recesses are on average 4 mm, behind 3.8 mm and medially 2.6 mm deep (as compared with the respective adjacent articular surfaces). In injection experiments it was possible to inject about 0.7 cm^3 of material into the atlanto-occipital joint. The anterior and upper recess was most markedly filled in extreme dorsal flexion, the lower and lateral in lateral flexion to the opposite side [36].

Atlanto-occipital joint. Thickened zones in the capsule

a) Anterior oblique atlanto-occipital ligament
From the lower part of the lateral mass of the atlas the ligaments spread radially outwards and anteriorly in the lateral part of the capsule.

b) Posterior atlanto-occipital ligament
The ligament spreads outwards from the superior tubercle of the atlas and is frequently blended with fibres arching over the vertebral artery.

c) Lateral accessory occipital ligaments
These thin ligaments run laterally in the side wall of the atlanto-occipital joint and are attached to the atlas behind the centre of its upper articular facet.

d) Anterior accessory occipital ligaments
These thin ligaments run in the anterior part of the capsule.

e) Accessory posterior ligaments
In the posterior part of the capsule thin ligaments extend downwards and laterally from the occiput.

Atlanto-occipital joints, capsules and ligaments (fig. 18)

Altogether there are four joint cavities between the atlas and the axis. The dens (odontoid process) [37] articulates with the "fovea dentis" of the anterior arch of the atlas and the transverse ligament of the atlas. The inferior articular facets of the atlas are related on each side to the upper ones of the axis.

a) Transverse ligament of the atlas (fig. 19)
The ligament arises on each side of the inner surface of the anterior arch of the atlas, from the tubercle of the transverse ligament and its fibres run almost parallel and broadly flattened over the posterior surface of the dens. It is slightly bowed dorsally. Thus, the dens of the axis fits in an osteofibrous socket. In its central portion the ligament is about 10 mm high and 2 mm thick. In sagittal section it is possible at times to identify a thicker portion above and below. Occasionally in our material foci of degeneration were found in the transverse ligament of the atlas. According to Macalister [86] it is only possible to rupture the ligament with a force of 130 kg. Fielding et al. [28] produced tears of the transverse ligament of the atlas and heard usually that the ligament ruptured with a loud crack. The force required to rupture the transverse ligament ranged from 12 to 180 kp (mean 84 kp) under slow loading. Under rapid loading the mean was 111 kp. Isolated cartilage cells are scattered on the anterior side of the ligament. On the posterior aspect of the dens there is a thin covering of cartilage.

b) Transverse occipital ligament (fig. 19)
From the inner aspect of the occipital condyle immediately above the transverse ligament of the atlas a transverse ligament runs from one side to the other. Some of its fibres blend with the alar ligament.

c) Cruciform ligament
Longitudinal bands of fibres (unevenly developed) lie on the dorsal aspect of the transverse ligament of the atlas: fasciculi longitudinales. When well developed

Fig. 18

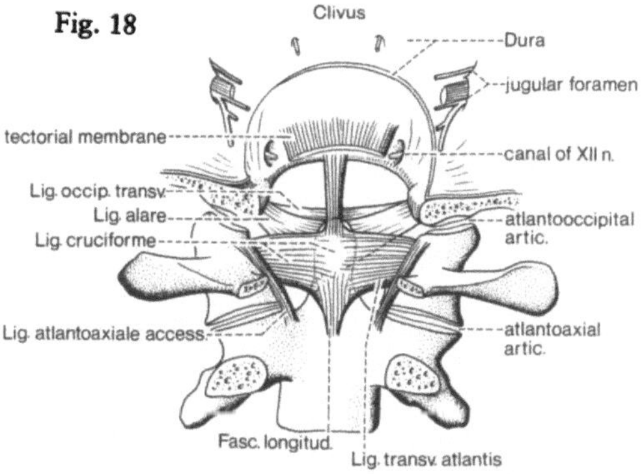

Fig. 19

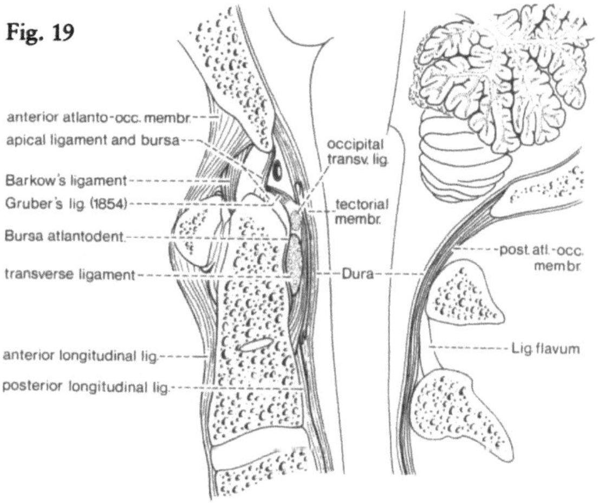

Fig. 18 Ligaments of the craniocervical junction from behind.

Fig. 19 Ligaments of the craniocervical junction on a median sagittal section.

the upper band extends up as far as the basion, the lower one down to the posterior surface of the body of the axis. Together with the transverse ligament of the atlas it produces a cruciform ligament whose transverse portion is much more strongly developed than its longitudinal.

d) Ligamentum apicis dentis (ligament of the apex of the dens) [23]
The ligamentum apicis dentis extends from the tip of the dens to the upper side of the basion. It is 2–5 mm wide and 2–8 mm long, and consists of a small amount of loosely arranged collagen and some elastic fibres. Foci of calcification and rods of cartilage have been identified in it [83]. This ligament does not appear to be of any mechanical significance, being only the continuation into the skull of the perinotochordal tissues.

e) Accessory atlanto-axial ligaments
Immedially dorsal to the tubercle for the transverse ligament of the atlas there is usually a further tubercle from which the accessory atlanto-axial ligament takes origin. The ligament runs behind the cruciform ligament, obliquely medially and downwards to the posterior surface of the body of the axis. It reinforces the medial aspect of the lateral atlanto-axial joint.

f) Alar ligaments
A strong ligament runs from the lateral and posterior surfaces of the dens obliquely laterally and upwards to the medial sides of the occipital condyles. This ounded ligament, about 8 mm wide, also strengthens the medial aspect of the capsule of the atlanto-occipital joint. It can be duplicated or be attached by

an accessory band to the cruciate ligament. According to Fielding et al. [28] the alar ligaments allow an anterior shift of the first cervical vertebra from three to five mm. Following failure of the transverse ligament, the force necessary to produce anterior shift, up to the endpoint of 12 mm ranged from 20 to 120 kp (mean 72 kp). During this procedure the alar ligaments did not break.

The ligament of Barkow, thinly developed, runs from the tip of the dens to the antero-lateral margin of the foramen magnum. The ligament of Gruber [42] goes from the transverse ligament of the atlas to the tip of the dens.

g) Lateral occipito-axial ligament

From the lateral margin of the occipital condyle a ligament about 20 mm long and 2 mm thick comes off and is attached to the lateral margin of the axis [92, 126].

h) Recesses

In our material the recesses of the lateral atlanto-axial joint were measured in joint injection preparations. On the anterior side the height of the recess (in a cranio-caudal direction) was on average 2.1 mm, on the posterior side it was about 7.1 mm, medially about 5 mm and laterally it showed heights of ca. 10 mm [111].

i) Capsular fibres

As a result of the stretching of the joint space, impressions can be detected on the outer surface of the cast, which are produced by the circular fibres of the capsule. Anteriorly, laterally and behind they are well-marked, but medially are scarcely apparent.

In the central region of the joint capsule there are decussations of the fibres at angles of $20° - 40°$, hence the collagenous capsular fibres which are first of all inside, run underneath to the outer surface of the capsule. On its inner aspect the joint capsule is covered by the synovial membrane, from which the circular synovial folds project into the joint space. A similar arrangement is apparent anteriorly. Laterally the capsular fibres run from above and dorsally to below and anteriorly as far as the level of the middle of the joint space, and then from anteriorly and above, to posteriorly and below. Here, there is likewise a decussation of the collagen fibres. On the medial side there are similar relationships. On the dorsal side the capsule is formed on its inner aspect by fibres which ascend from below and medially to above and laterally, and which correspond to the inner portions of the accessory atlanto-axial ligament. A decussation of the fibres can also be identified here.

j) Anterior and posterior atlanto-occipital membranes

The broad and powerful membrane stretches between the upper border of the posterior arch of the atlas and the posterior part of the clivus. It is continued downwards as the anterior longitudinal ligament (fig. 19). The posterior atlanto-occipital membrane consists of several layers. In contrast to the anterior atlanto-occipital membrane, its fibres do not run longitudinally but obliquely and have special gaps for the vertebral artery and its accompanying veins and nerves.

k) Bursae

α) Atlanto-dental bursa
Strange to say the joint space between the posterior surface of the dens and the anterior aspect of the transverse ligament of the atlas, is described as the atlanto-dental bursa. The joint space forms very extensive recesses of varying size, bilaterally and also above and below.

β) Cruciate tectorial bursa
In our material there is, not uncommonly, a bursa between the posterior aspect of the cruciate ligament and the tectorial membrane, or else loose sliding tissue.

γ) Bursa apicis dentis
Between Gruber's ligament and the dens there is a diverticulum of the atlanto-dental bursa – the bursa of the apex of the dens. This can also exist as a separate entity.

δ) Cruciate bursa
A bursa may also be developed between the cranial longitudinal fasciculi of the cruciate ligament.

l. Ligaments and their function
The ligaments of the cranio-cervical junction protect the central nervous system from injuries, and limit the range movement of the joints of the head.

First of all the transverse ligament of the atlas prevents any dorsal displacement of the dens, and on the other hand allows movements of the dens upwards and downwards, by means of the recesses of the anterior and posterior joints of the dens.

The alar ligaments are stretched in dorsi-flexion of the head and are relaxed in forward flexion. They also check the dens anteriorly and above, and prevent any excessive posterior displacement. With lateral tilting at the atlanto-occipital joint (only possible to a slight degree as an isolated movement) the ipsilateral alar ligament is relaxed, particularly with flexion of the head posteriorly. The thinner transverse occipital ligament likewise checks any forward movement of the dens. The cruciate ligament and the tectorial membrane form the posterior wall of the atlanto-dental joint and also produce a posterior deviation of the dens. The powerful anterior atlanto-occipital membrane prevents a downward displacement of the anterior arch of the atlas, while the posterior atlanto-occipital membrane on account of its oblique fibres, particularly restricts rotation movements of the atlas in relation to the occiput. At the same time, an excessive lateral tilting is prevented by the controlateral lateral occipito-axial ligament.

m) Head joints. Function
The head joints taken together form a sort of ball-and-socket joint, by which forward and retroflexion can be undertaken, particularly at the atlanto-occipital joint – around 5–6° forward flexion and 11°–21° dorsiflexion. In forward flexion the atlas together with the occiput tips forwards on the axis. Some lateral flexion to each side, of around 4° is possible in the upper joints, particularly with slight forward flexion (combined with forced rotation). In the atlanto-axial joints rotation [119] movements are particularly performed (up to ca. 30°–35° in each direction). In this the head and the atlas as a rule rotate together (figs. 15, 16).

Rotation movements are restricted in particular by the alar ligaments, as well as by the posterior atlanto-occipital membrane.

Lateral movements of the atlas takes place in association with lateral flexion of the head: if the head is tilted towards the left, the occipital condyles slide about 5° from left to right on the upper joint surface of the atlas. At the same time the atlas slides to the left on the left upper articular facet of the axis, so that the right articular facet climbs medially onto the lateral atlanto-axial joint. The atlas turns with the skull 2°–3° to the left and the head about 10° in relation to the axis. It must be emphasised that in flexion and extension movements at the atlanto-axial joints, movements of 8.5 to 19.5° can be achieved [120]. According to Bakke [5] lateral movements of between 3 and 4° are possible at the atlanto-axial joints.

Atlas and axis. Vascular supply

It should be stressed, that in the region of the cranio-cervical junction the various arteries vertebral, deep cervical, ascending pharyngeal and occipital – partly through muscular arteries – anastomose extensively with each other. The arteries over the anterior aspect of the axis and atlas come most frequently from the vertebral artery in the interspace between C3/C4 or C2/3, and run upwards and medially. Their bony branches enter the anterior aspect of the body of the axis and the base of the odontoid process (dens). A branch (the anterior dental artery) runs upwards close to the dens and forms at its apex, a so-called anterior axis arcade. The anterior aspect of the lateral atlanto-axial joint is supplied by branches from the anterior ascending artery of the axis.

There is likewise a branch from the vertebral artery between C3 and C4 or C2/C3, which reaches the posterior aspect of the axis, ascends close to the bone and becomes a posterior dental artery, which forms a posterior axis arcade. The two arcades on the dens lie close to the skull and from them branches are given off to the alar ligaments and to the other ligaments in this region. Proximally, portions of the bodies of C 2 and C 3 are supplied. The atlas receives its principal blood supply via the vertebral artery and its anastomoses. One can distinguish an artery of the posterior arch of the atlas (and anterior external) as well as corresponding branches on the inner aspect of both arches of the atlas, which were called by Rothman and Simone [98] the posterior and anterior arteries of the vertebral canal. Fischer et al. [29] emphasise that the left anterior ascending artery as a rule runs further distally from the vertebral than the right and it usually has a wider lumen than the right. Schiff et al. [101] particularly pointed out anastomoses with branches of the internal carotid. Accordingly numerous little twigs from the internal carotid run through the retropharyngeal space and across the midline of the axis to form anastomoses with the anterior ascending artery, and in the prevertebral musculature anastomoses exist with branches of the ascending pharyngeal artery. The joint capsules, the cruciate ligament and the tectorial membrane are also supplied by the posterior axis arteries.

Dura mater

At the cranio-cervical junction the cranial dura mater is directly continuous with the spinal dura mater. Apart from this, parts of the dura mater, very strongly developed, are attached around the margins of the foramen magnum, while other bundles of fibres pass outwards into the surrounding pericranium. The dura consists of a mixture of collagenous and elastic fibres, long stretches of which are longitudinally orientated. Particularly in the cervical region there are numerous transverse fibres [79]. This author described a cranial ligament of the dura mater (Ligamentum craniale durae matris), a strand of dura going to the posterior border of the atlanto-occipital joint, as well as fibres going to the posterior arch of the atlas. In our material a band of fibres up to 9 mm wide extended downwards from the posterior arch of the atlas to the spinal dura (fig. 20). Schürmann has particularly referred to the apparently reinforced dura mater which is seen during operations at the anterior margin of the foramen magnum and the posterior arch of the atlas, which e. g. in dislocations [104] is likely to cause damage to the spinal cord.

The central nervous system (spinal cord) and the mechanism of its fixation in the subarachnoid space

The most important mechanism of this sort is undoubtedly the dentate ligament (Ligamentum denticulatum). This frontally arranged layer consists predominantly of (inelastic) collagenous fibres and is fixed by 10 – 23 triangular tooth-like

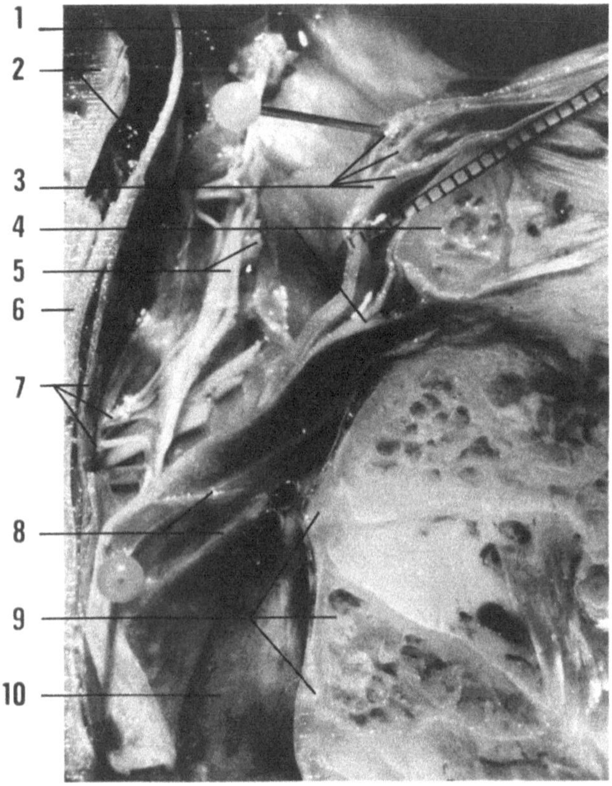

Fig. 20 Ligaments of the craniocervical junction in the posterior area, dura mater displaced ventrally. 1 = A. vertebralis; 2 = Dens axis (Lig. transversum removed); 3 = Dura mater displaced ventrally and fibres to opisthion; 4 = mm-graph, dorsal arch of atlas and lig. duro-atlantis dors; 5 = Lig. denticulatum and dorsal root fibres C_2; 6 = Membrana tectoria; 7 = Anterior dura and fila radicularia ventralia et dorsalia C_3; 8 = Dura-axial ligaments; 9 = l. flava C_2/C_3 and C_3/C_4 and proc. spinalis C_3; 10 = Cavitas epiduralis (faty tissues removed).

processes to the inner aspect of the dura mater. We were able to trace extensions of these fibres not only into the dura, but also into the pia mater (epipia) [74]. The most cranial process crosses behind the first intracranial portion of the vertebral artery and is attached to the dura an average of 3.55 (2 – 7) mm cranial and 2.1 (0 – 4) mm dorsal to the point where that vessel pierces the dura mater. On the left side the average cranial distance is 3.88 (1 – 8) mm. There is no difference between left and right for the average distance posterior to the average entry point of the vertebral artery. On rare occasions we have seen fibres of the uppermost denticulate ligament also running ventral to the vertebral artery. Stofft [108] found the processes completely ventral and caudal to the artery in 4%. In the upper cervical region the processes are as a rule attached 1.5 – 2 mm dorsal to the adjoining dural pockets in the dura mater [74].

Rhomboid ligaments (fig. 21)

Key and Retzius [58] were the first to describe a thin rhomboidal layer of fibres, which surrounds the spinal cord from in front. Their lateral fibres always run along with the second, and frequently also with the first process of the denticulate ligament in the dura. Numerous variations of this rhomboid ligament are seen.

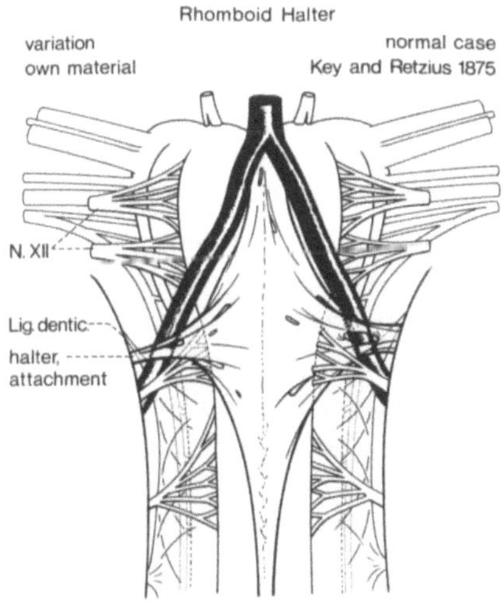

Fig. 21 Rhomboid halter on the ventral side of the medulla spinalis.

Septum posticum

As a rule a septum posticum stretches from the pia on the dorsal aspect of the spinal cord to the dura mater. In the uppermost cervical region it consists for the most part of sagittally arranged arachnoid fibres.

Biological significance

The dentate ligament and the other structures mentioned above may be regarded as a functional unit. Their purpose is certainly to keep the spinal cord and the lower part of the medulla oblongata away from the walls of the spinal canal and also to leave room for the vertebral artery to move, in displacements of the spinal cord [18].

Medulla oblongata and spinal cord

At the craniocervical junction the medulla oblongata merges imperceptibly into the spinal cord. From time immemorial anatomists have considered the upper limit of the spinal cord to be the exit point of the uppermost root fibres of C 1.

As the dorsal root fibres are frequently absent, only the ventral ones can be used for determining this boundary. Another suggestion for deciding this boundary was at the lower end of the decussation of the pyramids [59, 80, 99, 116, 117, 128].

Craniocervical junction. Approach from behind (fig. 22)

With a posterior approach, as a rule, the one through the ligamentum nuchae is preferred although in our material there are not infrequently relatively wide veins running through it. The ligamentum nuchae forms a layer of connective tissue, which in man consists principally of collagenous tissue with a few elastic fibres and which extends from the superficial muscle layers as far as the spinous processes. It must be noted that the "third occipital nerve", in our material passes through the trapezius muscle 7.4 mm from the midline, on average, and on a level with the lower border of the arch of the atlas, while the greater occipital nerve, enters the under surface of the trapezius, on average, 15.9 mm from the midline and leaves the muscle near the squama nuchalis an average of 23.5 mm from the midline. This point for the passage of the greater occipital nerve is, on the average, 18.1 mm below the external occipital protuberance. Afterwards the nerve runs obliquely laterally and upwards, and crosses the occipital artery on average about 40 mm from the midline. This region can be overlapped by a

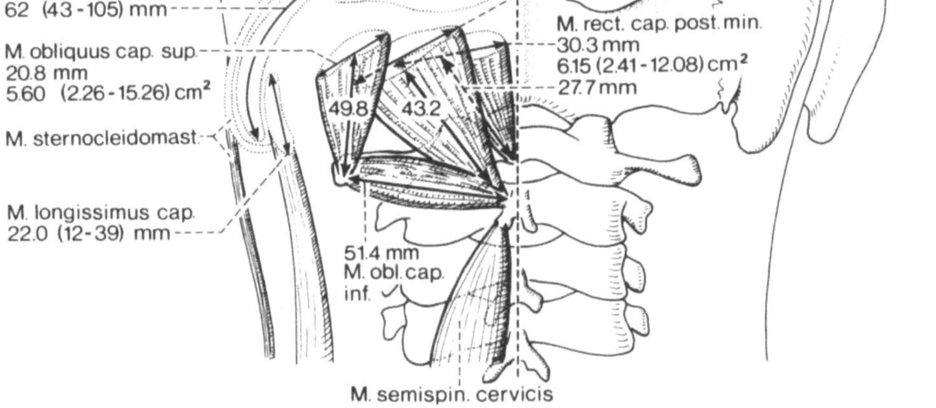

Fig. 22 Occipital muscles and insertion area of muscles on the dorsal area of the skull.

transverse occipital muscle or by a tendinous band and in collagen diseases can result in an incarceration or trapping. Attached to the occipital region near the midline, from above downwards are the trapezius, the semispinalis capitis and a little more laterally the obliquus capitis superior, the rectus capitis superior major and, near the midline the rectus capitis posterior minor. This muscle has its origin from the posterior tubercle of the atlas, while the rectus capitis posterior major and the obliquus capitis posterior minor come from the spinous process of the axis. Numerous variations of the origin and course of these short neck muscles exist [69]. The blood supply of the short neck muscles comes from the branches of the vertebral artery, which are mostly given off from the third part (pars atlantis), and from anastomoses with the deep cervical as well as with the occipital arteries. Their nerve supply is through the suboccipital nerve, from the posterior division of C1. According to the direction of these muscles they certainly have the possibilities of turning the cranial joints and of carrying out dorsi-flexion, but actually on account of their relatively slight power they just serve to correct the posture and positioning, in particular the correct adjustment, of the atlas. In addition the relatively numerous stretch receptors found in these muscles make them particularly suitable for the fine adjustment and the fixation of the cranial joints. When exposing the lateral part of the posterior arch of the atlas care must be taken of the muscular branches coming from the third part (pars atlantis) of the vertebral artery and the anastomoses of the vessels with the occipital and deep cervical arteries. In addition the extradural part of the vertebral artery is surrounded by a dense venous network that is, at present, called the suboccipital venous plexus on account of its connection with the adjoining veins. This takes place through various large veins in communication with the marginal sinus of the foramen magnum, the condylar emissary veins, internal jugular vein, occipital vein, the atlanto-occipital sinus, the venous plexus of the hypoglossal canal, the internal carotid plexus as well as with the vertebral bodies and the deep cervical veins. In our material the suboccipital nerve frequently goes through the gap between the third part of the vertebral artery (pars atlantis) and an accompanying vein which lies between this and the sulcus for the vertebral artery (fig. 152, in [69]). From the third part of the vertebral artery posterior meningeal branches run to the dura mater and floor of the posterior fossa and particularly to the falx cerebelli. These can be replaced by other meningeal branches e.g. from the occipital artery, which enter the skull by the mastoid emissary foramen. Lang [72] has described posterior inferior cerebellar arteries [106] which arise extradurally and after courses of varying length in the dura mater pass the vertebral artery dorsally. Also, during lateral retraction of the soft tissues on the posterior arch of the atlas particular care must be taken of these vessels which are important for the circulation of the central nervous system. At the point where the vertebral artery goes through the dura mater, or slightly proximal to this, small lateral medullary branches which supply the lateral surface of the

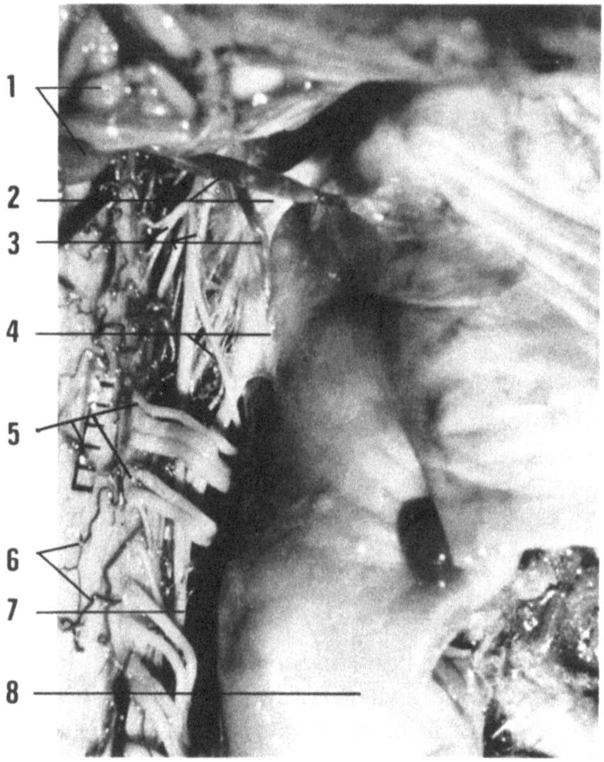

Fig. 23 Craniocervical junction, viewed from backwards.
1. Tonsilla cerebelli and PICA; 2. First serration of denticulate ligament and posterior transcisternal vein; 3. Lat. medullary branch and accessory nerve fibers; 4. 2nd serration of denticulate ligament and anastomoses with C_2; 5. Fila radic. dors. C_2 and mm-paper; 6. Post. spinal arteries; 7. Accessory nerve; 8. Dura mater, opened dorsally and fixed laterally.

medulla oblongata and the spinal cord, may be given off. However, these vessels as a rule anastomose with adjoining branches from the posterior inferior cerebellar artery and more distal sections of the radicular arteries.

Vertebral nerve in the upper cervical region

In 1981 we demonstrated in a dissection of the vertebral nerve, from the cervicothoracic ganglion and other neighbouring sympathetic ganglia of the cervical spine, which accompanies the vertebral artery in its canal within the foramina transversaria. These fibres accompany the vertebral artery in its upward course, and divide into even finer branches. Near C 1 and C 2 the upper cervical ganglion of the sympathetic trunk and its anastomosing plexus, with the adjoining lower cranial nerves gives off thin fibres to the vertebral artery, which accompany it into the cranial cavity. The fine branches of the nerve, are visible there in the adventitia of the vertebral artery and its branches. Corresponding to the developmental situation these branches take over the innervation of the cerebral arteries up to and including the superior cerebellar artery, as the posterior cerebral artery is regarded as one of the primitive branches of the internal carotid system. It is open to discussion whether lesions of the vertebral artery or constrictions of the vertebral artery at the craniocervical junction, or at other sites can be responsible for tinnitus, vertigo, loss of hearing, nystagmus and other symptoms.

When removing the posterior arch of the axis, to whose spinous process many muscles are attached, it may be noted that the multifidus muscles and the semispinalis cervicis muscles in this region can only be artifically distinguished from each other [54, 118]. The insertion of the multifidus can take place along the whole extent of the posterior arch of the axis as far as the inferior articular process of this vertebra.

After opening the dura mater and the arachnoid from behind, the medulla and the spinal cord, the posterior nerve roots and the posterior inferior cerebellar artery are visible as well as the vessels to the spinal cord and medulla (fig. 23). As a rule the accessory nerve runs dorsal to the dentate ligament and between this and the strands of the dorsal roots. The uppermost process of the denticulate ligament is then visible behind the vertebral artery. Rarely, the posterior inferior cerebellar artery has already arisen extradurally and has its own place of entry through the dura, dorsal to the vertebral artery. In these cases sometimes the upper process of the dentate ligament and the vertebral artery cannot be recognised without displacement of the PICA [72]. In our material, not uncommonly a vein runs out from the dorsal aspect of the medulla through the cisterna magna to the occipital sinus or to the maginal sinus of the foramen magnum and continues over the fibres of the posterior roots, the arteries to the medulla oblongata and the spinal cord, as well as the ganglia between the posterior roots of C 1, C 2 and C 3 and the accessory nerve [69, 70, 71].

Dorsolateral approach to the vertebral artery

After division of the splenius capitis and the semispinalis cervicis Küttner [64] palpates the upper border of the posterior arch of the atlas and afterwards exposes the vessel [65]. The occipital artery and the rectus capitis posterior major must be protected.

Elkin and Harris [27] expose the upper section of the vertebral artery – pars transversaria and pars atlantis by Henry's [49] approach. The incision is made along the anterior border of the sternocleidomastoid from the middle of the neck to the mastoid process. The muscle is then separated from its cranial attachment, retracted posteriorly and after protecting the accessory nerve, deepened to the transverse process of the atlas. The origin of the levator scapulae must be detached from the atlas and axis and retracted downwards. Afterwards the vertebral artery is protected. By this approach the greater auricular nerve and the cervical plexus should also be handled with care. The occipital artery can be ligated without any trouble.

Transoral approaches to the craniocervical junction, according to my knowledge were described for the first time by Chipault [22] and then by Le Fort [81]. The soft palate is retracted towards the base of the skull, the posterior wall of the pharynx divided in the midline for a distance of 5 cm, from the upper border of the anterior tubercle of the atlas to C 2 – C 3. At the lower border of the body of the axis and the upper border of C 2, the exposure should not stray much from the midline as medial displacements of the vertebral artery are occasionally encountered (Regarding the distances of the foramina transversaria v. s.).

Harms and Schmelzle [45] employ a transoral-transpalatine approach to clivus and the upper cervical vertebrae. The palate is incised to a variable extent and in the posterior part is retracted laterally. One must pay attention to its blood supply from the greater palatine, lesser palatine and ascending palatine arteries. Afterwards the posterior part of the hard palate and the vomer can be removed. The posterior pharyngeal wall, as well as the longus capitis can be resected from the base of the skull and retracted downwards. Care must be taken of its blood supply, particularly through the ascending pharyngeal which is given off further caudally and supplies branches to these structures. The vessels from the vertebral artery in the upper segments must be ligated. As a rule, a fixation of the atlanto-occipital joint can be successfully achieved by this route, using bone chips between the clivus and C 2 – C 3. The submandibular approach can be used, going either above or below the hyoid. With the suprahyoid approach the mylohyoid and geniohyoid are separated from the hyoid bone. These approaches have the advantage of going through a sterile field to reach the upper cervical spine.

References

[1] Abel, M. S.: Clinical and roentgenological aspects of "occult" fractures of the smaller elements of the cervical vertebrae. Am. J. Surg. **97** (1959) 530 – 542.

[2] Ackermann, J. R.: Über die Kretinen, eine besondere Menschenart in den Alpen. Ettinger'sche Buchhandlung, Gotha 1790.

[3] Adson, A. W., J. W. Kernohan, H. W. Woltman: Cranial and cervical chordomas. A clinical and histologic study. Arch. Neurol. Psychiat. **33** (1935) 247 – 261.

[4] Albrecht, P.: Über das zwischen dem Basioccipitale and dem Basipostsphenoid liegende Basi-Oticum. Zbl. med. Wiss. **16** (1878) 593.

[5] Bakke, S. N.: Röntgenologische Beobachtungen über die Bewegungen der Wirbelsäule. Acta Radiol. (Stockh.) Suppl. **13** (1931) 75.

[6] Barge, J. A. J.: Probleme im Craniovertebralgebiet. Verh. K. Akad. Wissensch. **20** (1918).

[7] Becker, E.: Messungen der Keilbeinhöhlen der Sella turcica, der Basiswinkel und des Sulcus fasciculi optici am seitlichen Röntgenbild des Schädels bei Kindern und Jugendlichen. Inaug. Diss., Rostock 1960.

[8] Behrens, M.: Über Volumen und Öffnungen der hinteren Schädelgrube. Med. Diss., Würzburg 1975.

[9] Bergerhoff, W., R. Stilz: Die Beugung der Schädelbasis im Röntgenbild. ROEFO **80** (1954) 618–622.

[10] Bergmann, C.: Einige Beobachtungen und Reflexionen über die Skeletsysteme der Wirbelthiere. Göttingen 1846.

[11] Bersch, W., W. Reinbach: Das Primordialcranium eines menschlichen Embryo von 52 mm Sch.-St.-Länge. Zur Morphologie des Cranium älterer menschlicher Feten. II. Z. Anat. Entwickl.-Gesch. **132** (1970) 240–259.

[12] Bertrand, G., J. Blundell, R. Musella: Electrical exploration of the interna capsule and neighbouring structures during stereotaxic procedures. J. Neurosurg. **22** (1965) 333–343.

[13] Bharucha, E. P., H. M. Dastur: Craniovertebral anomalies (A report on 40 cases). Brain **87** (1964) 469–480.

[14] Bodechtel, G., H. U. Guizetti: Pseudotumor cerebri, bedingt durch eine röntgenologisch faßbare Anomalie des Hinterhauptloches mit Verlagerung der beiden oberen Halswirbel. Z. f. d. g. Neur. u. Psych. (Berlin) **143** (1933) 470–477.

[15] Bonorden, B.: Über die allgemeine und spezielle Morphologie des menschlichen Foramen jugulare. Med. Diss., Würzburg 1976.

[16] Boogard, J. A.: De Indrukking der Grondvlakte van den Schedel door de wervelkolom, hare oorzaken en gevolgen. Ned. Tijdschr. Geneesk **1** (1865) 81–108.

[17] Bošković, M., V. Savić, J. Josifov: Über die Sinus petrosi und ihre Zuflüsse. Gegenbaurs Morphol. Jahrb. **104** (1963) 420–429.

[18] Breig, A.: Biomechanics of the central nervous system. Almqvist & Wiksell, Uppsala 1960.

[19] Bystrow, A. P.: Assimilation des Atlas and Manifestation des Proatlas. Z. Anat. Entwickl.-Gesch. **95** (1931) 210–242.

[20] Cave, J. E.: On the occipito-atlanto-axial articulations. J. Anat. **68** (1933/34) 416–428.

[21] Chamberlain, W. E.: Basilar Impression (Platybasia). A bizarre developmental anomaly of the occipital bone and upper cervical spine with striking and misleading neurologic manifestations. Yale J. Biol. Med. **11** (1939) 487–496.

[22] Chiapault (1894).

[23] Cramer, A.: Dens bicornis (Entwicklungsstörungen am Dens axis). In: Wirbelsäule in Forschung und Praxis, vol. 28. Hippokrates, Stuttgart 1964.

[24] Dahlin, D. C., C. S. MacCarty: Chordoma. A study of fifty-nine Cases. Cancer **5** (1952) 1170–1178.

[25] Dietemann, J. L., J. Lang, J. P. Francke et al.: Anatomy and Radiology of the Sellar Spine. Neuroradiology **21** (1981) 5–7.

[26] Debreuil-Chambardel, L.: Variations sexuelles de l'Atlas. Bull. Soc. Anthropologie de Paris. Ser. **5**, **8** (1907) 399.

[27] Elkin, D. C., M. H. Harris: Arteriovenous aneurysm of the vertebral vessels. Ann. Surg. (Philadelphia) **124** (1946) 934–951.

[28] Fielding, J. W., G. B. van Cochran, J. F. Lawsing et al.: Tears of the transverse ligament of the atlas. J. Bone Joint Surg. **56** (1974) 1683–1691.

[29] Fischer, L. P., J.-P. Carret, G. P. Gonon et al.: La vascularisation artérielle de l'axis. Bull. Assoc. Anat. (Nancy) **60** (1976) 335–346.

[30] Fischgold, H., J. Metzger: Etude radio-tomographique de l'impression basilaire. Rev. Rheum. **19** (1952) 261–264.

[31] Francis, C. C.: Variations in the articular facets of the cervical vertebrae. Anat. Rec. **122** (1955) 589–602.

[32] Froriep, A.: Über ein Ganglion des Hypoglossus und Wirbelanlagen in der Occipitalregion. p. 279, Arch. Anat. Physiol., 1882.

[33] Froriep, A.: Zur Entwicklungsgeschichte der Wirbelsäule, insbesondere des Atlas und Epistropheus und der Occipitalregion. I. Beobachtungen an Hühnerembryonen, pp. 177 – 234. Arch. Anat. Physiol. (1883).
[34] Froriep, A.: Zur Entwicklungsgeschichte der Wirbelsäule, insbesondere des Atlas und Epistropheus und der Occipitalregion. II. Beobachtungen an Säugethierembryonen. Arch. Anat. Physiol. (1886) 69 – 150.
[35] Froriep, A.: Die occipitalen Urwirbel der Amnioten im Vergleich mit denen der Selachier. Verh. Anat. Ges. **19** (1905) 111 – 120.
[36] Fuchs, E.: Untersuchung über die Gelenkflächen der Articulatio atlanto-occipitalis. Med. Diss., Würzburg 1980.
[37] Fullenlove, T. M.: Congenital absence of the odontoid process. Radiology **63** (1954) 72 – 73.
[38] Ganguly, D. N., K. K. Singh-Roy: A study on the craniovertebral joint in the man. Anat. Anz. **114** (1964) 433 – 452.
[39] Ganguly, D. N., K. K. Singh-Roy: A study on the craniovertebral joint in the vertebrates. (Guinea pig and Talpa) Anat. Anz. **117** (1965) 421 – 429.
[40] Geipel, P.: Zur Kenntnis der Spaltbildung des Atlas und Epistropheus. Part III. Fortschr. Röntgenstr. **52** (1935) 533.
[41] Gruber, W.: Neue Anomalien als Beiträge zur physiologischen, chirurgischen und pathologischen Anatomie. A. Förstner, Berlin 1849.
[42] Gruber, W.: Abhandlung aus der menschlichen und vergleichenden Anatomie. Petersburg 1854.
[43] Gruber, W.: Über den anomalen Canalis basilaris medianus des Os occipitale beim Menschen. Mém. Acad. Imp. Sci. St. Pétersburg (Sér. 7) 27/9 (1880).
[44] Gutmann, G.: Die Wirbelblockierung und ihr röntgenologischer Nachweis. In: Wirbelsäule in Forschung und Praxis, vol. XV (H. Junghanns, ed.). Hippokrates, Stuttgart 1960.
[45] Harms, J., R. Schmelzle: Persönliche Mitteilung 1985.
[46] Hasebe, K.: Die Wirbelsäule der Japaner. Zeitschr. f. Morph. u. Anthrop. **15** (1913) (zitiert nach Tsusaki, 1924).
[47] Hayek, H. v.: Über den Proatlas und die Entwicklung der Kopfgelenke beim Menschen und bei Säugetieren. S.-B. Akad. Wiss. Wien 1923.
[48] Hayek, H. v.: Untersuchungen über Epistropheus, Atlas und Hinterhauptsbein. Gegenbaurs Morphol. Jahrb. **58** (1927) 269 – 347.
[49] Henry, A. K.: Exposures of long bondes and other surgical methods. Wright & Sons, Bristol 1927.
[50] Hori, T.: Über die Anomalien des Hinterhauptbeines. Folia Anatomica Japonica **3** (1925) 291 – 312.
[51] Ingelmark, B. E.: Über das craniovertebrale Grenzgebiet beim Menschen. Acta Anat. (Suppl.) **6** (1947) 1 – 116.
[52] Issing, P.: Wissenschaftliche Arbeit am Anatomischen Institut Würzburg, 1985.
[53] Kalenscher, I.: Über den sogenannten dritten Gelenkhöcker und die accessorischen Höcker des Hinterhauptbeins. Inaug. Diss., Königsberg i. Pr. 1893.
[54] Kasche, F.: Die verschiedenen Formen des Epistropheusdornes in ihren Beziehungen zur Muskulatur. Anat. Anz. **56** (1923) 165 – 175.
[55] Keats, T. E.: The inferior accessory ossicle of the anterior arch of the atlas. Am. J. Roentgenol. **101** (1967) 834 – 836.
[56] Keller, H. L., A. Neiss: Abnorme Beweglichkeit der Occipito-Zervikalgegend beim Os odontoideum. Acta Radiol. **57** (1962) 145 – 155.
[57] Kertesz, A., N. Geschwind: Patterns of pyramidal decussation and their relationship to handedness. Arch. Neurol. **24** (1971) 326 – 332.
[58] Key, A., G. Retzius: Studien in der Anatomie des Nervensystems und des Bindegewebes. Nordstadt, Stockholm 1875.

[59] Keyserlingk, D. Graf v., U. Schramm: Diameter of axons and thickness of myelin sheaths of the pyramidal tract fibres in the adult human medullary pyramid. Anat. Anz. **157** (1984) 97–111.

[60] Knese, K.-H.: Kopfgelenk, Kopfhaltung und Kopfbewegung des Menschen. Z. Anat. Entwickl.-Gesch. **114** (1949/50) 67–107.

[61] Kohler, A., F. A. Zimmer: Borderlands of the normal and early Pathologic in Skeletal Roentgenology, Tenth ed. Grune & Straton, New York 1956.

[62] Kollmann, J.: Varianten am Os occipitale, besonders in der Umgebung des Foramen occipitale magnum. Anat. Anz. **27** (Suppl.) (1905) 231–236.

[63] Krauss, J.: Wissenschaftliche Arbeiten am Anatomischen Institut Würzburg 1985.

[64] Küttner, E.: Die Verletzungen und traumatischen Aneurysmen der Vertebralgefäße am Halse und ihre operative Behandlung. Beitr. Klin. Chirurgie **108** (1917) 1–60.

[65] Küttner, H.: Die Operation des Vertebralisaneurysmas und ihre Erleichterung durch lebende Tamponade. Zentralbl. Chir. (Leipzig) **57** (1930) 1025–1033.

[66] Lamberty, B. G. H., S. Zivanovic: The retro-articular vertebral artery ring of the atlas and its significance. Acta Anat. (Basel) **85** (1973) 113–122.

[67] Landzert, Th.: Der Sattelwinkel und sein Verhältnis zur Pro- und Orthognathie. Abh. Senckenberg. Nat. Forsch. Ges. **6** (1866) 145–165.

[68] Lang, J.: Structure and postnatal organization of heretofore uninvestigated and infrequent ossifications of the sella turcica region. Acta Anat. **99** (1977) 121–139.

[69] Lang, J.: Praktische Anatomie: e. Lehr- u. Hilfsbuch d. anat. Grundlagen ärztl. Handelns (founded by Lanz, W. Wachsmuth, edited by J. Lang and W. Wachsmuth), vol. 1, part 1, chapter B: Gehirn- und Augenschädel. Springer, Berlin–Heidelberg–New York 1979.

[70] Lang, J.: Klinische Anatomie des Kopfes – Neurokranium, Orbita, kraniozervikaler Übergang. Springer, Berlin–Heidelberg–New York 1981.

[71] Lang, J.: Clinical Anatomy of the Head. Neurocranium Orbit Craniocervical Regions (Translated by R. R. Wilson and D. P. Winstanley). Springer, Berlin–Heidelberg–New York 1983.

[72] Lang, J.: Anatomie der BWS und des benachbarten Nervensystems. In: Brustwirbelsäulenerkrankungen (D. Hohmann, B. Kügelgen, K. Liebig, eds.); Neuroorthopädie 3. Springer, Berlin–Heidelberg–New York–Tokyo 1985.

[73] Lang, J., B. Brückner: Über dicke und dünne Zonen des Neurocranium, Impressiones gyrorum und Foramina parietalia bei Kindern und Erwachsenen. Anat. Anz. **149** (1981) 11–50.

[74] Lang, J., A. Emminger: Über die Textur des Ligamentum denticulatum und der Pia mater spinalis. Z. Anat. Entwickl-Gesch. **123** (1963) 505–522.

[75] Lang, J., E. Heilek: Anatomisch-klinische Befunde zur A. pharyngea ascendens. Anat. Anz. **156** (1984) 177–207.

[76] Lang, J., K. Schäfer: Über Ursprung und Versorgungsgebiete der intracavernösen Strecke der A. carotis interna. Gegenbaurs morphol. Jahrb. **122** (1976) 182–202.

[77] Lang, J., O. Schafhauser, S. Hoffmann: Über die postnatale Entwicklung der transbasalen Schädelpforten: Canalis caroticus, Foramen jugulare, Canalis hypoglossalis, Canalis condylaris und Foramen magnum. Anat. Anz. **153** (1983) 315–357.

[78] Lang, J., M. Weigel: Nerve-vessel relations in jugulari foramen region. Anat. Clin. **5** (1983) 1–16.

[79] Lanz, T. v.: Über die Rückenmarkshäute. I. Die konstruktive Form der harten Haut des menschlichen Rückenmarks und ihrer Bänder. Arch. Entwickl.-Mech. Org. **118** (1929) 252–307.

[80] Lassek, A. M.: The pyramidal tract. A study of retrograde degeneration in the monkey. Arch. Neurol. Psychiatr. **48** (1942) 561–567.

[81] LeFort (1948).

[82] Luschka, H. v.: Die Altersveränderungen der Zwischenwirbelknorpel. Virchows Arch. f. path. Anat. **9** (1856) 311.

[83] Luschka, H. v.: Die Anatomie des menschlichen Kopfes. Laupp, Tübingen 1867.
[84] Mabrey, R. E.: Chordoma. A study of 150 cases. Cancer **25** (1935) 501 – 517.
[85] Mathews, W., C. B. Wilson: Ectopic intrasellar chordoma. J. Neurosurg. **39** (1974) 260 – 263.
[86] Macalister, A.: Notes on the development and variations of the atlas. J. Anat. Physiol. **27** (1893) 518 – 542.
[87] McGregor, M.: The significance of certain measurement of the skull in the diagnosis of basilar impression. Br. J. Radiol. **21** (1948) 171 – 181.
[88] McRae, D. L.: The significance of abnormalities of the cervical spine. Am. J. Roentgenol., Rad. Therap. and Nuclear Med. **84** (Springfield/Ill.) (1960) 3 – 25.
[89] Melsen, B.: A histological study of the influence of sutural morphology and skeletal maturation on rapid palatal expansion in children, pp. 499 – 507. Transactions of the European Orthodontic Society, 1972.
[90] Mizuno, N., M. Yoshida, M. Okamoto: Helweg's triangular fasciculus in anencephalic fetuses. J. Comp. Neurol. **132** (1968) 167 – 188.
[91] Müller, H.: Über das Vorkommen von Resten der Chorda dorsalis bei Menschen nach der Geburt und über die Verhältnisse zu den Gallertgeschwülsten an Clivus. Ztschr. f. rat. Med. **2** (1858) 202 – 229.
[92] Nordqvist, L.: The sagittal diameter of the spinal cord and sub-arachnoid space in different age groups. Acta Radiol. Suppl. **227** (1964) 1 – 96.
[93] Oehmke, H.-J.: Die Bedeutung des Canalis basilaris und seine Darstellung im Röntgenbild. Gegenbaurs Morphol. Jahrb. **104** (1963) 459 – 475.
[94] O'Rahilly, R., F. Müller, D. B. Meyer: The human vertebral column at the end of the embryonic period proper. 2. The occipitocervical region. J. Anat. **136** (1983) 181 – 195.
[95] Poppen, J. L., A. B. King: Chordoma: Experience with thirteen Cases. J. Neurosurg. **9** (1952) 139 – 163.
[96] Psenner, L.: Beitrag zur Klinik und zur Röntgendiagnostik des Chordoms der Schädelbasis. ROEFO **77** (1952) 425 – 433.
[97] Rathke, H.: Entwicklungsgeschichte der Natter (coluber natrix). Verlag der Brueder Borntraeger, Königsberg 1839.
[98] Rothman, S. L. G., J. F. Simeone.
[99] Russel, I. R., W. de Myer: The quantitative cortical origin of pyramidal axons of Macaca rhesus. With some remarks on the slow rate of axolysis. Neurology **11** (1961) 96 – 108.
[100] Schäfer, W.: Messungen zur Stufung der menschlichen Schädelbasis und Winkelbestimmungen. Gegenbaurs morph. Jahrb. **121** (1975) 1 – 25.
[101] Schiff, D. C. M., W. W. Parke: The arterial supply of the odontoid process. J. Bone Surg. A (Boston) **55** (1973) 1450 – 1456.
[102] Schmidt, H., E. Fischer: Die okzipitale Dysplasie. Thieme, Stuttgart 1960.
[103] Schoen, D.: Über eine vorgetäuschte Frakturlinie im Dens epistrophei. ROEFO **82** (1955) 52 – 54.
[104] Schürmann, K.: Atlanto-axial dislocation in rheumatoid arthritis with cervical cord compression (Myelopathy). Advances in Neurosurgery 7 (1979) 151 – 159.
[105] Schumacher, S. v.: Ein Beitrag zur Frage der Manifestation des Occipitalwirbels. Anat. Anz. **31** (1907) 145 – 165.
[106] Scotti, G.: Anterior inferior cerebellar artery originate from the cavernous portion of the internal carotid artery. Radiology **116** (1975) 93 – 94.
[107] Sensenig, E. C.: The development of the occipital and cervical segments and their associated structures in human embryos. Contr. Embryol. Carneg. Instn. **36** (1957) 141 – 151.
[108] Stofft, E.: Zur Morphologie des Aufhängeapparates der Medulla spinalis im HWS-Bereich. Radiologe **12** (1973) 531 – 540.
[109] Stofft, E.: Zur Morphometrie der Gelenkflächen des oberen Kopfgelenkes (Beitrag zur Statik der zerviko-okzipitalen Übergangsregion). Verh. Anat. Ges. 70 (1976) 575 – 584.

[110] Strecker, C.: Über die Condylen des Hinterhauptes. Arch. Anat. Entwickl.-Gesch. Anat. Abt. **301** (1887).

[111] Sturm, R.: Gelenkspalt und Gelenkkapsel der Articulatio atlanto-occipitalis lateralis. Inaug. Diss., Würzburg 1981.

[112] Török, I., L. Szebe: Untersuchungen über die Frage der Assimilation und Manifestation des Atlas. Z. Anat. Entwickl.-Gesch. **111** (1942) 186 – 200.

[113] Torklus, D. v.: Okzipitale und subokzipitale Dysplasie. Tagung, Vereinig. Nordwestdtsch. Orthop., Hannover 1964.

[114] Torklus, D., W. v. Gehle: Die obere Halswirbelsäule, 2nd rev. ed. Thieme, Stuttgart 1975.

[115] Tsusaki, T.: Über den Atlas und Epistropheus bei den eingeborenen Formosanern. Folia Anatomica Japonica **2** (1924) 221 – 246.

[116] Verhaart, W. J. C.: Hypertrophy of pes pedunculi and pyramid as result of degeneration of contralateral corticofugal fiber tracts. J. Comp. Neurol. **92** (1950) 1 – 17.

[117] Verhaart, W. J. C., W. Kramer: The uncrossed pyramidal tract. Acta Psychiat. Neurol. Scand. **27** (1952) 181 – 200.

[118] Virchow, H.: Die sagittale Flexion am Hinterhauptsgelenk von Säugetieren. S.-B. Ges. Naturforsch. Freunde Berlin (1907) 43 – 69.

[119] Virchow, H.: Über die sagittal-flexorische Bewegung im Atlas-Epistropheusgelenk des Menschen. Separat-Abzug aus Archiv für Anatomie und Physiologie. Anatomische Abteilung 1909.

[120] Virchow, H.: Die sagittal-flexorische Bewegung der menschlichen Halswirbelsäule. Arch. orthopäd. u. Unfall-Chir. **24** (1928) 1 – 42.

[121] Virchow, R.: Untersuchungen über die Entwicklung der Schädelgrube im gesunden und krankhaften Zustande und über den Einfluß derselben auf Schädelform, Gesichtsbildung und Gehirnbau. Reimer, Berlin 1857.

[122] Wackenheim, A.: La ligne médiane de la charniére cervico-occipitale. Ètude d'un ligne intervestibulaire. Sem. Hôp. (Paris) **42** (1966) 32, 1448.

[123] Wackenheim, A.: Visualization of the choroid plexuses of the lateral ventricles in the frontal projection in vertebral angiography. Neuroradiology **6** (1973) 231 – 232.

[124] Wackenheim, A.: Occipitalization of the ventral part and vertebralization of the dorsal part of the atlas with Insufficiency of the transverse ligament. Neuroradiology **24** (1982) 45 – 47.

[125] Wackenheim, A.: Roentgendiagnosis of the craniovertebral region. Springer, Berlin – Heidelberg – New York 1974.

[126] Wackenheim, A., J. P. Braun: Weichteile, Stürze und Erweiterung am Atlas. Thieme, Stuttgart 1968.

[127] Weigner, K.: Über die Assimilation des Atlas und Variationen am Os occipitale beim Menschen. Anat. Hefte **45** (1911) 81 – 195.

[128] Yakovlev, P. I., P. Rakic: Patterns of decussation of bulbar pyramids and distribution of pyramidal tracts in two sides of the spinal cord. Trans. Am. Neurol. Assoc. **91** (New York) (1966) 366 – 367.

[129] Zaaijer, T.: Die Persistenz der Synchondrosis condylo-squamosa am Hinterhauptsbeine des Menschen und der Säugetiere. Anat. Anz. **9** (1894) 337 – 342.

The pathogenesis of two distinct cervico-occipital malformations

A. Wackenheim

Introduction

The great number of malformations of the cervico-occipital region makes it very difficult to assume a single developmental mode causing these malformations. In the past, we had the opportunity to demonstrate a mechanism in two malformations which we summarize in this paper.

The first mechanism concerns the basilar invagination and the second the odontoideum mobile.

Basilar invagination

The development of the basilar part of the occipital bone, called basi-occipital, may be easily disturbed, especially by hypoplasia. This hypoplasia was described in 1926 by J. Déjérine [2]. A large number of cases was published in the literature after this first case. It consists in a very thin basi-occiput i. e. the posterior part of the clivus behind the synchondrosis spheno-occipitalis (fig. 1). In such cases,

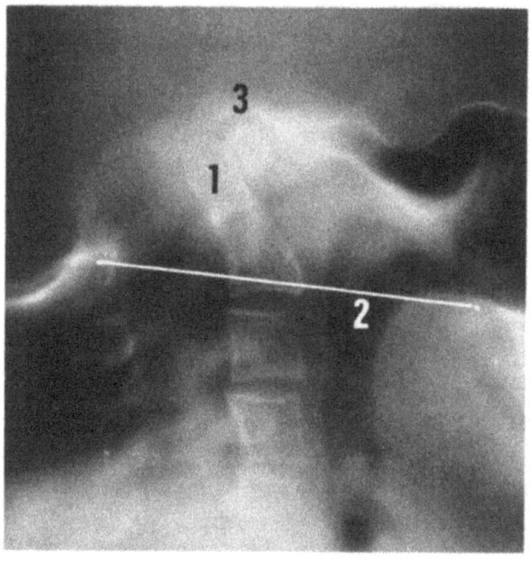

Fig. 1 Basilar invagination characterized by the overlapping of the atlas and axis (1) cranially to Chamberlain's line (2). The origin of this situation is a single hypoplasia of the basi-occipital (3) which is schematized in figure 3 b.

the pathology of the basilar invagination is easily understood, for it is a matter of reduced ossification leading to underdevelopment. Recently we had the opportunity to publish a further developmental cause for basilar invagination [3]. In this patient, the lower part of the clivus developed as an independant ossicle, corresponding to the basi-occipital bone. This free ossicle is then responsible for too high a location of the odontoid process, i. e. for the basilar invagination. In figure 2 we recall the development of this type of basilar invagination from the age of 2 years up to 20, and figure 3 illustrates the terminal stage of this malformation.

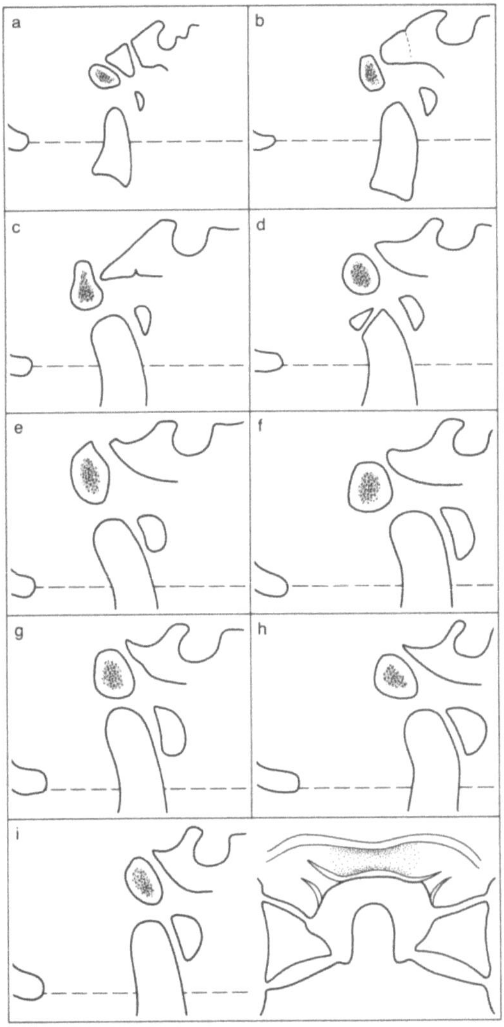

Fig. 2 Development from 2 years (a) to 20 years (i) of an original mechanism of basilar invagination: the non fused rounded ossicle corresponding to the basi-occipital, schematized in figure 3 b.

Odontoideum mobile

The odontoideum mobile is generally considered to be a result of a lack of ossification in the middle third of the odontoid process. There is however no explanation of the etiology of this lack of ossification which separates the odontoid process into 2 parts, the free odontoid mobile (cranial part) and the epistropheal stump (caudal part). In a recent case of odontoideum mobile [4], it

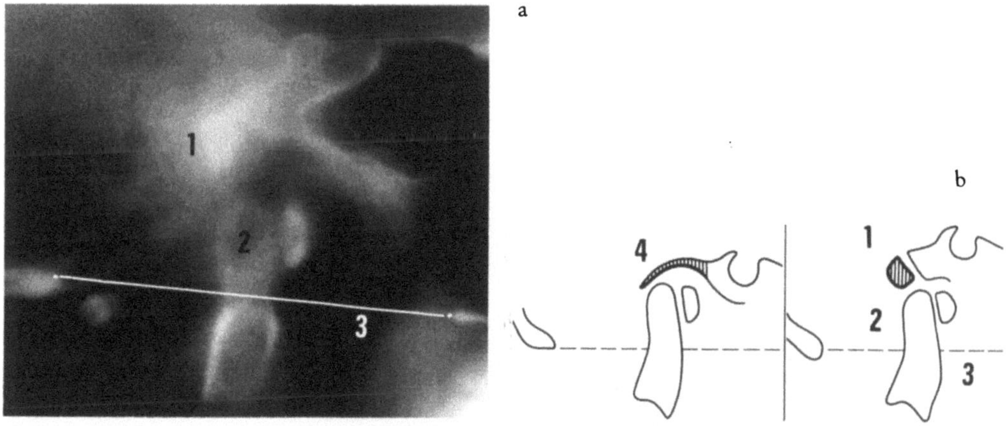

Fig. 3 At a age of 20 years, our patient has a free ossicle (1) at the place of the basi-occipital. This free ossicle is responsible for the overlapping of the atlas and axis (2) cranially to Chamberlain's line (3) [a]. Note the comparison with Déjérine's form of basilar invagination (4) [b].

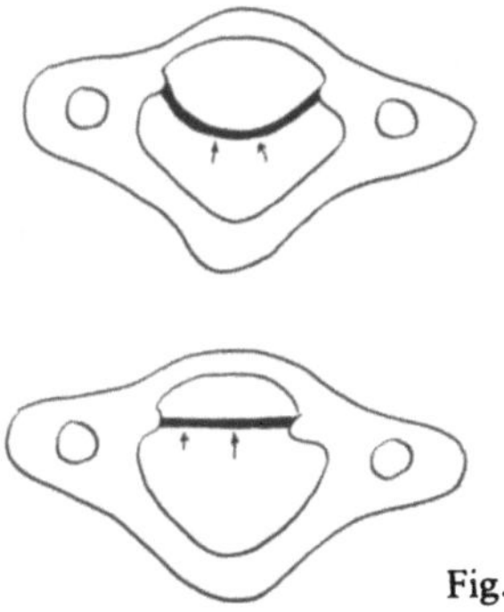

Fig. 4

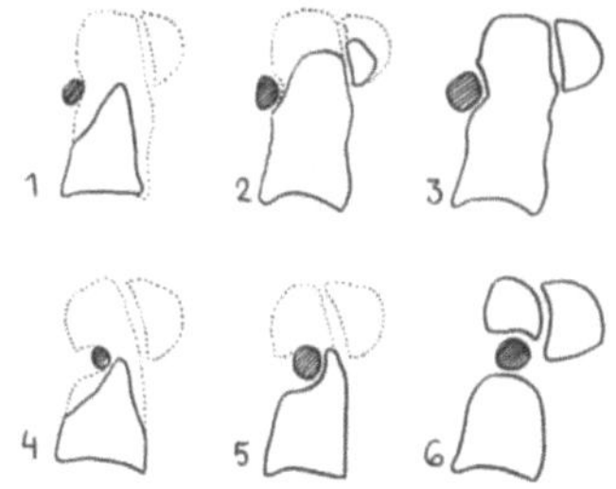

Fig. 5

Fig. 4 Above: Normal transverse ligament in an axial cut of the atlas.
Below: A too short transverse ligament.

Fig. 5 Above: Normal ossification of the axis.
1 = new born; 2 = during childhood; 3 = adulthood.
Below: The development of an odontoideum mobile malformation by a too short transverse ligament.
4 = in the new born, the transverse ligament is located too frontally; 5 = during childhood, the transverse ligament separates the odontoid process into 2 parts; 6 = in adults, the too short transverse ligament lies between the 2 fragments of the odontoid process.

was possible to demonstrate a too short transverse ligament which we consider to be responsible for the separation of the odontoid process into 2 parts. Figure 4 illustrates our view of this pathogenic condition. The transverse ligament is anteriorly concave in normal conditions. In the proposed explanation we assume that a too short transverse ligament, as depicted in figure 4, extends transversely, from one tuberculum to the other. In figure 5, we schematize the normal development above and the constitution of the odontoideum mobile below. The computer tomography enables the demonstration of the course of the transverse ligament [1], in normal as in pathological conditions. In our case, it was possible to demonstrate the transverse ligament between the 2 parts of the odontoid process (fig. 6).

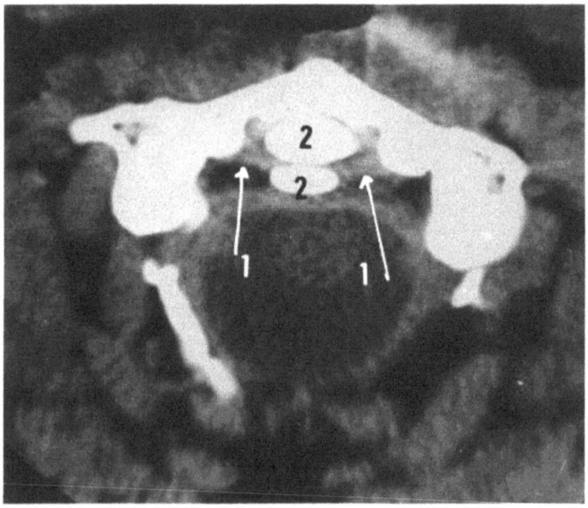

Fig. 6 The short transverse ligament (1), as seen in the axial cut, lying between the 2 fragments of the odontoid process (2).

Summary

A mechanism for 2 malformations of the cervico-occipital junction is proposed explaining the basilar invagination by a separate hypoplastic ossicle displacing the basi-occipital bone and the odontoideum mobile by a too short transverse ligament.

References

[1] Burguet, J. L., H. Sick, Y. Dirheimer et al.: CT of the main ligaments of the cervico-occipital hinge. Neuroradiology 27 (1985) 112–118.

[2] Dejerine, J.: Dystrophie osseuse par aplasie de la substance spongieuse du corps basilaire de l'occipital. Rev. Neurol. 2 (1926) 281–300.

[3] Wackenheim, A.: Hypoplasia of the basi-occipital bone and persistance of the spheno-occipital synchondrosis in a patient with transitory supplementary fissure of the basi-occipital. Neuroradiology 27 (1985) 226–231.

[4] Wackenheim, A., J. L. Burguet, H. Sick: Section of the odontoid process by a shortened transverse ligament (a possible etiology for the mobile odontoid). Neuroradiology (1986 in press).

Basilar processes — visualized in radiographs and CT scans

F. Hilgenstock

The basilar processes are remnants of the hypochordal arches in early embryonic development corresponding to each segment of the spine and forming the ventral rim of the foramen magnum. Only the hypochordal arch or brace of C 1 is fully developed to form the anterior arch of the atlas. If involution of the hypochordal arch of the proatlas is incomplete the ventral parts of the foramen magnum will show extracranial alterations in its appearance. With the involution of the lateral parts of the brace a tertiary condyle persists. After involution of the medial parts the basilar processes are formed.

Bony alterations of the ventral extracranial margin of the foramen magnum are not readily visible on radiographs. On the lateral view of the skull, the malformation often lies behind the petrous bones and mastoid processes. Additional

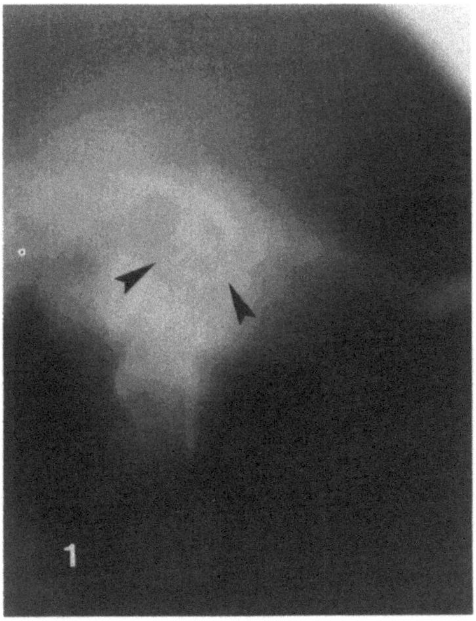

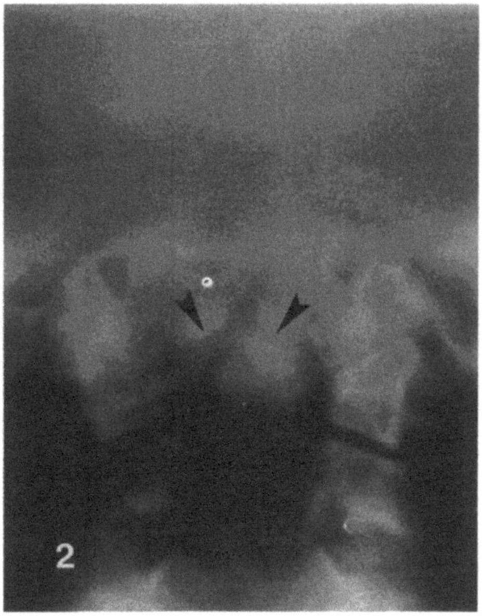

Fig. 1 The tomography shows a distinct bony protuberance above the tip of the odontoid process.

Fig. 2 Paramedian symmetrical protrusions with an central notch.

malformation – like basilar impression – may draw the observer's attention towards the area of the foramen magnum. Even in median sagittal-plane tomography, basilar processes are not visualized easily. With their little extension, they may not show up on a CT scan, either. Fischer [1] showed basilar processes on X-ray tomography; visualisation on CT scan has not been shown.

Case: A 45-year-old female patient suffering from a persistent cephalgia was sent for a CT scan of the skull. The tomogram of the base of the skull shows dome-shaped protrusions in the medial parts of the foramen magnum. The anteroposterior diameter of the foramen magnum measuring 23 mm is significantly lower than the mean of 35 mm known for adults [2]. The CT scan shows that the tip of the odontoid process appears ventrally removed from the foramen magnum.

The above CT scan findings of the base of the skull initiated a search for a malformation in the cervico-occipital transition.

On the lateral view of the skull, an interpretation of the cervico-occipital transition is unclear, due to a marked platybasia with a basal angle of 170 degrees. The odontoid process protrude McGregor's line by 20 mm on lateral tomography and the digastric line of Fischgold by 18 mm in sagittal tomography.

Median-sagittal plane tomography shows a narrow bony structure between the tip of the clivus and the anterior rim of the foramen magnum, which is unusual in this area. The neighbouring plane, 3 mm lateral off the median, shows a distinct bony protuberance above the tip of the dens, not to be mistaken for the occipital condyle (fig. 1).

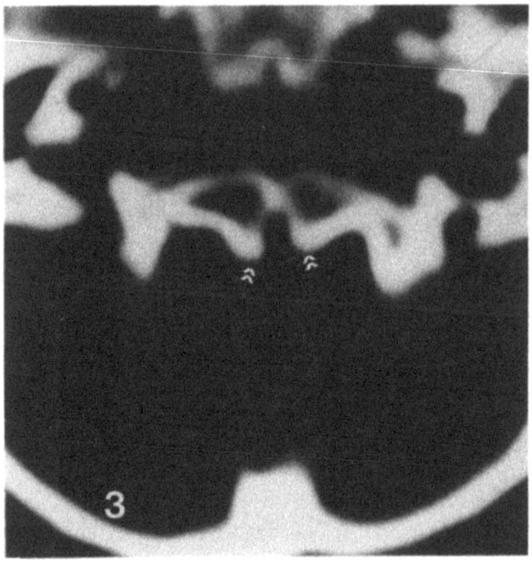

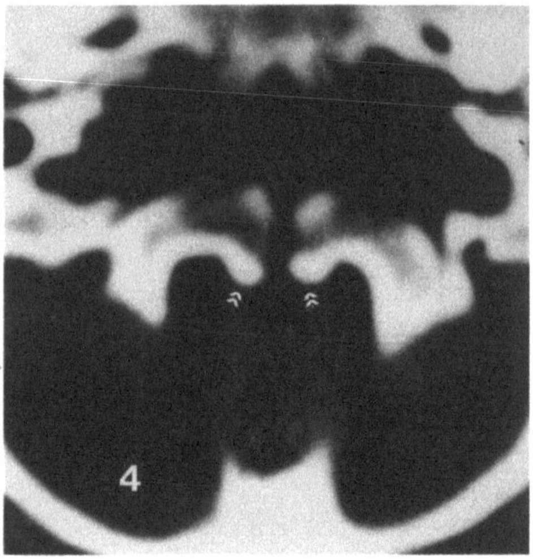

Fig. 3 CT scan shows bilateral protrusions of the basion with a dorsal notch.

Fig. 4 3 mm caudally a complete fissure is shown.

Sagittal tomography reveals paramedian symmetrical protrusions of the anterior margin of the foramen magnum with an central notch (fig. 2). CT scan shows this bilateral paramedian protrusions of the basion with a dorsal notch (fig. 3), and 3 mm caudally a complete fissure is shown (fig. 4). Since the anterior arch of the atlas is completely visible in lower tomographs this fissure should not to be mistaken for a dehiscence of the anterior arch of the atlas.

The combined interpretation of X-ray tomography and CT scan allows a reliable diagnosis of persistent basilar processes seen as a manifestation of a occipital vertebra. Despite the coincidence of basilar processes with a narrow foramen magnum and a marked basilar impression, the clinical neurological examination has not revealed any pathological signs.

References

[1] Fischer, E.: Akzessorische freie Knochenelemente in der Umgebung des Foramen occipitale magnum. Röntgenstr. **91** (1959) 638.

[2] Wackenheim, A.: Roentgen Diagnosis of the Craniovertebral Region. Springer, Berlin – Heidelberg – New York 1974.

Radionuclide imaging of the cranio-cervical region

A. Roesler, K. Hahn, G. Gutjahr, Th. Schaub

Introduction

Similar to other diagnostic procedures a specific nuclear investigation should be chosen according to the clinical problem.

In the following we give a survey of nuclear medical diagnostic procedures for assessing the cranio-cervical region followed by a discussion of their relevance.

Skeletal imaging

Bone scanning is the most frequently requested nuclear test. The radiopharmaceuticals used are 99 m-Tc labeled phosphate complexes which are absorbed by the calcium apatite crystals of bone reflecting the bone blood flow and metabolism.

Bone scans can be carried out as three-phase studies. The first phase is the radionuclide angiogram. In a second phase static images of the "blood pool" are made. The third phase are static images made 2 – 3 hours later which reflect the bone metabolism.

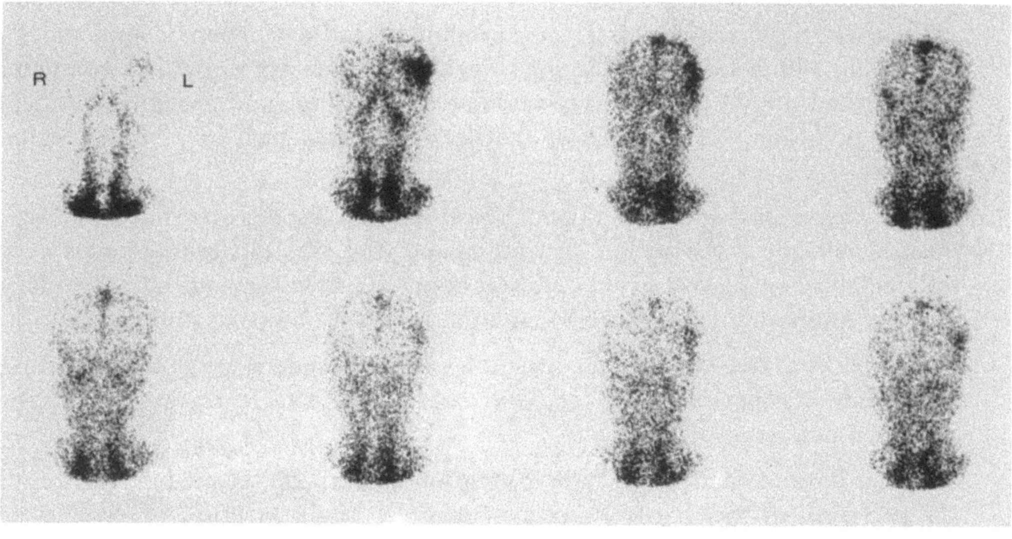

Fig. 1 a Anterior cerebral radionuclide angiogram showing an intracerebral angioma on the left.

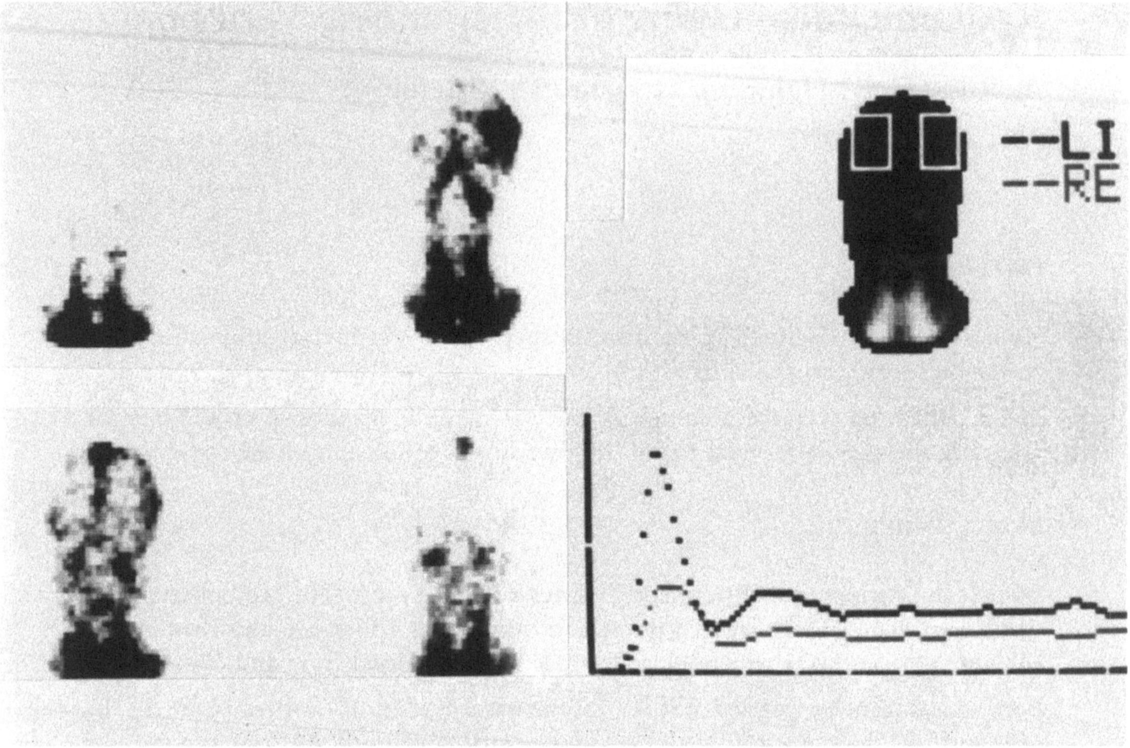

Fig. 1 b Computer assisted analysis of perfusion over the cerebral hemispheres in a case of intracerebral angioma on the left (see fig. 1 a).

First phase: Immediately after the injection of the technetium compound an angiogram with 2 seconds per frame is made. The data are stored in a computer system which allows an analysis of vascular abnormalities and a rough quantification of perfusion, for example of the neck region as such or a tumor region (fig. 1 a).

Second phase: During the blood-pool phase 30 to 60 seconds after injection static images are made of the specific skeletal regions (fig. 2). A differentiation between inflammatory or degenerative processes, between soft tissue and bone disorders, also the determination of blood circulation in a bony lesions can be made [6].

Third phase: 2 to 3 hours after injection a radionuclide skeletal survey with a total body scanner is performed with subsequent camera images of specific regions if necessary (fig. 3).

With the data of the radionuclide angiogram a computer assisted evaluation of the perfusion in specific neck areas is possible. Major stenoses of the carotid arteries or even occlusion can be detected. The intracranial perfusion can also be assessed (fig. 1 b).

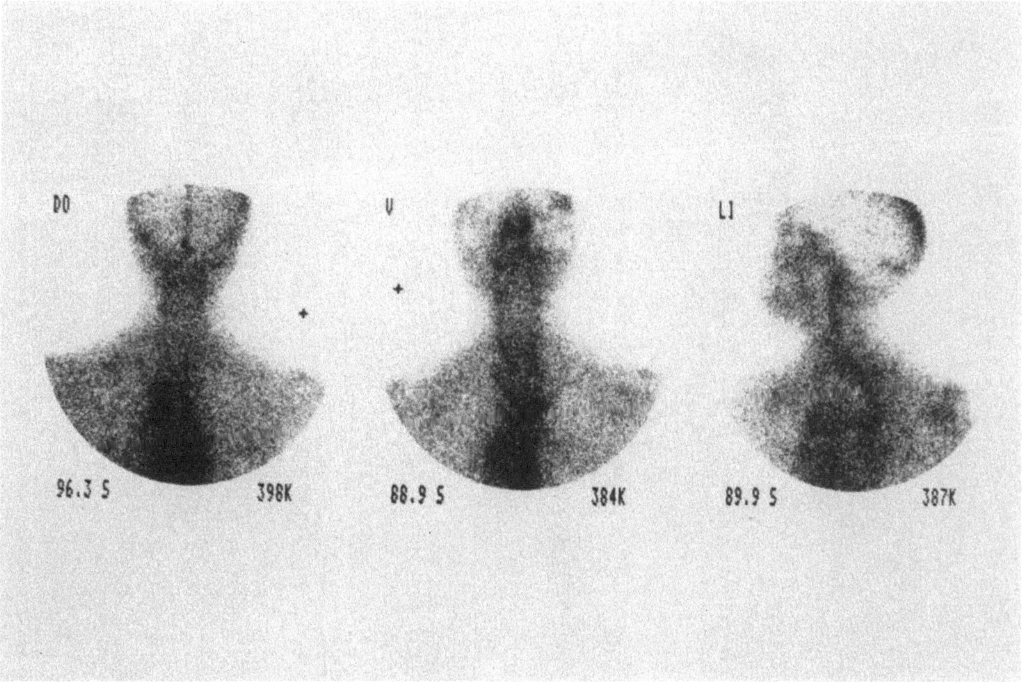

Fig. 2 Normal "blood-pool" phase of the cranio-cervical region.

Hyperaemia in the blood-pool images is seen in inflammatory processes which can be differentiated from degenerative processes in the cervical spine. Hypervascular and angiomatous tumors show hyperaemia too. The vascularity of bone lesions is sometimes of decisive importance in differential diagnosis.

Bone scanning is a highly sensitive procedure in trauma cases [2]. In the cervical region whiplash injuries with associated microtraumas are positive in bone scans while radiographs can be negative. In case of radiologically evident structural loosening even small osseous tears within the ligamentous insertions are detectable. This investigation is also indicated to exclude osseous lesions in cases with normal X-ray but with persistant pain in the cranio-cervical or cervical region after previous trauma (fig. 4). In case of a bony trauma, experimental studies [7] have shown a pathologic bone scan in approximately 90% of cases at 24 hours after trauma and almost 100% in cases at 48 hours after trauma. After 72 hours all fractures show increased bone metabolism i.e. an increased radionuclide accumulation. In radiographs osseous reaction is not seen until day 6 or 8.

According to our protocols in cases of suspected osseous trauma we radiograph the clinically suspicious area immediately after the trauma. If the radiographs

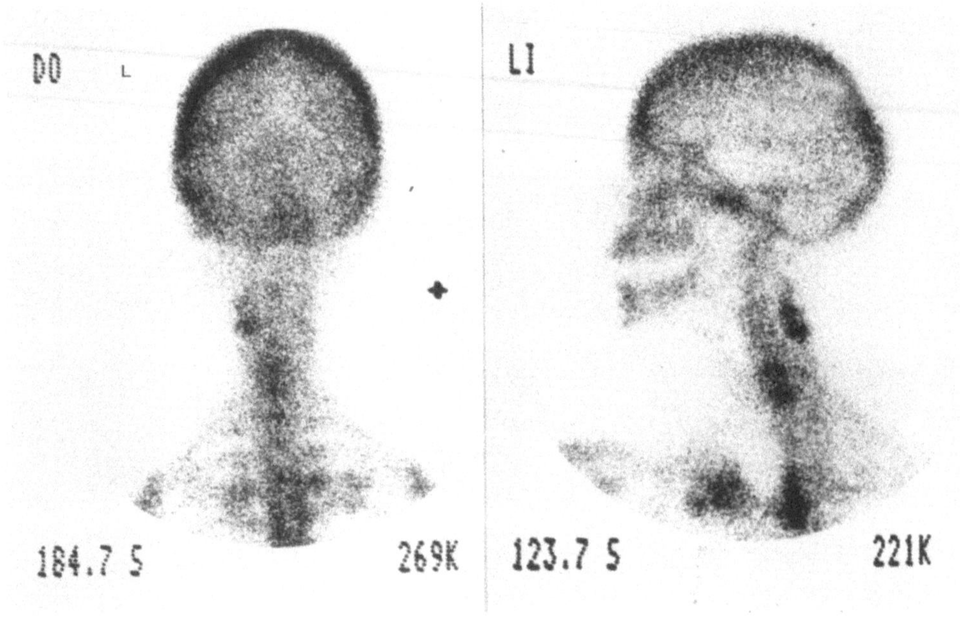

a

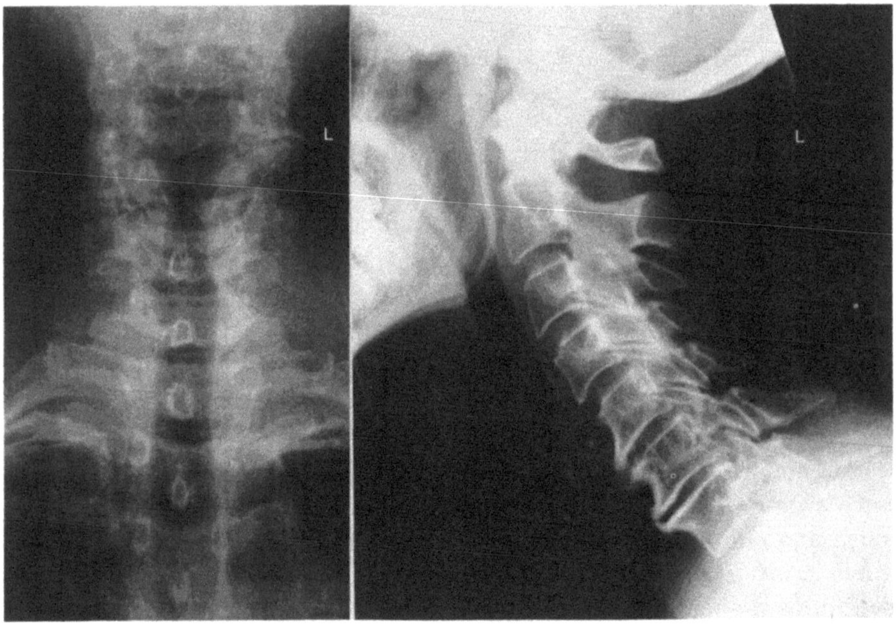

b

Fig. 3 a + b Degenerative processes of the cervical spine.

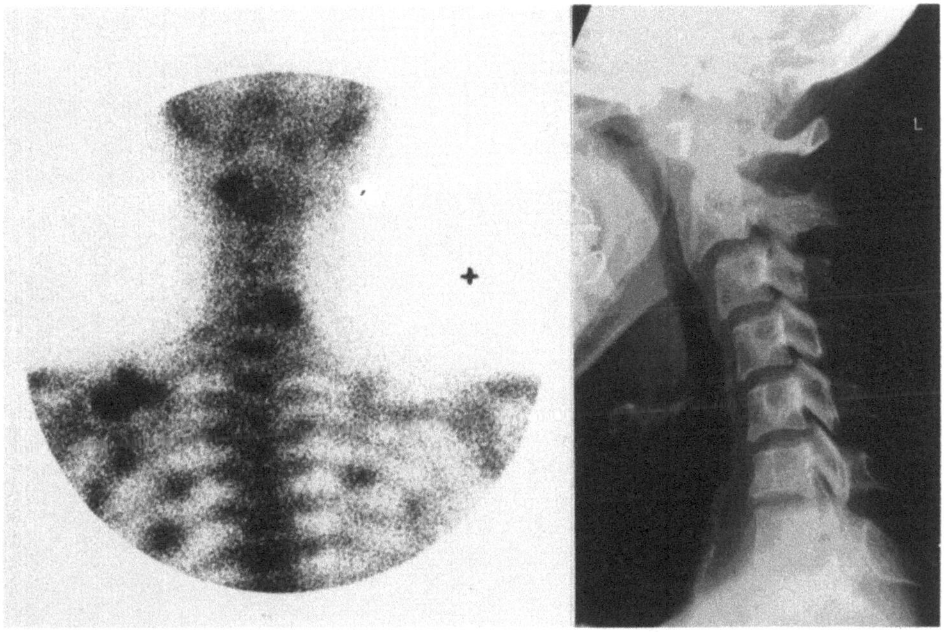

Fig. 4 Bone trauma after whiplash injury.

are negative but there is a strong clinical reason a bone scan is carried out 48 to 72 hours later. Scintigraphically abnormal regions are correlated with radiographs.

Due to the high sensitivity of the bone scan primary and secondary bone tumors can be detected early and reliably before radiographs show abnormality. Skeletal regions with increased bone metabolism are detectable on bone scan by a local accumulation of the radionuclide (fig. 5). In case of absent blood flow or in case of bone replacement by tumor, decreased or absent activity is seen, also known as "cold-lesions".

The specifity of the bone scan is relatively low as the majority of bone disorders will show increased uptake. However with the radiographs, clinical history and findings, the bone scan is valuable in the differentiation of bone disorders. Particulary in tumor diseases with an early metastatic spread to bone [3], the role of bone scanning is well established. In these cases bone scanning is used as a screening procedure of the whole skeletal. Regions with an increased bone metabolism which are suspicious are further examined by radiographic methods. Bone scanning shows not only the presence but also the extent of osseous metastases. It is also used in follow-up and restaging of tumor patients (fig. 6).

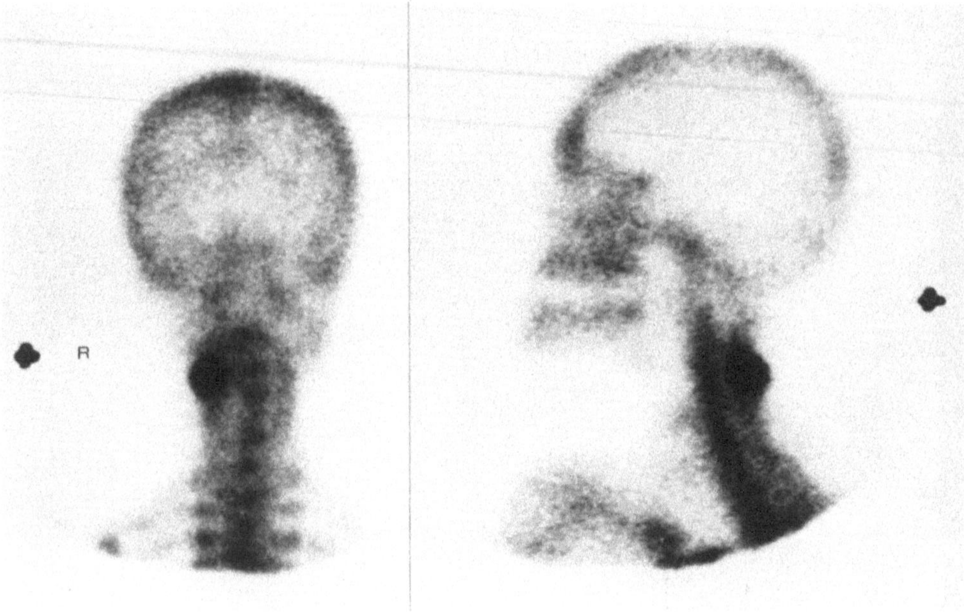

a

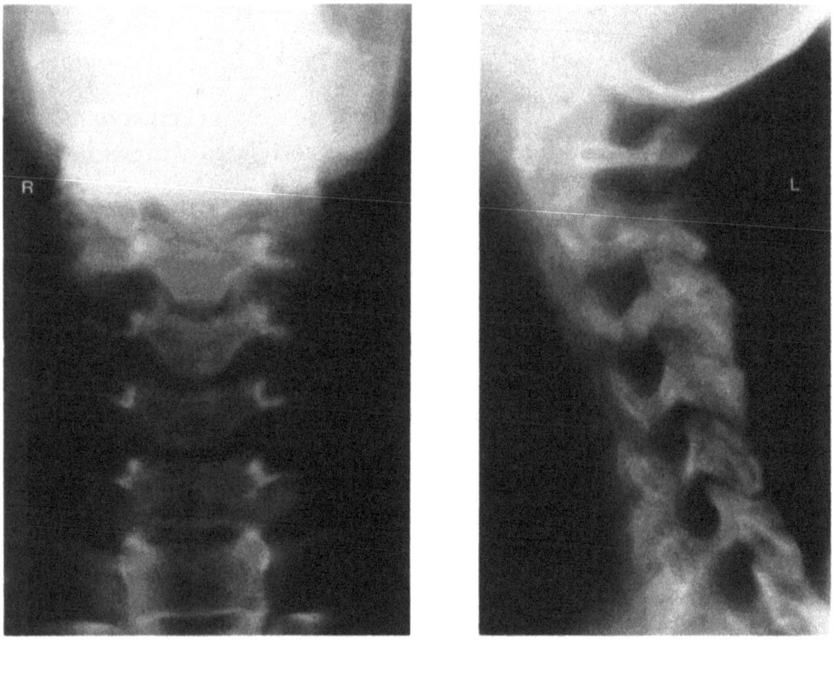

b

Fig. 5 a + b Osteoid osteoma of the cervical spine.

Inflammation imaging

Local infections can be detected with 67-gallium-citrate as well as with 111-indium-labeled leukocytes.

67-Gallium-citrate [1] accumulates in infectious lesions and tumors. 24, 48 and 72 hours after injection imaging is done. The 67-gallium uptake reflects the infectious activity of a lesion. 67-Gallium can be used in cases with fever of unknown origin. Since there is also 67-gallium-citrate uptake in malignant tumors, metastases and sarcoidoses, there can be problems with their differentiation.

Imaging with 111-indium-labeled leukocytes [3] is carried out at 4 hours and if necessary at 24 to 48 hours. The location and extent of a suspected infection can be determined. In contrast to 67-gallium-scans, tumors and inflammations can be differentiated.

With the introduction of single photon emission computer tomography (SPECT) a more precise anatomic localisation of the lesion is possible [4], which can be difficult with the conventional planar images especially in the cranial-cervical region and at the base of the skull (fig. 7).

The potential of the scintigraphy with radioactive-labeled (123-iodine, 131-iodine, 111-indium) monoclonal antibodies in the head and neck region is still to be determined.

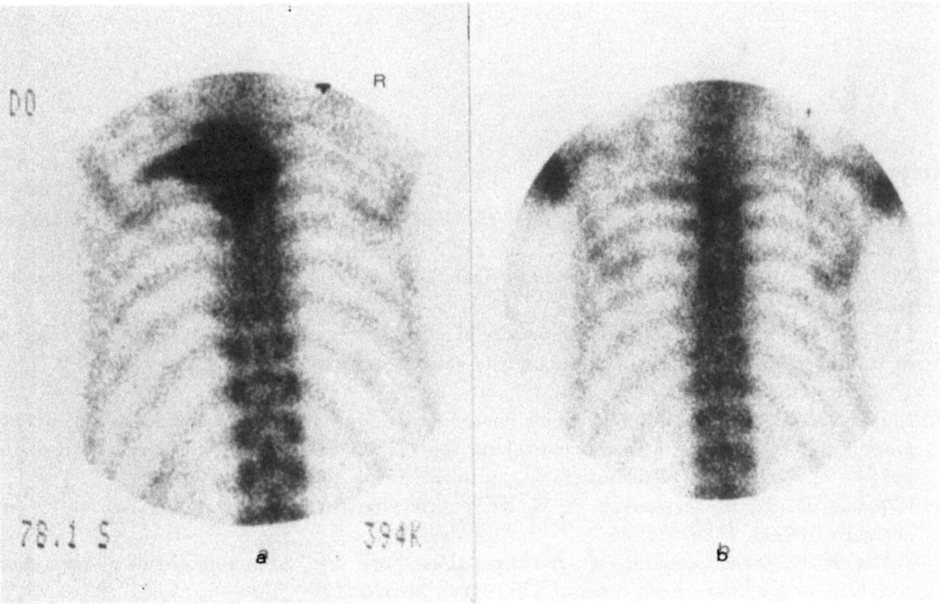

Fig. 6 Spinal metastases before (a) and after (b) chemo-therapy.

Since nuclear clinical studies are easy to perform and non-invasive, they are well tolerated by the patient. If used appropriately nuclear medical studies permit early diagnoses and are a major contribution to cost reduction in health services.

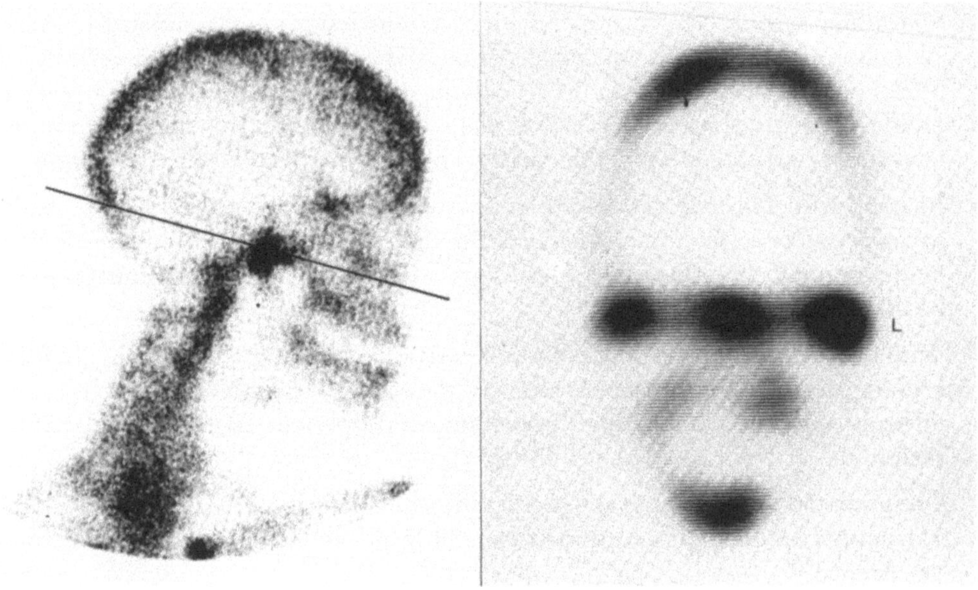

Fig. 7 SPECT: degenerative disease of the left tempero-mandibular joint.

References

[1] Hayes, R. L.: The medical use of gallium radionuclides: A brief history with some comments. Semin. Nucl. Med. **8** (1978) 183.

[2] Kim, H.-R., J. H. Thrall, J. W. Keyer: Skeletal scintigraphy following incidential trauma. Radiology **130** (1979) 447–451.

[3] Lane, A., U. Heinken, D. Schulz-Heinken et al.: Leukocyte scanning: Preparation and labelling of leukocytes with 111-indium oxine and its clinical application. Eur. J. Nucl. Med. **9** (1984) 17–22.

[4] Müller-Schauenburg, W., U. Feine: Single Photon Emission – Tomographie in der Knochenszintigraphie. In: U. Feine, W. Müller-Schauenburg (eds.): Nuklearmedizinische Knochendiagnostik, pp. 84–92. Verlag D. E. Wachholz K. G., Nürnberg 1985.

[5] Pistenma, D. A., R. McDougall, J. W. Kriss: Screening for bone metastasis: Are only scans necessary? JAMA **231** (1975) 46.

[6] Shafer, R. B., G. F. Edebara: Can the three-phase bone scan differentiate osteomyelitis from metabolic or metastatic bone disease? Clin. Nucl. Med. **9** (1984) 373.

[7] Tröger, B., O. Schofer: Traumatische Skelettveränderungen. In: K. Hahn (ed.): Pädiatrische Nuklearmedizin, Band III, pp. 85–90. Verlag Kirchheim, Mainz 1985.

Magnetic resonance imaging in the cranio-cervical region: Experiences in 194 cases

F. Koschorek, H.-P. Jensen, B. Terwey

Introduction

Since the introduction of nuclear magnetic resonance imaging (NMR) in the neurosurgical and neurological diagnostic this new imaging modality has shown to be of high diagnostic value – especially in disease processes of the cranio-vertebral junction. Other imaging modalities such as x-ray CT and myelography are of inferior quality as the images are degraded by bone artefacts and superposition of other structures. NMR can reveal many aspects of the cranio-vertebral region in a single examination without artefacts from surrounding structures. A further improvement of NMR is the introduction of para-magnetic agents, such as gadolinium-DTPA, as it increases the specifity by dynamic magnetic resonance imaging. The following is a review of our clinical experience based on 194 cases.

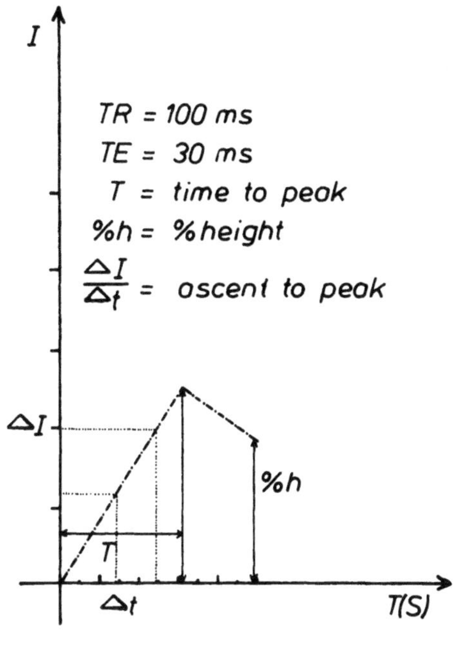

Fig. 1 Dynamic magnetic resonance imaging.

Clinical cases

Magnetic resonance measurements were performed by a 0.35 and 0.5 Tesla superconducting magnet respectively. Since (1985) we have used in some cases gadolinium-DTPA for detailed information about the kind of lesion.

We performed dynamic magnetic resonance imaging using a series of 9 images through 2 minutes and 40 sec. with TR 100 ms. and TE 30 ms, so one is able to obtain information about the change of signal-intensity in the lesion as related to time of measurement. As shown in figure 1 the time to peak, the percentage of height in the end of measurement and the ascent to peak are measured.

As table 1 shows 51 patients had malformations, 18 had inflammatory – degenerative diseases. 33 had lesions in the midline and the posterior fossa, 90 had vascular lesions and 60 patients were examined for lesions in the upper cervical canal and spinal cord.

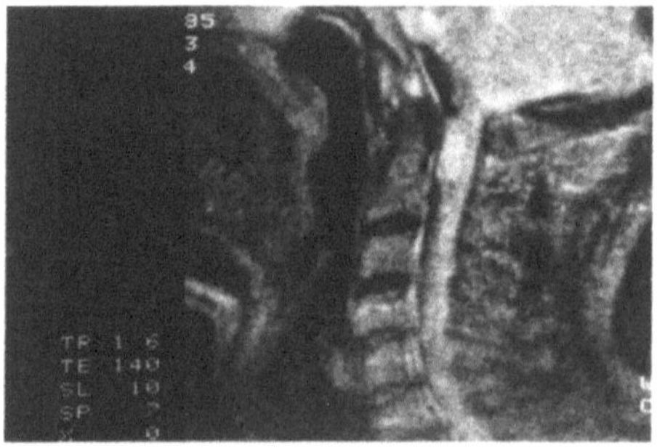

Fig. 2 T 2-weighted image in a male patient with 3 neurinomas (arrows) in the region of foramen magnum.

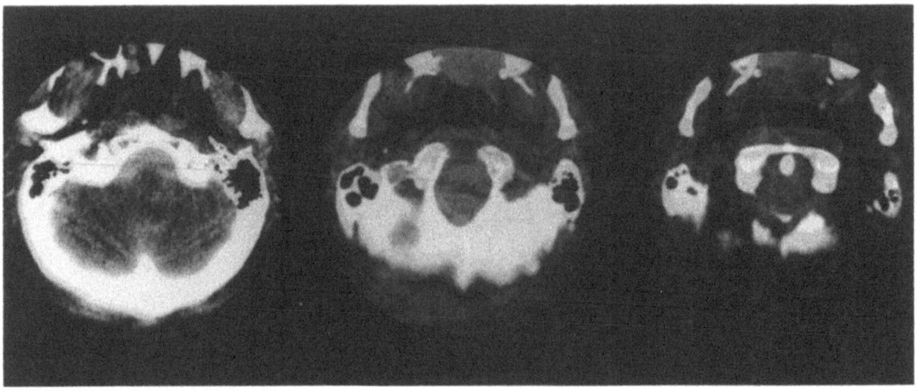

Fig. 3 CT of the same patient. The image-quality is degraded by bone-artefacts.

Table 1 Destribution of patients in 194 cases of nuclear magnetic resoncance imaging in the cranio-vertebral region

Malformations		*51*
Arnold-Chiari	8	
Arnold-Chiari and Syringomyelia	5	
Arnold-Chiari, Syringomyelia and basilar impression	2	
Syringomyelia/Hydromyelia	31	
Basilar impression	2	
Assimilation of atlas	1	
Dandy-Walker-Syndrom	2	
Inflammatory/degenerative diseases		*18*
Multiple sclerosis	16	
Ponto-olivar atrophy	1	
Central-pontine myelinolysis	1	
Vascular lesion		*19*
AV Angioma in pons/IV ventricle	3	
Infarct in brainstem	8	
Infarct in cerebellum	8	
Lesions in the midline and posterior fossa		*33*
Tumors in medulla oblongata	8	
Tumors in pons	3	
Tumors in cerebellum	8	
Metastasis in cerebellum	1	
Arachnoidalcysts	5	
Haematoma in pons	2	
Lindau tumors	3	
Tumors in IV ventricle	3	
Lesions in the upper cervical canal and spinal cord		*60*
Intromedullary tumors	25	
Meningioma	2	
Neurinoma	4	
Bone tumors	3	
Disc herniation (soft and hard)	26	
Normal findings		*13*
Sum total		*194*

Results

In agreement with other authors [2, 3] we find that magnetic resonance imaging has a high value in the diagnostics of lesions of the foramen magnum, the cranio-vertebral region and the posterior fossa. Meningeomas and neurinomas are well depicted in T 2-weighted images as high signal intensity areas and we refer to a case of 3 neurinomas of the cranio-vertebral junction (fig. 2) which x-ray CT and myelography failed to show (fig. 3).

Our results in respect to gadolinium-DTPA are as good as those reported by other authors [1, 4). The increase in signal-intensity was similar in magnitude to the contrast enhancement observed in CT, and permitted differentiation of solid tumor tissue from a surrounding cerebral edema on magnetic resonance images. Direct visualisation of otherwise iso-signal-intensitive lesions was also demonstrated [4]. Dynamic magnetic resonance imaging provide further information about the nature of a lesion as the change of signal-intensity is related to time of measurement. The percentage of height of signal-intensity at the end of measurement and the ascent to the peak of signal-intensity seems to be different in benign, malignant and vascular tissue.

Discussion

In our series of 194 cases magnetic resonance images of the cranio-vertebral region have proved to be far superior in anatomical detail when compared to x-ray computer-tomography (CT). In a single examination magnetic resonance

Table 2 Distribution of histological findings compared with the results of dynamic magnetic resonance imaging

Lesion	Time to peak	% Height	Ascent
Oligodendroglioma	80	64.7	0.66
Glioblastoma	140	79.5	1.04
Glioblastoma	160	100.0	1.90
Ependymoma	140	97.2	0.67
Plexuspapilloma	60	78.5	5.78
Angioblastoma	20	66.7	2.48
Meningioma	60	21.7	4.20
Meningioma	120	84.4	2.26
Meningioma	80	56.5	1.68
Angioma	40	0	2.47
Infarction	80	92.0	1.05
Angioma with bleeding	30	69.2	3.78

Table 3 Early result seems to increase likehood of specific diagnosis with respect to benign and malignant tissue

	Tumor		Vascular
	benign	malignant	
Time to peak	68.0 ± 36.3	*130.0 ± 34.6*	50.0 ± 26.4
% Height	61.6 ± 24.7	85.3 ± 16.5	53.7 ± 47.9
Ascent to peak	*3.3 ± 1.7*	1.1 ± 0.6	2.4 ± 1.4

imaging can reveal many aspects of the cranio-vertebral region without artefacts from surrounding structures. This method of image modality is more accurate than conventional CT and myelography.

The current criterion for identifying a genuine lesion is the presence of abnormal signals that are reproduceable on multiple pulse sequence images [1].

Dynamic magnetic resonance imaging is a step forward in order to get more information about lesions as the change of signal intensity, related to time of measurement allows further discrimination of benign and malign tissue. First results of our current dynamic magnetic resonance imaging study point in this direction. But further investigations will be needed, as our present case-numbers are small.

Conclusions

1. Magnetic resonance imaging is the imaging modality of first choice in the diagnostic analysis of lesions in the cranio-vertebral junction.

2. Dynamic magnetic resonance imaging with gadolinium-DTPA seems to allow more information about the nature of a lesion. But this impression has to be confirmed on a larger number of cases.

References

[1] Gadian, D. G., I. A. Paque, D. I. Bryant et al.: Gadolinium-DTPA as a contrast agent in magnetic resonance imaging – Theoretical projections and practical observations. J. Comp. Ass. Tomogr. 9 (1985) 242–251.

[2] Han, J. S., C. T. Bonstelle, B. Kaufman et al.: Magnetic resonance imaging in the evaluation of the brain-stam. Radiology **150** (1984) 705–712.

[3] Modic, M. T., R. W. Hardy, M. A. Weinstein et al.: Nuclear magnetic resonance of the spine: Clinical potential and limitations. Neurosurgery **15** (1984) 583–592.

[4] Runge, V. M., W. Schörner, H. P. Niendorf et al.: Initial clinical evaluation of Gadolinium-DTPA for contrast-enhanced magnetic resonance imaging. Magn. Res. Imag. **3** (1985) 27–35.

Space-occupying, inflammatory and dysplastic lesions of the cranio-cervical junction seen in nuclear magnetic resonance imaging (MRI)

H. G. Friedburg, M. Schuhmacher, J. Jennig

Introduction

Lesions of the cranio-cervical junction have acquired a special place amongst lesions of the posterior cranial fossa and the upper cervical region. This is due to the unusually long period between the appearance of the first symptoms [3] and reaching a conclusive diagnosis.

Frequently such lesions cannot be detected by either normal X-rays or conventional tomographic techniques. Even the improved myelographic techniques which employ C 1/2 puncture do not succeed in achieving a very clear demonstration of the medullary region this is the result of the inevitable dispersion of contrast media. The introduction, however, of computer tomography (CT) and, in particular, magnetic resonance imaging (MRI) [9, 10, 13, 15, 16] has meant that the examination of the critical zone of the cranio-cervical junction is so much easier and the diagnosis of thee lesions has now become largely dependent upon those techniques.

Because soft tissue contrast is intrinsic to MRI this technique, in particular, has made possible substantial improvements in the quality of images of ligaments and soft tissue than those provided by standard CT. In the following sections the advantages which are provided by MRI in the context of the diagnosis of non-bony lesions in the cranio-cervical region are first presented and then discussed.

Results

In 133 MRI examinations, from a total of 906 patients examined within the last year, a lesion of the cranio-cervical junction was suspected. The tentative diagnoses are listed in table 1. 68 patients had pathological findings (tab. 2).

Table 1 Clinical reason for employing MRI

Space occupying lesion (general)	68
Syringomyelia	12
Multiple sclerosis, infratentorial plaques	10
Extension of a tumor (medullo-cervical)	7
Chronic polyarthritis of the atlanto-dental-joint	7
Acute trauma	7
Cranio-cervicale dysplasia	6
Bleeding	4
Degeneration of the vertebral discs	4
Traumatic scar	3
Myelitis	3
Tumor of intramedullar location	2
Total	133

Table 2 133 MR examinations of the cranio-cervical junction: Pathological findings

Multiple sclerosis: Plaques of the medulla oblongata and upper cervical myelon	7
Syringomyelia, Syringobulbia	6
Acute trauma (C I respectivly II fracture, Contusion of the myelon)	5
Sequela of trauma (glial scar)	2
Neurogenic tumors of the posterior fossa	7
Bony tumors with relationship to the foramen magnum	5
Tumors of the cervical spinal cord	3
Extramedullary tumors of the upper cervical region	4
Cranio-cervical dysplasia	3
Subarachnoidal and arachnoidal cysts	4
Bleeding	4
Encephalomyelitis (except MS)	3
Chronic polyarthritis of the atlanto-dental joint	7
Malum suboccipitale (Abscess formation by staphylococci)	1
Degeneration of a cervical disc	6
Thickening of the ventral collateral ligament with narrowing of the subarachnoidal space	1
Total	68

65 examinations without pathological findings including one case of a not diagnosed meningeoma.

Discussion

In contrast to the inflexible system of X-ray tubes-detectors in CT, MRI offers a free choice of slice planes and provides multi-dimensional imaging of the complicated spatial conditions of the cranio-cervical junction. No other imaging method directly demonstrates soft tissue structures so well and identifies intramedullary fluid-containing spaces so clearly without, any strain on the patient. MRI has therefore become the method of choice [7, 9] for establishing the presence of syringomyelia (fig. 1) and syringobulbia.

Although bony abnormalities in the presence of cranio-cervical dysplasia can be identified by conventional X-ray techniques their effects on soft tissue structures, especially those of compression or displacement of the cervical spinal cord and the medulla oblongata, can be directly detected only by MRI. The secondary effects of chronic pressure on the spinal cord, for instance, such as pressure atrophy, edema, or ischemia, cannot be determined by any other method. Complex deformities such as Arnold-Chiari syndrome [1] in conjuction with platybasia and basilar impression can be diagnosed conclusively on the basis of just a few slices (fig. 2).

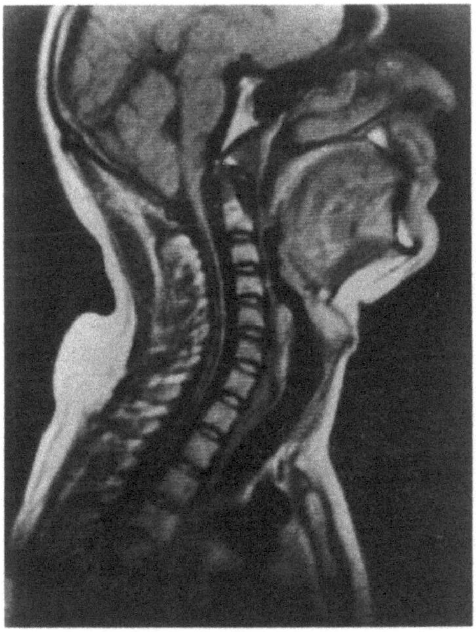

Fig. 1

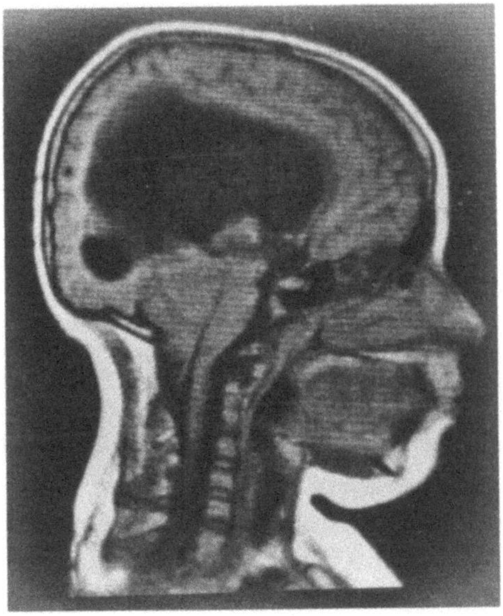

Fig. 2

Fig. 1 T 1-weighted sagittal slice (400/33 NEX = 4). MR image of a syringomyelia of the cervical cord with simultaneous partial descent of the tonsil. The central, intramedullary collection of liquid is dark (= hypointensive) due to the long T 1 time.

Fig. 2 T 1-weighted sagittal slice (500/33 NEX = 4). Image of an Arnold Chiary syndrome with platybasia, cerebellar tonsil prolapse and secondary hydrocephalus.

The effects of trauma on bones, such as fractures of the upper cervical vertebral column, are not well shown by MRI in contrast to hematomas, spinal cord lesions caused by compression or edema and the late sequelae, such as glial scars, of cervical vertebral column whiplash injury. Those lesions, particularly hematomas, are prone to display marked alterations with time as a result of variations in signal intensity dependent upon the state of plasma resorption, red cell lysis or the presence of methemoglobin.

With MRI, the diagnosis of intramedullary and extramedullary tumors [6] of the cranio-cervical junction has been made considerably easier and faster [4]. Intramedullary gliomas or spongioblastomas, which are usually very difficult to diagnose, appear in MRI as hyperintensive zones (fig. 3). Combining MRI with

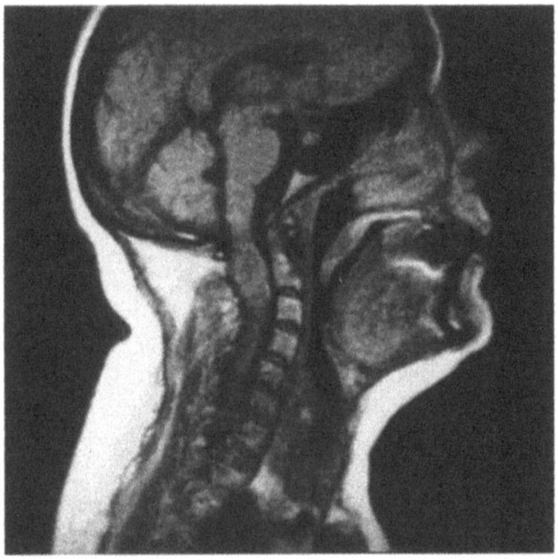

Fig. 3 T 1-weighted sagittal slice (300/33 NEX = 4). Image of an extramedullary tumor (Meningioma: confirmed by histology) directly below the foramen magnum.

RARE myelography, a method we have recently developed [5], the effects of intramedullary tumors and the space-occupying signs of extramedullary space-occupying lesions such as meningiomas and neurinomas generate images similar to those obtained by myelography. We can perform data acquisition of images with and without slice selection. The time required for imaging and reconstruction for this type of MRI-myelogram in two planes is less than one minute. Although matrix improvements and compensation programs for artefacts in CT have improved imagory of the posterior crania fossa [3], MRI is still superior in terms of the exact demarcation of tumors, by being able to provide images of tumors which extend caudally (fig. 4). Morever MRI can provide information valuable for planning the treatment of bony lesions near the foramen magnum: which we were able to demonstrate in the case of a chondrosarcoma of the occipital bone, a caudally infiltrating clivus-chordoma, and a metastasis of the cranial base.

Only in isolated cases do available native MRI-techniques fail to achieve an exact demarcation of a tumor and require the performance of contrast enhanced MRI.

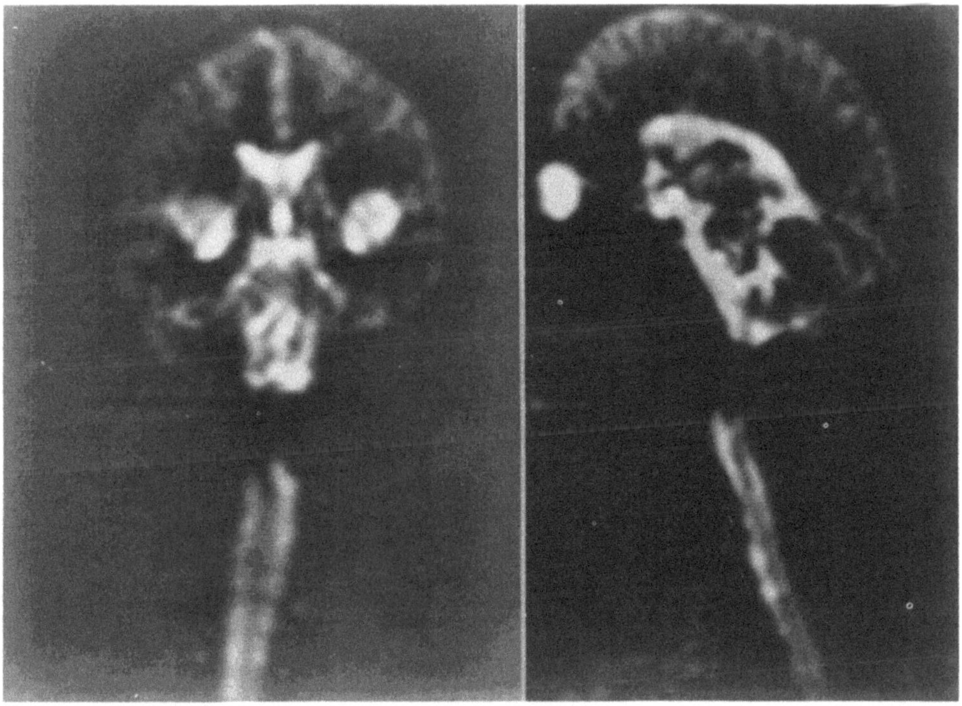

a b

Fig. 4 a, b Heavily T2-weighted MR – myelogram acquired with RARE-technique [5]. Total acquisition and reconstruction time for the two projection is less than 1 min. The antero-postero and lateral images show the CSF blocked out by the tumor (same case as fig. 3): comparable to conventional myelography.

In our series the application of MRI contrast material was necessary in only 3 out of 19 of our tumor patients. In those patients the tumor could not be defined, even after acquiring a T1-weighted sequence and a multi-echo sequence (3 slices at 12 echoes each 2000/33,66.99,133 ...) (figs. 5 a – c). Our experiences have shown that if the T1 and T2 of tumor tissue, edema and necrotic tissue is of about the same level then Gadolinium-DTPA allows a better delineation of tumors in the cervical part of the medulla. Meves et al. [12] claim that one can achieve a better contrast-resolution without using contrast material by means of a T-1/2 grid sequence with subsequent digital processing. We have not yet had any experience with that method.

Inflammatory and demyelinizing foci can be located exactly with MRI and can be identified in their early stages on the basis of their hyperintensity in T2-weighted images. We were able to prove this in three patients with myelitides and three patients with cervical plaques in the presence of multiple sclerosis. As for us such plaques are concerned Maravilla et al. [11] have already pointed out

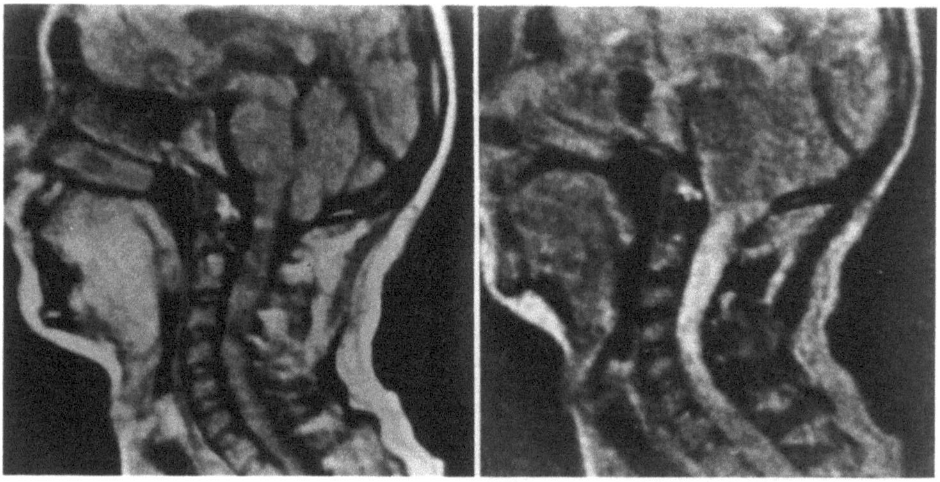

a b

Fig. 5 a T 1-weighted sagittal slice (500/33 NEX = 4). Extensive medullary space-occupying lesion from the foramen magnum to the first thoracic vertebra. Multiple hypointensive zones. Tumor demarcation cannot be determined.

Fig. 5 b T 2 weighted image (1800/99 NEX = 2). Prolonged T 2 in the cervical myelon corresponding to tumor tissue and reactive edema.

Fig. 5 c T 1-weighted sagittal slice (500/33 NEX = 4) after intravenous injection of gadolinium-DTPA (0.1 ml/kg BW). Clear enhancement of the tumor tissue at the level of the first and second cervical vertebrae.

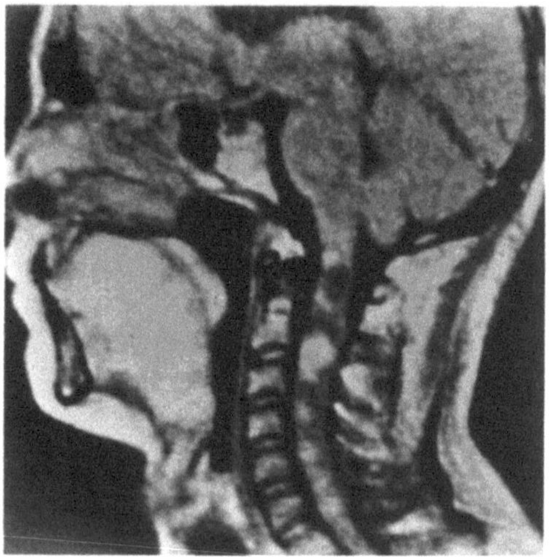

c

the usefulness of magnetic resonance imagining. In two of our patients with myelitis, the therapeutic effect of cortisone could be clearly observed during follow up examinations.

In the case of rheumatic arthritis bone changes can be demonstrated in the cranio-cervical junction by convention X-ray methods [2, 14, 16] supplemented if necessary by CT [2, 9]. MRI, however, provides further information on this disease, particularly with regard to soft tissue changes. Indeed, in seven of our cases the extent of the space-occupying lesion stemming from the pannus tissue could be determined only upon the basis of MRI. The manifestation of threatening ventral atlas dislocation in the case of chronic polyarthritis can be identified in its functional position in MRI. In contrast to conventional tomography, MRI has the additional advantage that patients suffering from polyarthritis do not have to be positioned on their side, which can be very painful, and that the relationship between dislocation and myelon compression can be assessed (fig. 6). In a patient with rapidly progressing symptoms of a high transverse lesion, we were able to demonstrate the advantages of being able simultaneously to demonstrate the dislocation, bone destruction, space-occupying lesion in the soft tissue and compression of the spinal cord by means of MRI. In this patient, the diagnosis suboccipital malum was confirmed by biopsy as a staphylococcal abscess (fig. 7).

Fig. 6

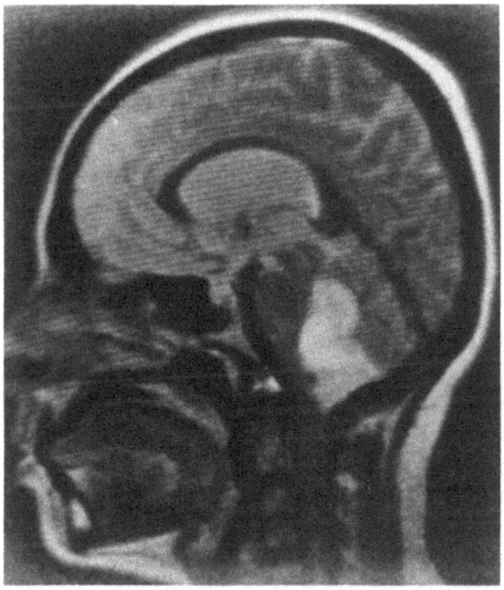

Fig. 7

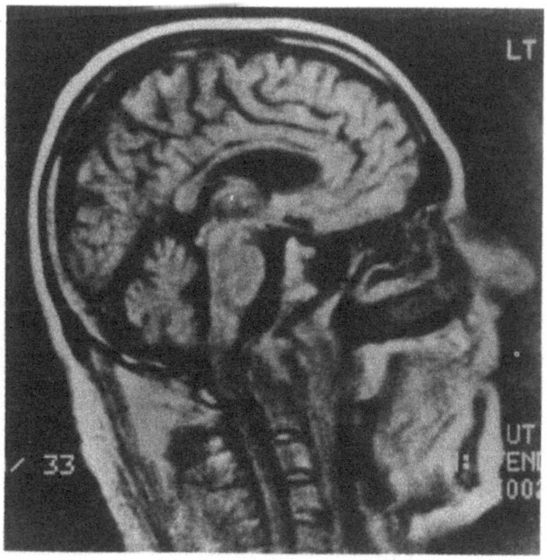

Fig. 6 T 1-weighted sagittal slice (1800/33-132) NEX = 2. The caudal boundary of the tumor (surgically confirmed medulloblastoma) reaches to below the level of the foramen magnum.

Fig. 7 T 1 weighted sagittal slice (300/33 NEX = 4). Destruction of the dens axis and compression of the upper cervical spinal cord caused by a destructive and space occupying lesion (= malum suboccipitale). Peroral biopsy revealed a staphylococci abscess.

Cervical disc prolapses are still being diagnosed by myelography, in some cases combined with CT-myelography [8]. Nevertheless MRI would be an excellent screening method since soft disc prolapses can be detected at an early stage and the method gives information concerning the onset of degeneration of the cartilage substance of the disc. Furthermore, the combination of T 1- and T 2-weighted images, the last in the time saving RARE-myelography, will allow definite decisions as to whether spondyloses or disc prolapses have already led to compression of the spinal cord.

Summary

MRI is already considered to be the diagnostic method of choice when symptoms and clinical findings indicate a lesion of the cranio-cervical junction. With this method it is always possible to define and localise space-occupying, inflammatory demyelinizing and degenerative changes. Only in isolated cases it is necessary to administer MRI contrast media. The minimum stress to the patient and the fast examination time inherent in the use of MRI present considerable advantages over the time-consuming conventional methods of myelography and high resolution CT.

References

[1] DeLaPaz, R. L., T. J. Brady, F. S. Buonanno: Nuclear magnetic resonance (NMR) imaging of the Arnold-chiari type I malformation with hydromyelia. J. Comput. Assist. Tomogr. 7 (1983) 126 – 129.

[2] Dihlmann, W.: Röntgenatlas rheumatischer Krankheiten. Georg Thieme Verlag, Stuttgart – New York 1985.

[3] Ersting, M.: Vergleich der Kernspintomographie der hinteren Schädelgrube mit der hochauflösenden Computertomographie. In: MR-'85 (J. Lissner, J. L. Dopman; eds.), pp. 391 – 393. Schnetztor-Verlag, Konstanz (1985).

[4] Hawkes, R. C., G. N. Holland, W. S. Moore, et al.: Craniovertebral Junction Pathology: Asssessment by NMR. AJNR **4** (1983) 232 – 233.

[5] Hennig, J., H. Friedburg, B. Ströbel: MR-Myelographie. J. Comput. Assist. Tomogr. (in press).

[6] Holland, G. N., R. C. Hawkes, W. S. Moore: NMR tomography of the brain: coronal and sagittal sections. J. Comput. Assist. Tomogr. **4** (1980) 429 – 433.

[7] Köhler, D., J. Treisch, G. Hertel, et al.: Die magnetische Resonanztomographie der Syringomyelie. Fortschr. Röntgenstr. **143** (1985) 617 – 770.

[8] Krause, D., D. Mairot, F. Buchheit, et al.: Soft cervical herniations, CT and surgery. 10. Oberrheinische Radiologentagung, Badenweiler 1985.

[9] Laasonen, E. M., U. Kankaanpää, J. Sandelin, et al.: Computed tomographic myelography (CTM) in atlanto-axial rheumatoid arthritis. Neuroradiology **27** (1985) 119 – 122.

[10] Lee, B. C. P., M. D. F. Deck, J. B. Kneeland, et al.: MR Imaging of the Craniocervical Junction. AJNR **6** (1985) 209 – 213.

[11] Maravilla, K. R., J. C. Weinreb, R. Suss, et al.: Magnetic Resonance Demonstration of Multiple Sclerosis Plaques in the Cervical Cord. AJNR **5** (1984) 685 – 689.

[12] Meves, M., G. Bielke, P. Higer, et al.: Kontrastoptimierung bei der MR-Diagnostik cerebraler Läsionen. In: MR-'85 (J. Lissner, J. L. Dopman, eds.), pp. 267 – 273. Schnetztor-Verlag, Konstanz (1985).

[13] Skalpe, I. O., O. Sortland: Cervical myelography with metrizamide (Amipaque). A comparison between conventional and computer-assisted myelography with special reference to the upper cervical and foramen magnum region. Neuroradiology **16** (1978) 275 – 278.

[14] Schilling, F., J. P. Haas, M. Schacherl: Die spontane atlanto-axiale Dislokation (Ventralluxation des Atlas) bei chronischer Polyarthritis und Spondylitis ankylopoetica. Fortschr. Röntgenstr. **99** (1963) 518 – 538.

[15] Schörner, W., R. Felix, C. Claussen, et al.: Kernspintomographische Diagnostik von Hirntumoren mit dem Kontrastmittel Gadolinium-DTPA. Fortschr. Röntgenstr. **141** (1984) 511 – 519.

[16] Wackenheim, A.: Roentgen diagnosis of the craniovertebral region. Springer, Berlin – Heidelberg – New York 1974.

NMR-finding in a case of Morquio's syndrome with syncope

T. Treig, D. Claus, W. Huk, B. Nüsslein

Introduction

Acute or chronic cervical myelopathies are well known neurological complications of mucopolysaccharidoses [1, 3, 5, 7, 8]. This paper deals with a case of a mild form of Morquio's disease which appeared with syncope.

NMR-imaging of the cranio-spinal region demonstrated a high intensity echo in the medulla oblongata before and after spinal decompression.

Case report

The 46 year-old patient of Italian origin was referred to the Neurological Clinic because of three occurences of loss of conciousness accompanied by tonic extension movements of all extremities.

One month before admission, he had a sudden weakness in his legs and arms which lasted a quarter of an hour and which forced him to sit down before

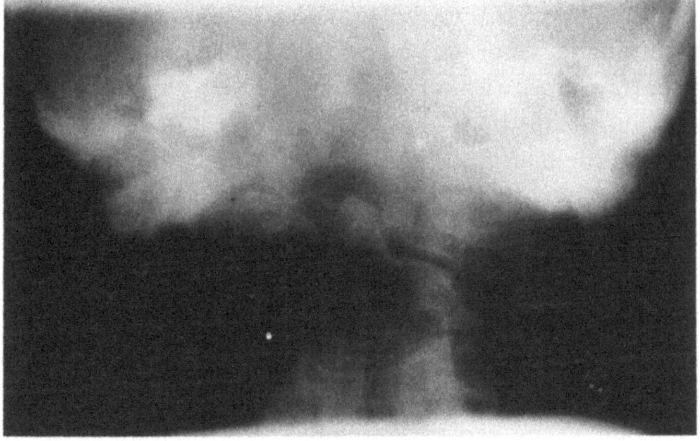

Fig. 1. Conventional tomography showes a normal odontoid process.

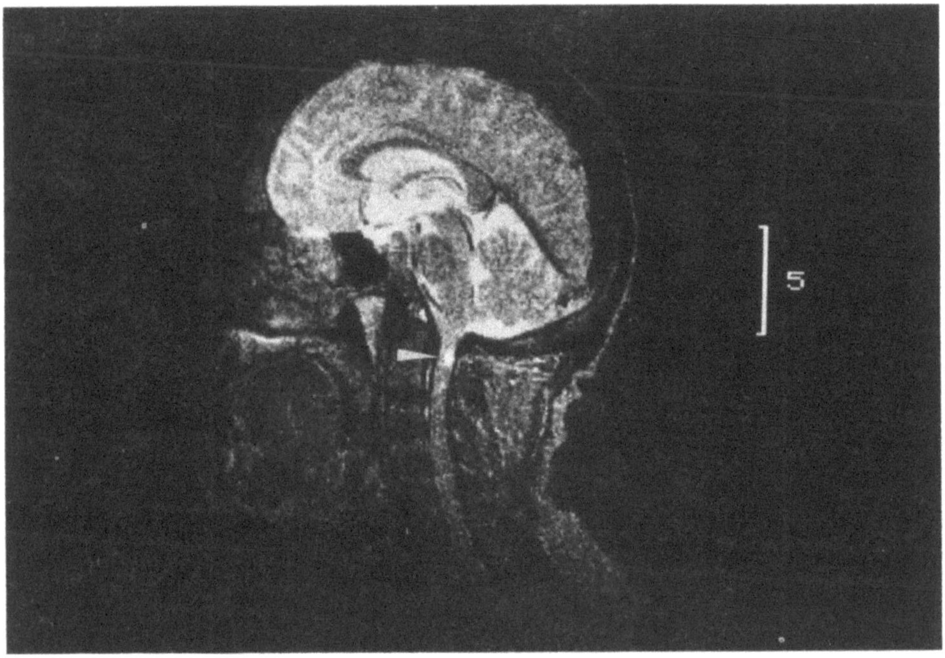

Fig. 2 NMR-scan taken before surgical intervention. The white arrow indicates the zone of enhanced echo.

continuing his way home. Furthermore he complained about numbness on the distal left arm and loss of strengh in the first to third fingers of his left hand. Headache, pain in the neck, hips and knees were long-standing complaints in his medical history.

Family history is non-contributory as far as the Morquio syndrome is concerned.

Initial physical examination gave the following data: height 152 cm, short neck, barrel trunk, relatively long limbs, reduced mobility of the cervical spine, genu valgum. A grade 3/6 systolic murmur was heard over the second intercostal space of the right chest, no corneal opacities were found. On neurological examination tendon reflexes were diminished, the triceps reflexes were absent. There were no pyramidal tract responses. He had mild paralysis when extending and flexing his left hand, and medium paralysis in the fingers of the left hand. Thumb muscles of the left hand were atrophic.

Sensory function was impaired in the dermatome corresponding to the cervical roots C 8 to Th 1 where our patient complained of hypalgesia and hypesthesia.

Echocardiography revealed a clinically insignificant aortic stenosis and regurgitation. The EEG recording showed bifrontally theta-activity. The other electrophysiological examinations, including evoked potentials and the long latency reflex, were normal.

Laboratory data: no abnormal finding in the routine investigation. There was a slight decrease in leucocyte β-galactosidasis (44% of normal controls). Ceratansulfaturia was not present, suggesting a mild form of the disease [6].

X-radiographic features: The spine radiographs demonstrated flattening of the vertebral bodies and anterior wedging which results in kyphosis and a short neck. The spinal canal was narrow (anterior posterior diameter at C6 less than 10 mm). The intervertebral foramina at C6 down to Th1 were narrow and oblique on both sides.

Conventional tomography of the cranio-spinal region showed a normal odontoid process. The top of the odontoid process laid 17 mm beyond a line drawn between the two mastoid processes (fig. 1).

NMR-imaging obtained an increased echo signal in the lower medulla (fig. 2). After laminectomy (C1 and C2) and enlargement of the foramen magnum, the NMR-scan still displayed enhanced intensity in the same region five month later. In addition, a zone of high echo had developed extending posteriorly which presumably consists of cerebrospinal fluid (fig. 3).

The postoperative recovery was uncomplicated and the patient experienced no more syncopal attacks.

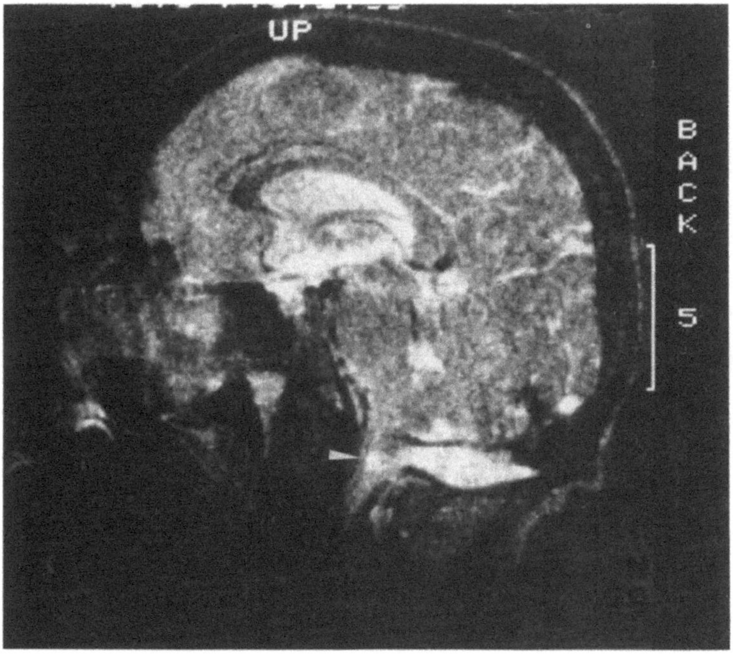

Fig. 3 NMR-scan obtained after spinal decompression. Posteriorly to the lesion (white arrow) there is another area of intensified signal.

Discussion

Acute tetraplegia with respiratory arrest as the most serious neurological complication of Morquio's disease, develop as a result of atlantoaxial dislocation. Contributing factors may be a narrow spinal canal and mucopolysaccharide deposits in the spinal dura.

We have reported a case of Morquio's disease with syncopes which are not of cardiac or cerebral origin.

NMR-imaging disclosed a lesion in the lower medulla oblongata found on re-examination five months after surgical intervention. The lesion site was sensitive to the regulation of blood pressure and played a role in respiratory control.

We do not know the histological correlation of this finding, however on macroscopic examination by the surgeon no pathological condition was seen. The dura in particular was not thickened. Regional storage of mucopolysaccharides in the diencephalon and cerebellum has been reported in Morquio's disease [4] and other mucopolysaccharidoses [2]. We do not suspect storage of this material as a pathogenetic factor in our patient since his clinical picture improved considerably.

The spinal echo probably corresponds to a chronic ischaemic lesion caused by the narrow spinal canal. The syncopes resulted then from an additional functional deficit which was brought about by an unusual movement of the neck.

References

[1] Blaw, M., L. O. Langer: Spinal cord compression in Morquio – Brailford's disease. J. Pediatr. **74** (1969) 593–600.

[2] Doshi, R., S. A. Sandry, A. W. Churchill, et al.: The cerebellum in mucopolysaccharidosis. J. Neurol. Neurosurg. Psychiatry 37 (1974) 1133–1138.

[3] Edwards, M. K., D. C. Harwood-Nash, C. R. Fitz, et al.: CT metrizamide myelography of the cervical spine in Morquio syndrome. AJNR **3** (1982) 666–669.

[4] Gilles, F. H., R. Deuel: Neuronal cytoplasmatic globules in the brain in Morquios syndrome. Arch. Neurol. **25** (1971) 393–403.

[5] Kaufman, H. H., H. S. Rosenberg, C. I. Scott, et al.: Cervical myelopathy due to dural compression in mucopolysaccharidosis. Neurology **17** (1982) 404–410.

[6] Maroteaux, P., V. Stanescu, R. Stanescu, et al.: Hétérogénité des formes frustes de la maladie de Morquio. Arch. Fr. Pédiatr. **39** (1982) 761–765.

[7] Scully, R. E., E. J. Mark, B. U. McNeely (eds.): Case 44 – 1983. N. Engl. J. Med. **309** (1983) 1109–1117.

[8] Wald, S. L., H. H. Schmidek: Compressive myelopathy associated with type VI mucopolysaccharidosis (Maroteaux-Lamy syndrome). Neurosurgery **14** (1984) 83–88.

The dynamic evaluation of the cervical spinal canal and spinal cord by magnetic resonance imaging during movement

F. Koschorek, H.-P. Jensen, B. Terwey

Introduction

Since the introduction of the ventral approach in treatment of chronic cervical myelopathy by Smith and Robinson and Cloward the discussion about the best way of surgical treatment – dorsal or ventral approach – is controversial. According to a review of literature by Epstein and Janin the dorsal approach seems to be slightly more favourable. Our own results point in the same direction.

By magnetic resonance imaging it is possible to study the relationship of the spinal canal to the spinal cord during movement without using contrast material. For the first time biomechanical factors, which may be responsible for the development of chronic cervical myelopathy, can be shown. This factors have been earlier investigated by Breig [1] in post mortem studies.

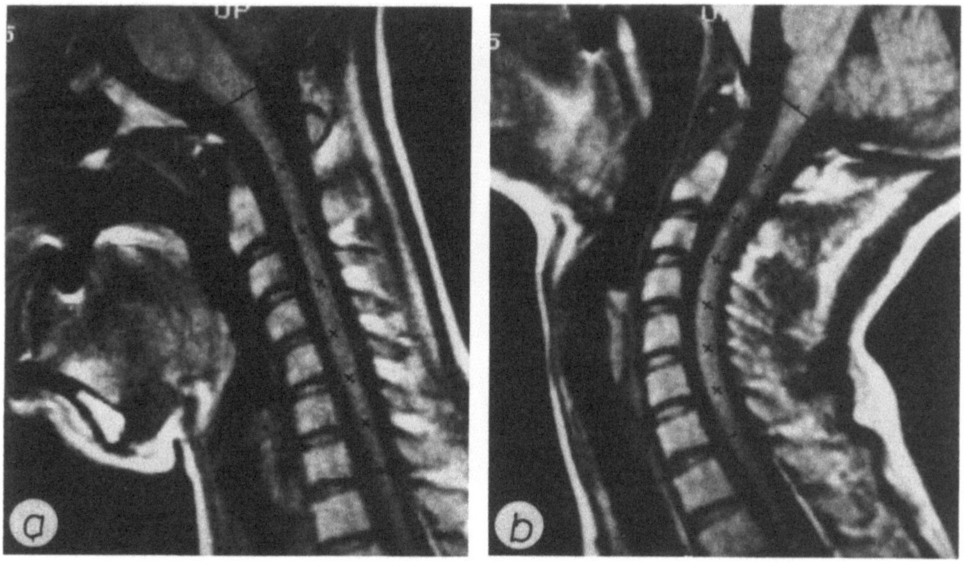

Fig. 1 T 1-weighted image of cervical spinal canal and spinal cord in flexion (a) and extension (b).

Methods

For the present study we used a 0.35 T and 0.5 T respectively super-conducting magnet. As described earlier [5] magnetic resonance measurements of the cervical spinal canal and the cervical spinal cord in flexion and extension were performed (fig. 1).

Additionally measurements of the complete spinal cord in flexion and extension were done (fig. 2).

The imaging procedure was as follows: At first we did a rapid axial scan using a 128 × 128 matrix to measure the midline. After a sagittal scan, an axial scan in the level of the ground plate of C7 and in the level of the foramen magnum the midline could be determined exactly. By exactly determining the midline a sagittal scan was performed using a matrix of 256 × 256 with 4 averages. On this scan the length of cervical canal and also the spinal cord were measured in flexion and extension position.

a b

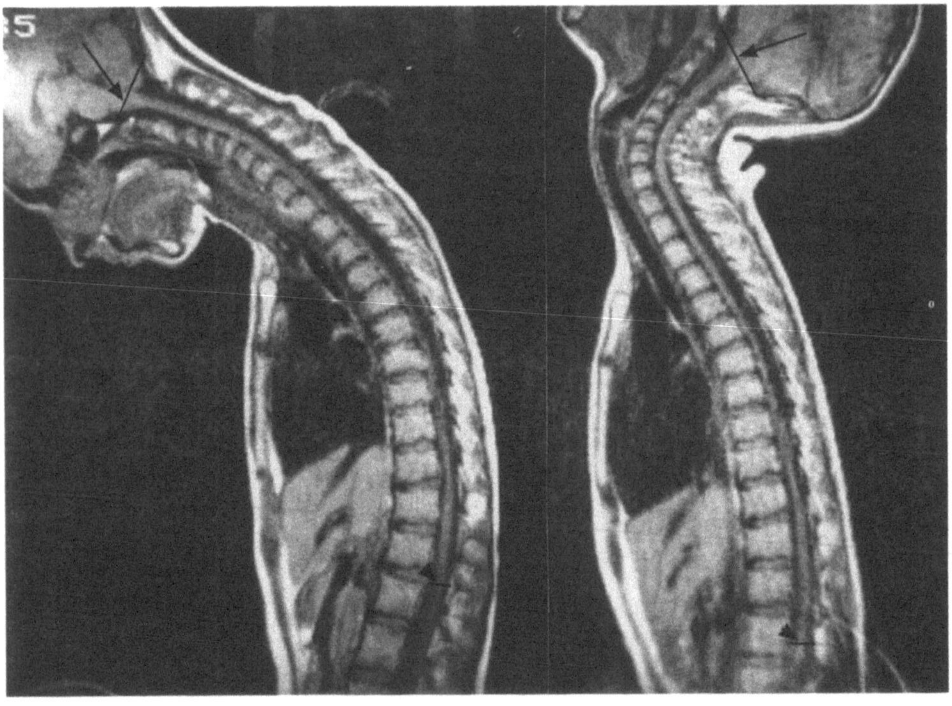

Fig. 2 T1-weighted image of spinal canal and spinal cord in flexion and extension. Points of measurements: From conus medullaris (arrow head) to the height of the foramen magnum (arrow).

For measurements of the complete length of the spinal cord we used the same technique. The measure-points were the conus medullaris and the spinal cord at the level of the foramen magnum.

Results

Table 1 shows the results of measurements of the cervical canal and spinal cord in 5 volunteers and 10 patients. On the average the lengthening of the cervical canal and spinal cord during flexion as compared to extention is 12.7 cm ± 0.23 cm and 11.5 cm ± 0.23 cm respectively. The difference is 1.2 cm. Table 2

Table 1 Results of measurement of the cervical canal and spinal cord in 5 volunteers and 10 patients

Case	Anteflexion (cm)	Standart Mean Deviation	Retroflexion (cm)	Standart Mean Deviation	Difference (cm)
K. G.	14.6	0.07	12.1	0.22	2.5
S. K.	12.6	0.33	10.4	0.31	2.2
R. J.	13.8	0.16	11.7	0.28	2.1
R. H.	14.0	0.22	12.0	0.20	2.0
W. C.	13.0	0.24	11.5	0.19	1.5
S. H.	11.8	0.20	10.7	0.10	1.1
P. M.	12.2	0.30	11.1	0.10	1.1
A. F.	12.3	0.20	11.3	0.22	1.0
K. C.	10.3	0.22	9.4	0.22	0.9
H. R.	12.8	0.19	12.0	0.29	0.8
E. H.	12.4	0.21	11.6	0.36	0.8
K. F.	12.7	0.30	12.0	0.29	0.7
S. H.	12.3	0.21	11.7	0.35	0.6
Z. U.	13.9	0.45	13.4	0.19	0.5
J. H.	11.7	0.17	11.3	0.09	0.4

Table 2 Results of measurement of the whole spinal cord

Case	Anteflexion (cm)	Retroflexion (cm)	Movement of Conus Medullaris (cm)	Difference (cm)
P. M.	50.9	47.4	1.5	3.5
V. H.	52.5	49.1	1.4	3.4
H. P.	52.8	51.4	1.4	1.4
G. S.	53.9	52.2	1.0	1.7
B. J.	52.2	48.3	0.9	3.9
Mean	52.5	49.7	1.24	2.8

demonstrates the results of the additionally performed measurements of the complete spinal cord. On the average the spinal canal lengthens during flexion as compared to extention 2.8 cm ± 1.0 cm. The conus medullaris rises during movement in average 1.24 cm ± 0.24 cm.

Discussion

Breig demonstrated in measurements of post mortem cases that the lengthening of cervical spinal cord during flexion and extension is 8 – 10 mm [2]. Our measurements in vivo of the cervical spinal canal and spinal cord show the same range: a lengthening averaging 12 mm. The measurement of the whole spinal cord points in the direction that the spinal canal lengthens more than the spinal cord, which changes in length on the average 12 mm. That appears to us that the axial tension of the spinal cord increases during flexion and that malposition and especially pathological kyphosis leads to increased tension in the spinal cord, which may result in a decrease of bloodflow as the small vessels become stretched. This results in an increase of clinical signs of chronic cervical myelopathy. In the ventral approach the malposition of cervical spine up to a kyphosis increases frequently (fig. 3). In such cases the surgical procedure fails to correct malposition of the cervical spine [4]. According to Breig the dorsal approach avoids these disadvantages and furthermore the increased tension of the spinal cord will diminish.

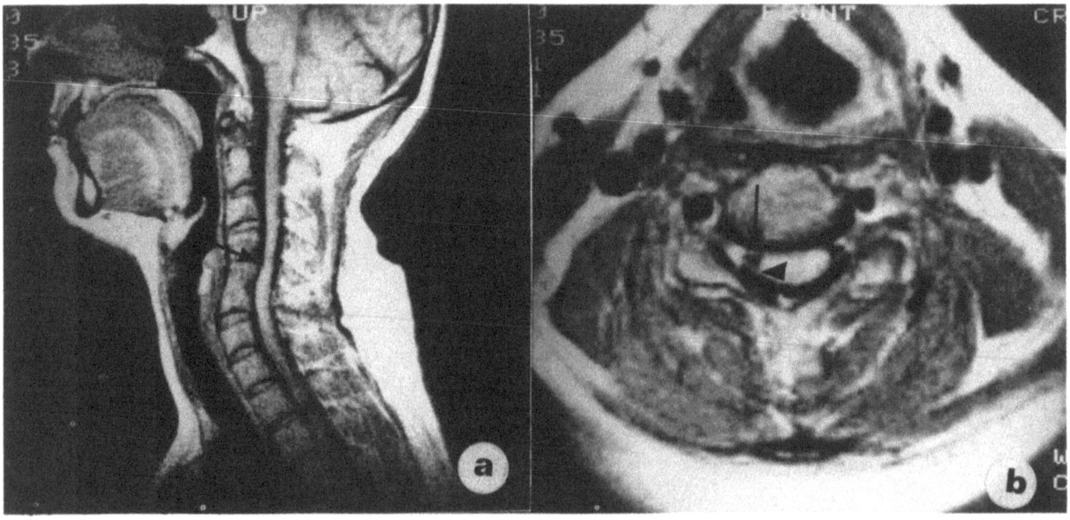

Fig. 3 T1-weighted image of spinal canal and spinal cord after Cloward procedure. a) Sagittal scan: Compression of spinal cord due to collapsed Cloward-dowel (arrow); b) Axial scan: Compression of spinal cord. Ventral nerve-root (arrow), dorsal nerve-root (arrow head).

Conclusion

1. The first results of in vivo measurements of the cervical canal and spinal cord indicate that tension in the spinal cord increases during flexion.
2. As the dorsal approach avoids this increased tension of the spinal cord the surgical treatment in chronic cervical myelopathy using this route seems to be preferable.

References

[1] Breig, A.: Effect of histo-dynamic tension on the function of the central nervous-system; with special reference to its analysis in spinal cord injury and a skulltraction. In: H. Kuhlendahl, V. Haensel (eds.): Proceedings of the German Society for Neurosurgery, vol. 3, pp. 36–54. Excerpta Medica, Amsterdam, American Elsevier Comp., Inc., New York 1973.
[2] Breig, A.: Adverse mechanical tension in the central nervous-system. p. 130. Almqvist and Wiksell International, Stockholm 1978.
[3] Breig, A.: Biomechanische Verfahren zur Wiederherstellung neuraler Funktion bei posttraumatischen Para- und Tetraplegien. In: Neuro-Orthopädie (D. Hohmann, B. Kügelgen, K. Liebich, M. Schirmer, eds.), vol. 2, pp. 1975–1987. Springer Verlag, Berlin – Heidelberg – New York – Tokyo 1984.
[4] Galera, R., D. Tovi: Anterior disc excision with interbody fusion in cervical spondylotic myelopathy and rhizopathy. J. Neurosurg. **28** (1968) 305–310.
[5] Koschorek, F., B. Terwey: Kernspintomographie im Bereich der HWS: Erleichterung der Indikation zur Operation und Beeinflussung der Wahl des Operationsverfahrens. Vortrag gehalten auf der 36. Jahrestagung der Deutschen Gesellschaft für Neurochirurgie in Berlin 1985.

Somatosensory evoked potentials in cervical myelopathy

R. Besser, H. C. Hopf

Introduction

Somatosensory evoked potentials (SEP) are usually elicted by electrical stimulation of peripheral nerves, i. e. the median or ulnar nerve at the upper limbs and the tibial nerve at the lower limb. The evoked responses can be recorded from

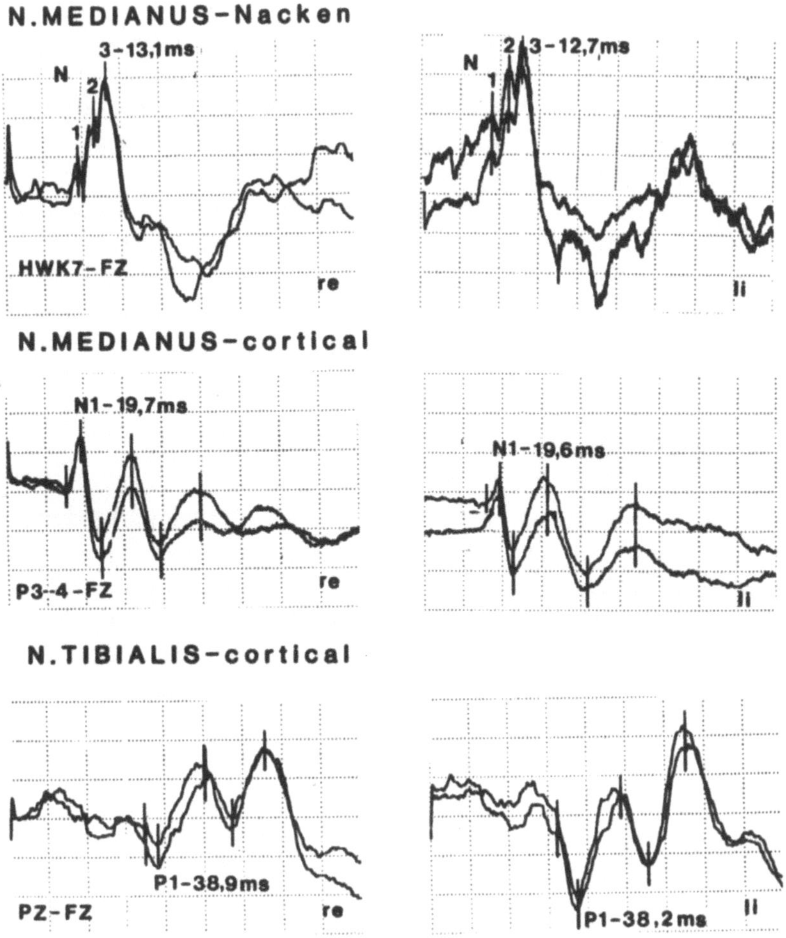

Fig. 1 Normal SEP from the neck and cortex after median and tibial nerve stimulation in a patient with sensory and motor deficit due to a rightsided radiculopathy C_6.

the 7th cervical vertebra (C 7) and the contralateral cortical sensory hand area (median and ulnar nerve) or the vertex (tibial nerve). The sensory pathways responsible for the different SEP's seem to be the posterior columns. Clinical studies have found that SEP abnormalities are mostly associated with those signs. Demyelination produces a marked delay of the potentials, but does not change its shape, while compression by space occupying lesions leads to small amplitude at normal latency.

The cervical SEP consists of three negative peaks: N 1 (N 9), N 2 (N 11) and N 3 (N 13) which are attributed to the activities of the brachial plexus, the dorsal roots and the ascending fibres of the posterior columns. A negative wave (N 1) at 18 to 21 ms is the first cortical reaction after median nerve stimulation followed by several positive and negative waves. The beginning of the cortical complex from tibial nerve stimulation is P 1 at 40 to 43 ms (fig. 1).

Discogenic and spondylotic radiculopathy of the cervical spine is characterized by a low incidence of SEP abnormalities to median or ulnar nerve stimulation despite severe sensory deficits (Fig. 1). It might be argued, that the large diameter fibres responsible for the SEP are relatively spared [5]. Cervical spondylosis however may result from spinal cord compression and secondary vascular alterations which exceed the level of spondylotic abnormalities. Clinically cervical myelopathy is characterized by slow progressive involvement of the corticospinal and posterior column tracts and occasional radiculopathy. The high incidence of cervical spondylosis in elderly patients requires exclusion of other diseases such as multiple sclerosis, amyotrophic lateral sclerosis and vitamin B 12 deficiency.

Patients and methods

Clinical evaluation comprises 17 patients with cervical myelopathy due to spondylosis or disc protusion with the diagnosis being confirmed by a myelogram. There was no hint of other diseases such as MS, combined tract degeneration, amyotrophic lateral sclerosis or luetic myelopathy by CSF analysis, B 12 and folate serum levels, resorption tests and TPHA tests. 15 of the 17 patients underwent surgical treatment. The severity of spondylotic compression was estimated from the relation (quotient) between the minimal and the maximal sagittal diameters of the contrast band of the positive myelography at the C 4 to C 7 level.

SEP's were recorded by surface electrodes from the neck (C 7) and contralaterally from the sensory cortical hand area (P 3/P 4) after median nerve stimulation at wrist and from the vertex (Pz) after tibial nerve stimulation at ankle. All electrodes were referred to Fz. Square wave stimuli of 0.2 ms duration were delivered at 3/sec to produce moderate twitches of the appropriate muscles. The bandpass of

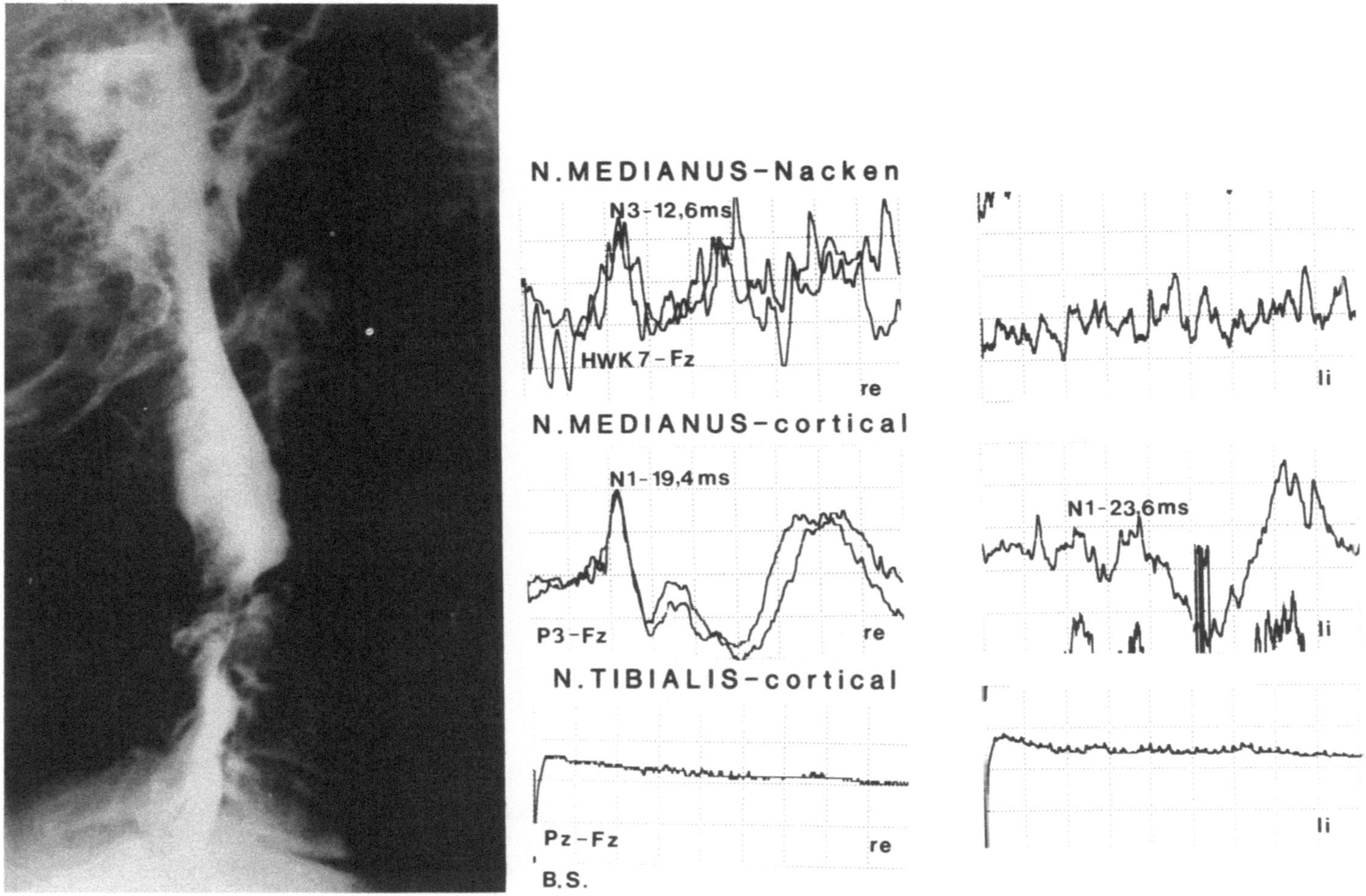

Fig. 2 Left side: Myelogramm with severe entrapment of the cervical spine due to spondylosis and subluxation. Right side: SEP after median and tibial nerve stimulation (see text).

the amplifier was set 20 to 2000 Hz. Analysis times were 100 msec for the cortical and 50 msec for the cervical responses. 256 sweeps were summed for each response. The criteria for abnormalities were absence or increased latencies. The upper range were 15.5 ms (N 1/C 7), 22.8 ms (N 1/cortical) and 45.5 (P 1/cortical).

Results

The investigations of a representative case are shown in figure 2. The patient was wheel chair bound due to myelopathy with severe impairment of the corticospinal and posterior column tracts. Myelography reveals marked compression of the spinal cord. Tibial SEP's were absent on both sides. The left median SEP showed absence of N 1 (C 7) and slightly late cortical N 1, while right median nerve stimulation exhibited normal potentials from the neck and the cortex.

The findings in the total of 17 cases with cervical myelopathy form three different categories of electrophysiological abnormalities irrespective of the nerves tested. The most severe changes were a bilateral absence of any responses. The milder cases showed bilateral abnormalities either absence on one side and a delay on the other or bilaterally delayed responses. The less pronounced abnormality was a delay on only one side, with normal responses on the other.

With tibial nerve stimulation the SEP were abnormal without exception. With median nerve stimulation N 3 (C 7) was abnormal in 14 cases, whereas N 1 (cortical) was always present but delayed in 5 (fig. 3).

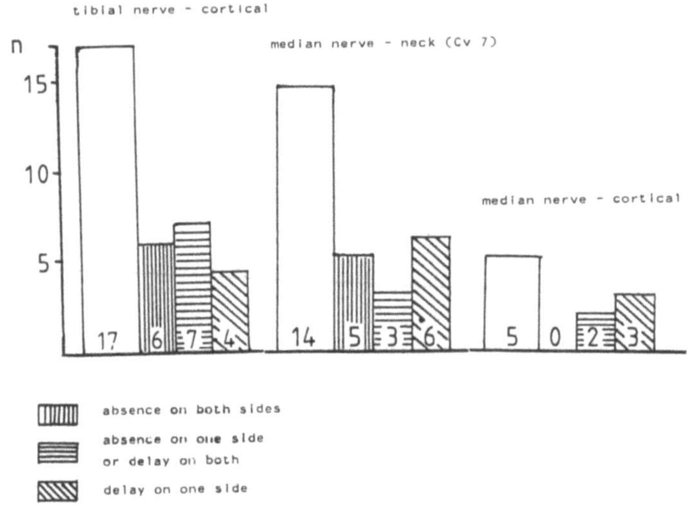

Fig. 3 Result of SEP investigations in 17 patients with cervical myelopathy. White columns: number of pathological SEP.

Of the total 17 cases 10 with posterior column signs showed absence or bilateral delay of tibial nerve SEP 10 (fig. 4). In 7 patients without those signs the SEP were abnormal, but to a much lesser degree.

Myelograms were available in 11 cases. The amount of cord compression (minimal/maximal sagittal cervical diameter) corresponded to the electrophysiological data (tab. 1). With minimal diameters less than 60% of the normal segments, the SEP responses predominantly were absent. In cases with minor compression bilateral SEP loss was never observed.

Table 1 Results of tibial nerve SEPs in relation to narrowing of the cervical spinal canal (n – 11)

% of narrowing	absence on both sides	absence on one side or delay on both	delay on one side	normal
less than 60%	0	3	1	0
more than 60%	5	2	0	0

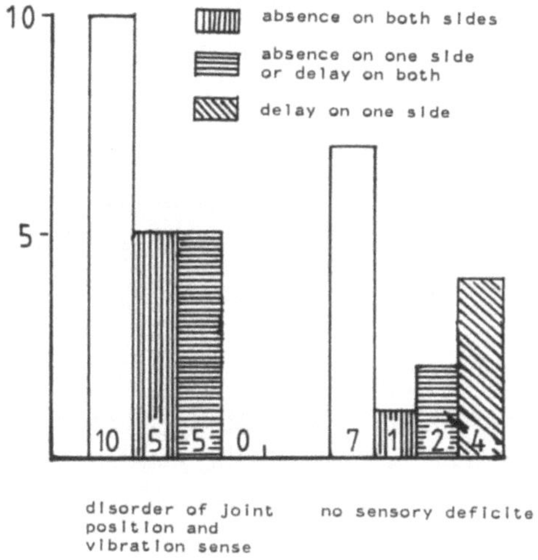

Fig. 4 Correlation between abnormality of tibial nerve SEP and posterior column signs.

Discussion

The outstanding electrophysiological feature of cervical myelopathy due to cervical spondylosis are abnormalities of tibial nerve SEP. The degree and frequency of SEP abnormalities were correlated to posterior column signs. Absence of every response was only found in cases with severe disturbances of joint position and vibration sense in the feet. But slightly abnormal tibial SEP were also recorded in patients without posterior column signs. Thus, SEP appear to be more sensitive for detecting posterior column impairment than a clinical examination. The latency of P 40 never exeeded 50 msec and a marked delay characteristic for demyelination, predominantly in MS [4] was never seen. Our findings are in agreement with those of Yu and Jones [5] in their series of 34 patients. We do not rely on the amplitude of the tibial nerve SEP. We believe that an appropriate and reproducible nerve stimulation is uncertain in severe myelopathy. Spasticity and spinal automatisms sometimes interfere with the examination, and may result in artefact contaminated responses. But it can be assumed that in accordance to other space occupying lesions of the spinal cord [4] reduction in amplitude is a common feature.

Although myelograms were available in only 11 of our 17 patients cervical spine width measurements reveal a correlation between the radiographicly established cord compression and the tibial SEP abnormalities. Despite that this finding is in contrast to the series of Yu and Jones [5], our results confirm the report of Nurick [3], who stated that the clinical signs increase with increasing compression of the spinal cord.

Absence or delay of cervical potentials following median nerve stimulation was observed in 14 cases, which corresponds to the study of El-Negamy and Sedgwick [1]. It was difficult to identify N 1 of the neck potentials so that valid results on the peripheral conduction time (N 1 – N 3) are not available in our cases. Ganes [2] reported long intervals between N 1 and N 3 in cases with radiculopathy and sometimes in patients with additional myelopathy. None of our cases had delayed central conduction time (N 3 – N 1). This finding seems to be of great value to discriminate cervical myelopathy from MS.

The lowest incidence of SEP abnormalities were found in cortical responses following median nerve stimulation. Only 5 patients had slightly delayed responses, whereas absence was never found. The input from the median nerve seems to be sufficient to generate cortical responses even if the cervical potentials are absent.

In conclusion there are three points of diagnostic significance of SEP in cervical myelopathy. 1. SEP abnormalities are correlated with the severity of posterior column involvement, even if clinical signs are missing. 2. they are correlated with the amount of spinal cord compression due to spondylosis. 3. they can be differentiated from other cases of spinal cord disease, such as MS and amyotrophic lateral sclerosis. In all instances tibial nerve SEP are most sensitive and superior to median nerve testing.

References

[1] El Negamy, E., E. M. Sedgwick: Delayed cervical somatosensory potentials in cervical spondylosis. J. Neurol. Neurosurg. Psychiat. **42** (1979) 238 – 241.

[2] Ganes, T.: Somatosensory conduction times and peripheral, cervical and cortical evoked potentials in patients with cervical spondylosis. J. Neurol. Neurosurg. Psychiat. **43** (1980) 683 – 689.

[3] Nurick, S.: The pathogenesis of spinal cord disorder associated with cervical spondylosis. Brain **95** (1972) 87 – 100.

[4] Riffel, B., M. Stöhr, F. Petruch, et al.: Somatosensory evoked potentials following tibial nerve stimulation in multiple sclerosis and space occupying spinal cord disease. In: J. Courjon, F. Mauguiere, M. Revol (eds.): Clinical applications of evoked potentials in Neurology, pp. 493 – 500. Raven Press, New York 1982.

[5] Yu, Y. L., S. J. Jones: Somatosensory evoked potentials in cervical spondylosis. Brain **108** (1985) 273 – 300.

Spontaneous eye movements in cranio-cervical abnormalities

R. Thümler, R. Besser, R. Hasselbach

Introduction

The anatomical substrates of ocular motor control are lower brainstem structures and cerebellum and lesions at the level of the cranio-spinal region should not normally be associated with eye movement disorders. However in craniocervical junction abnormalities resulting in a caudal displacement oculomotor pathways can be involved. Downbeat nystagmus and periodic alternating nystagmus are two specific oculomotor disorders highly suggestiv of an abnormality at the craniocervical junction, occuring in the Arnold-Chiari malformation, basilar invagination and platybasia.

Methods

Downbeat nystagmus is characterized by vertical jerk nystagmus in primary position with the fast phase beating in the downward direction. The eye movements of patients shown in the following figures were recorded by A. C. electro-oculographie (EOG) with a bandwidth 0 to 30 Hz and time constant of 5 s. For monocular horizontal recordings electrodes were placed at the inner and outer canthi. Vertical movements were recorded with electrodes placed above the eyebrow and below the lower eyelid.

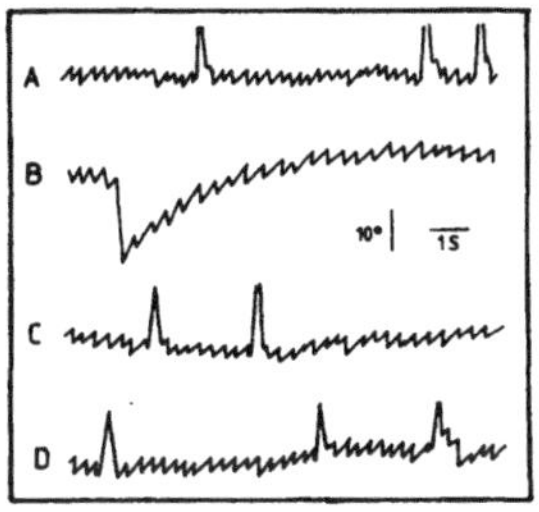

Fig. 1

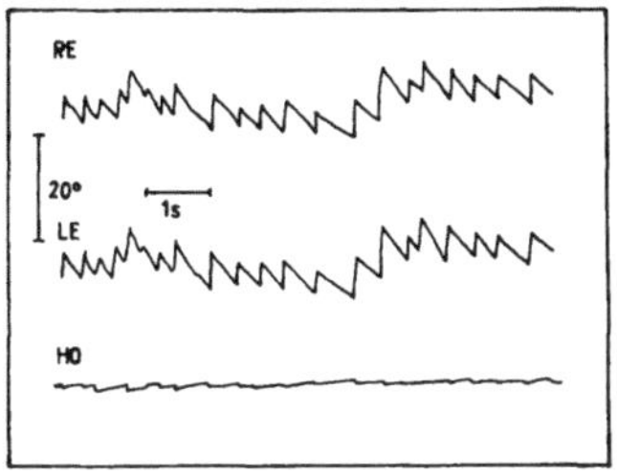

Fig. 2

Fig. 1 Vertical electro-oculogramm of a patient with basilar invagination. Downbeat nystagmus: A = in primary position; B = gaze down; C = gaze left; D = gaze right.

Fig. 2 Vertical electro-oculogramm of a patient with upbeat nystagmus. RE = right eye; LE = left eye; HO = horizontal EOG.

Case histories

Figure 1 shows the EOG of a 59-year-old patient who was admitted for investigation of headache, imbalance on walking and visual blurring. On examination he had downbeat nystagmus in the primary position and mild truncal ataxia. The rest of the neurological examination was normal. On specific questioning he reported that the world appeared to be moving up and down. The downbeat nystagmus persisted in all gaze positions, there was no accentuation on lateral gaze. CT scan, skull and cervical spine x-ray showed basilar impression.

About one-third of the patients with downbeat nystagmus have a Chiari-malformation. Usually (but not in our patient) the nystagmus increases on lateral gaze [1] and is not maximal at downward gaze. Rather, downbeat nystagmus on downgaze is usually associated with nystagmus in all directions of gaze and commonly cause of sedative or anticonvulsant medication. The pathophysiologic mechanism or the anatomical substrate is still unknown, but most authors suggested a dysfunction of the vestibulo-cerebellum. Zasorin and Baloh [7] reported a case of downbeat nystagmus in a patient with alcoholic cerebellar degeneration and concluded that associated floccular damage caused the downbeat nystagmus. Bogousslavsky and Regli [2] described a strictly monocular downbeat nystagmus in a patient with probable sporadic (olivo)ponto-cerebellar atrophy. They suggested that monocular downbeat nystagmus is due to dysfunction of the ipsilateral brachium conjunctivum.

Figure 2 shows another type of spontaneous vertical jerk nystagmus but with the fast phase beating upward (upbeat nystagmus). The upbeat nystagmus has also been correlated with lesions of the caudal brainstem and the cerebellar vermis, but is not a typically sign of craniocervical abnormalities [3]. The EOG shown in fig. 2 is of a patient with multiple sclerosis, who developed first primary position unbeat nystagmus and after recovery internuclear ophthalmoplegia.

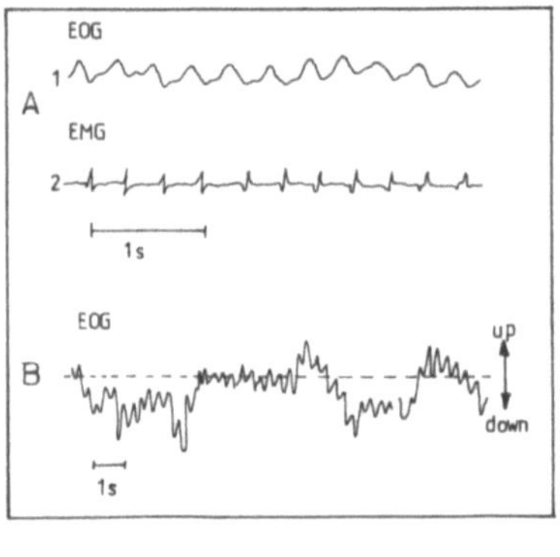

Fig. 3 Patient with ocular myoclonus ("locked in syndrome"). A 1 = vertical EOG; A 2 = facial muscle; B = vertical EOG during pursuit in the vertical plane.

Non-mystagmic vertical ocular oscillations should be differentiated from up- and downbeat nystagmus. Figure 3 shows the EOG-tracings of a patient with occlusion of the basilar artery at the midpontine level ("locked in syndrome"). His only possibility of communication are voluntary eye movements in the vertical plane. In Figure 3 b the patient is asked to look up- and downward. The upper tracing (A 1) shows continuous, rhythmic up-and-down pendular oscillations with a rate of 3 to 4 beats per second. This pendular vertical oscillations (ocular myoclonus) are associated with rhythmic movements of the facial muscles in synchrony with the eye movement (A 2). Clinically the patient has associated rhythmic contractions of the palate, pharynx, larynx and facial muscles. This myoclonus developed several month after an acute lesion and persisted until the death of the patient.

Another rare form of spontaneous nystagmus suggestiv of craniocervical junctional abnormalities is periodic alternating nystagmus (PAN). PAN is occasionally associated with downbeat nystagmus [4]. This extraordinary ocular motor phenomenon is manifested as a horizontal jerk nystagmus witch periodically changes directions after a short pause. Figure 4 shows PAN in a patient with trimethyltin

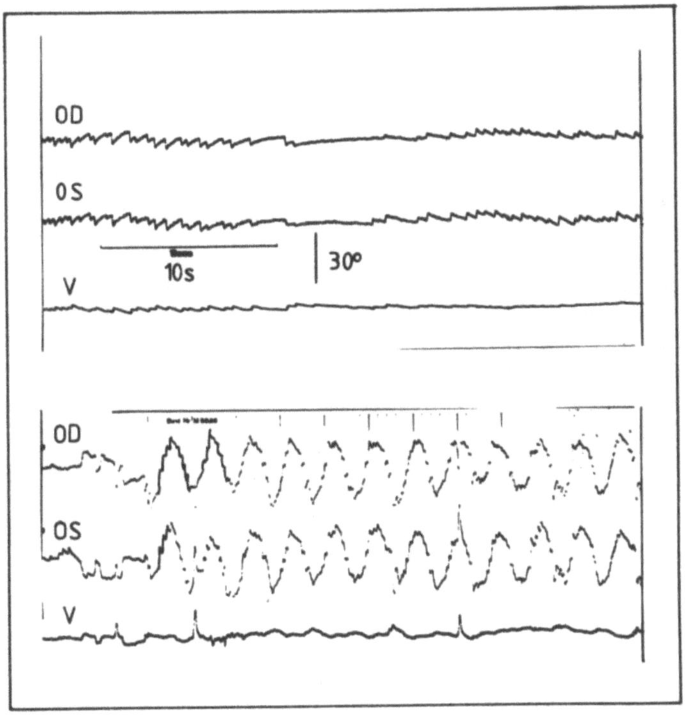

Fig. 4 Monocular electro-oculogramm of a patient with periodic alternating nystagmus. OD = right eye; OS = left eye; V = vertical EOG. Upper traces: recording in primary position; lower traces: recording during horizontal pursuit.

intoxication, published previously [6]. The upper two tracings are the monocular horizontal EOG tracings: in primary eye position there is horizontal jerk nystagmus with variable amplitudes and velocities of the slow phase. Nystagmus in one direction lasted for about 90 seconds by a non-nystagmic interlude of about 5 seconds. Then the similar sequence occurs with the rapid phase in the opposite direction. At the maximal height of nystagmus the patient showed oscillopsia. PAN was not significantly altered by eye closure, optokinetic or caloric stimulation. An autopsy of another patient with severe trimethyltin poisoning showed marked loss of Purkinje cells in the cerebellar cortex [6].

Conclusions

The described spontaneous eye movements indicate structural diseases in or near the medullary-cervical junction. In patients with downbeat nystagmus and/or periodic alternating nystagmus particular attention should be directed to the cranio-spinal region. Patients with Arnold-Chiari malformation and associated abnormalities of eye movement may benefit from surgical decompression [5].

References

[1] Baloh, R. W., J. W. Spooner: Downbeat nystagmus: A type of central vestibular nystagmus. Neurology **34** (1984) 304–310.

[2] Bogousslavsky, J., F. Regli: Monocular downbeat nystagmus. J. Neurol. **232** (1985) 99–101.

[2] Brandt, T., W. Büchele: Augenbewegungsstörungen. Fischer Verlag Stuttgart – New York 1983.

[4] Keane, J. R.: Periodic alternating nystagmus with downward beating nystagmus. Arch. Neurol. **30** (1974) 399–402.

[5] Spooner, J. W., R. W. Baloh: Arnold-Chiari Malformation. Improvement in eye movements after surgical treatment. Brain **104** (1981) 51–60.

[6] Thümler, R., R. Besser, H. Beuerbach: Periodic alternating nystagmus in a patient with trimethyltin poisoning. Electroenceph. Clin. Neurophysiol. **55** (1983) 3–184.

[7] Zasorin, N. L., R. W. Baloh: Downbeat Nystagmus with alcoholic cerebellar degeneration. Arch. Neurol. **41** (1984) 1301–1302.

Microsurgical aspects of the transoral and transcervical approach to the cranio-cervical junction

R. R. Renella, S. Hussein, H.-G. Höllerhage

Introduction

The main problem in surgical treatment of ventrally situated disease processes of the cranio-cervical junction is the operative access [2, 13]. The advantages of the transoral approach (direct anatomical access, possibility of increased extension cephalad) are outweighed by a high infection rate and problems in closing the posterior pharyngeal wall [1–4, 6, 7, 11, 14]. These complications are omitted when using the transcervical approach [8, 16]. However this access endangers neural and vascular structures of the upper lateral neck region and its usefulness is also limited. The aim of this anatomical study is to investigate the possibilities and limits of both approaches for epi- and intradural operation of the cranio-cervical junction.

Material and methods

The study was carried out in 8 bodies (3 male, 5 female). In 4 cases a transoral approach was performed in operative position, according to the technic of Franke and Clarisse [4]. In 2 unfixed bodies of this group the vertebral artery was selectively perfused with dye. The transcervical approach was investigated in 4 cases also using the operative position. In each specimen the right cervical region was exposed using the original technique of Stevenson [16] and the left side according to Lesoin [9]. In both cases the anterior arch of the atlas was dissected in 2 ways: in front of the external carotid artery and laterally to the internal jugular vein. In every specimen the distances between surgically important landmarks were measured and documented by photographes.

Results and discussion

Table 1 and 2 summarize the relevant measurements. The transoral approach (TOA) after splitting of the soft palate permits an optimal exposure of the cranio-cervical junction, the prebulbar and prepontine region and of the ventral cervical cord up to the middle of C3 (fig. 1). The operative field measures 36 – 40 mm in height from C1 up to the middle of C3 and 18.5 – 23 mm from the inferior edge of the clivus to the dorsum sellae. The width of the bony window is variable, the minimal values being found at the C1 level. Extending the bony resection to the margin of the atlanto-occipital joints a mean operative field of 17 mm width can be achieved, supposed the vertebral artery shows a normal course. With a 20° hyperextension of the neck, the anterior tubercle of the atlas (TAA) can be reached with an angle of 0 – 5° in a mean depth of 68 mm. The region of the clivus and the body of C3 are exposed with an angle of 35° in relation to the vertical plane. Since the mean operating distance in the epidural space of C2 – C3 is 122 mm, a 320 mm objective and bajonett-instruments of at last 20 cm lenght are required.

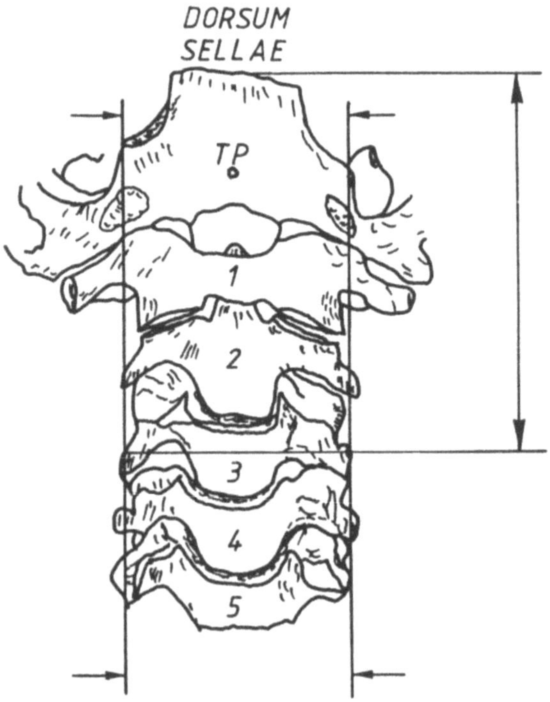

Fig. 1 Operative field by transoral approach to the cranio-cervical junction. Upper limit: dorsum sellae; lower limit: middle of the vertebral body C3; lateral limit: vertebral joints. TP = pharyngeal tubercle.

Landmark of the TOA is the TAA, which can be palpated easily above the retrolingual space. A paramedian longitudinal incision 25 mm cranially and 15 mm caudally from TAA splits the posterior pharyngeal wall down to the deep cervical fascia. The muscle layer (Mm. longus capitis et colli) are adherent to the anterior atlanto-occipital membrane (MAA) and to the anterior longitudinal ligament [12]. It can be dissected

Table 1 Relevant distance by transoral approach to the cranio-cervical junction

N	DS/LC	TA/TP	K(TP)	SPID	PB/LC
1	44	18.5	6.5	29.0	19.5
2	47	19.0	7.0	26.0	20.0
3	45	21.5	10.0	27.5	22.5
4	45	23.0	8.5	28.5	21.0

DS/LC = distance dorsum sellae/lower edge of the clivus; TA/TP = distance anterior tubercle of the atlas and pharyngeal tubercle; K(TP) = depth of the clivus at the level of the pharyngeal tubercle; PB/LC = distance basilar plexus/lower edge of the clivus.

Table 2 Relevant distance at the level of the foramen magnum (mm)

N	TFM	DFD	ICD	DHC	SPI(TP)
1	3.2	33	25.5	26.0	3.0/3.0
2	3.8	37	31.0	27.5	2.5/3.0
3	4.6	31	30.0	25.5	2.5/3.0
4	1.8	47	38.0	32.0	3.0/3.0
5	3.3	39	26.5	29.5	2.0/2.5
6	5.1	36	34.0	32.0	2.5/2.5
7	4.7	48	39.0	38.5	3.0/2.5
8	3.5	32	25.0	31.0	3.0/2.5

TFM = thickness of the anterior edge of the foramen magnum; DFD = distance from the anterior edge of the foramen magnum to the dorsum sellae; ICD = intercondylar distance (posterior edge); DHC = distance between the hypoglossal canals; SPI(TP) = diameter of the inferior petrosal sinuses at the level of the pharyngeal tubercle (right, left).

laterally with sharp instruments. During this phase heavy bleeding due to injury to the venous plexus of the vertebral artery may occur [12]. In our material this plexus was found 8 – 10 mm from the midline at the C 1 level. The pharyngeal tubercle (TP) is located 18.5 – 23 mm cranially from TAA and can be localized between the insertions of the longus capitis muscle. Since the TAA and the TP are frequently asymmetrical (3 of 4 cases in our material), the vertical line TAA/TP cannot be an orientation for the midline. This can be determined, however, by the midpoint of the distance between the atlanto-occipital joints [15]. The MAA (mean width 0.8 mm) is first incised cranially, 3 mm below the TP, then caudally at the edge of the anterior arch of the atlas. The bony window can be enlarged as required by drilling away the anterior edge of the foramen magnum or by removing the anterior arch of the atlas. This preparation exposes the dens axis with its ligaments. The frequent asymmetry of the dens (2 cases in our material) renders a preoperative frontal tomography of the cranio-cervical junction mandatory. A more extensive exploration of this level is possible only after removing the dens, which leads to problems of stability. After resection of the dens a tough layer of ligaments consisting of the ligg. transversum atlantis, cruciatum and membrana tectoria is exposed [12]. The different components of this layer cannot be separated from each other, with the exception of the transverse ligament. In order to increase the exposure upwards a bony window of 20 × 20 mm is cut above the TP. In this region the thickness of the clivus is variable (6 – 10 mm). After opening the dura in a Y-shaped manner, the subarachnoid space of the cranio-cervical junction becomes visible (fig. 2). For a short caudal extension, up to the middle of C 2, a partial C 2 spondylectomy is sufficient. Planning a deeper exploration, a discectomy C 2/C 3 with consecutive spondylectomy is recommended. The longitudinal ligament should be incised at the level of the intervertebral space, because here it is not adherent with the dura. The ventral dura is tough, its mean thickness being 0.3 mm at the C 2 level

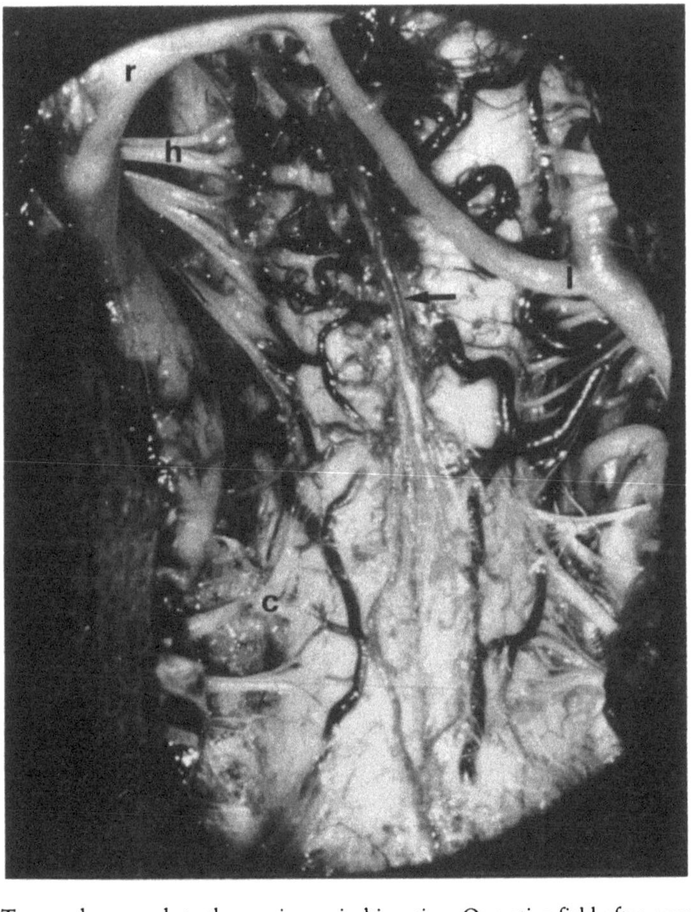

Fig. 2 Transoral approach to the cranio-cervical junction. Operative field after opening of the dura mater. r = right vertebral artery; l = left vertebral artery; h = XIth cranial nerve; c = ventral root of C 1; black arrow = anterior spinal artery.

and 0.5 at the foramen magnum. Venous epidural plexuses are normally observed, particularly at the cranio-cervical junction. In this area we regulary found tiny dural vessels with numerous anastomoses in the antero-lateral region. These branches are identical with the meningeal branches of the ascending pharyngeal and occipital arteries [7, 8, 10]. This pattern of vessels allows a dura incision in the midline without substantial blood loss.

The transcervical approach (TCA) is performed in the supine position with the neck hyperextended 10° and the head rotated 15° to the opposite side [10]. A further rotation or extension does not ease the preparation of the soft tissue of the neck and is unfavourable when retracting the muscle layer. Three different skin incision are possible (fig. 3).

The advantages of these variations can hardly be estimated when using fixed material. In our experience the L-shaped incision according to Lesoin [9] permits a more comfortable approach to the atlas in cases of a high located larynx. The superficial

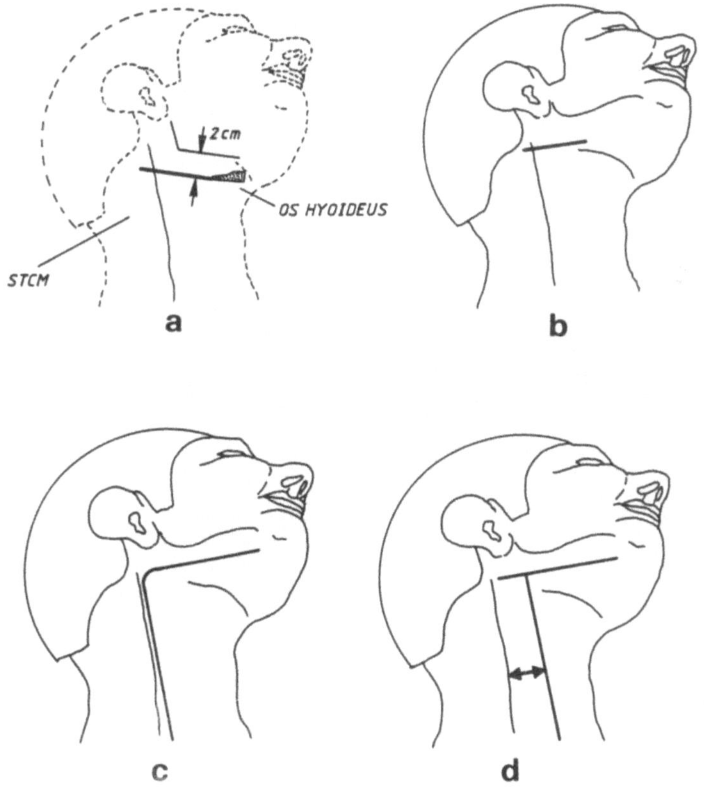

Fig. 3 Variants of skin incisions by the transcervical approach to the cranio-cervical junction. a = relationship of the horizontal incision to to the mandibula and hyoid bone. b = according to Seeger, c = according to Lesoin, d = according to Stevenson.

neck fascia is opened along the anterior border of the sternocleidomastoid muscle up to the level of the parotid gland. The inferior pole of the gland is slightly elevated in order to expose the posterior part of the digastric muscle without injury to the VIIth nerve (R. marginalis mandibulae). After lateral retraction of the sternocleidomastoid muscle the internal and external carotid arteries and the hypoglossal nerve become visible. The cranio-cervical junction can now be exposed using two different routes. The medial approach is performed in front of the big vessels. It requires ligation of the lingual, sometimes of the facial artery, retraction of the XIIth nerve and preparation of the stylopharyngeal muscle. The TAA is exposed below this muscle after a slight cranial retraction of the glossopharyngeal nerve (fig. 4).

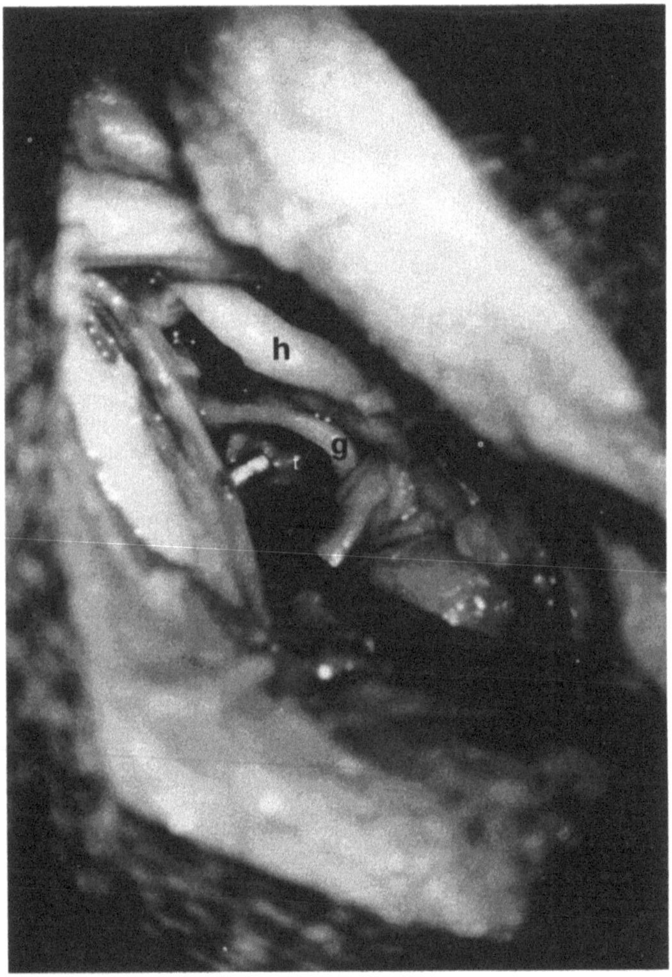

Fig. 4 Transcervical approach to the cranio-cervical junction. The anterior tubercle of the atlas is exposed after cranial retraction of the IXth cranial nerve. t = anterior tubercle of the atlas; g = IXth cranial nerve; h = XIIth cranial nerve.

Using the lateral approach a further retraction of the sternocleidomastoid muscle is necessary, while the Xth nerve and the internal jugular vein are exposed. The TAA is reached after medial retraction of the internal jugular vein up to the region of the upper cervical ganglion. The problems of both variants can be derived from the complex anatomical circumstances. Using the medial route the VIIth, IXth and Xth nerves become endangered. Moreover, according to the situs, 1–3 medial branches of the external carotid artery have to be sacrificied. In our material the facial, the lingual and the superior thyroid arteries had to be divided in two cases. Using the lateral approach, a venous congestion in the area of the internal jugular vein may become dangerous. With both variants the posterior pharyngeal wall can be injured by preparation to the opposite side. In one specimen we could show an unexpected connection with the prevertebral region after filling the oro-pharangeal space with water. An additional problem of the TCA poses the angle of exploration. The lateral region of the opposite side is hardly accessible without strong retraction. An increase of the exposure is possible only up to the region of the TP. Should a more cranial exploration be necessary, the difficulties will increase, depending on the higher level. According to our experience the limits of this approach should be at 15 mm above the TP (fig. 5).

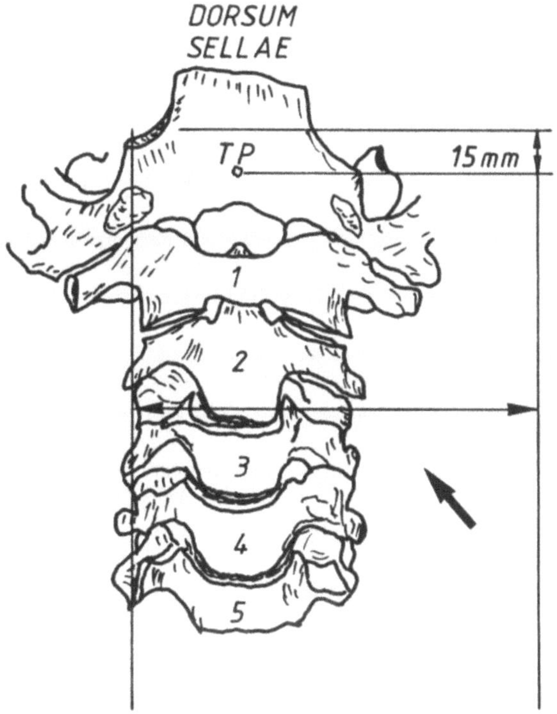

Fig. 5 Operative field by transcervical approach to the cranio-cervical junction. Upper limit: 15 mm above the pharyngeal tubercle. Lateral limit (opposite side): vertebral joints. TP = pharyngeal tubercle.

Conclusion

The transoral and the transcervical approaches permit a sufficient exploration of the cranio-cervical junction. The transoral approach is more direct, anatomically easier and presents a more comfortable angle of exploration. A cranial extension is possible up to the level of the dorsum sellae, the middle of the vertebral body C 3 being the caudal limit. The possibilities of exploration in the lateral areas are limited. This route is therefore specially indicated for midline processes with cranial extension.

The transcervical approach is anatomically difficult and presents an unfavourable angle of exploration. Furthermore the cranial extension and the lateral exploration to the opposite side are limited. On the other hand it permits an optimal preparation in the caudal and ipsilateral direction. This route is therefore specially indicated for ipsilateral processes with caudal extension.

References

[1] Delandsheer, J. M., J. P. Caron, M. Jomin: Voie trans-bucco-pharyngée et malformations de la charnière cervico-occipitale. Neurochirurgie **23** (1977) 276–281.

[2] Derome, P., J. P. Caron, M. Hurth: Indications de la voie trans-bucco-pharyngée et malformations de la charnière crânio-vertébrale. Neurochirurgie **23** (1977) 282–286.

[3] Fang, H. S. Y., G. B. Ong: Direct anterior approach to the upper cervical spine. J. Bone J. Surg. **44** a (1968) 1588–1604.

[4] Franke, J. P., J. Clarisse: Les bases anatomiques de l'abord trans-bucco-pharyngé du rachis cervical et du clivus. Neurochirurgie (Paris) **23** (1977) 250–258.

[5] Greitz, T., T. Lauren: Anterior meningeal branch of the vertebral artery. Acta Radiol. 7 (1968) 219–224.

[6] Jomin, M., J. M. Delandsheer, J. De Rougemont: Possibilités de la voie trans-bucco-pharyngée dans les lésions traumatiques ancienne des deux premières vertébres cervicales. Neurochirurgie **23** (1977) 271–275.

[7] Laujaunias, P., J. Moret: The ascending pharyngeal artery: normal and pathological radioanatomy. Neuroradiology **11** (1976) 77–82.

[8] Lazorthes, G., J. Poulhes, J. Gaubert: La dure mère de la charnière cranio-rachidienne. CR Ass. Anat. **78** (1954) 168–172.

[9] Lesoin, F., P. Pellerin, G. Lozes, et al.: Abord des lésions du clivus et du rachis cervical supérieur par voie intermaxillo-hyoidienne rétro-pharyngée. Neurochirurgie **31** (1985) 65–71.

[10] Manelfe, C., J. Roulleau, R. Combelles, et al.: La vascularisation de la dure mère du trou occipital. Neurochirurgie **17** (1971) 469–480.

[11] Mullan, S., R. Naunton, J. Hekmat-Panah, et al.: The use of an anterior approach to ventrally placed tumors in the foramen magnum et vertebral column. J. Neurosurg. **24** (1966) 536–543.

[12] Oliveira de, E., A. L. Rhoton, D. Peace: Microsurgical anatomy of the region of the foramen magnum. Surg. Neurol. **24** (1985) 293–352.

[13] Pech, A., M. Cannoni, J. Magnan, et al.: Les voies trans-orales en oto-neuro-chirurgie. Ann. Otolanygol. (Paris) **91** (1974) 281–292.

[14] Rougemont, J., M. De Abada, M. Barge: Les possibilités de la voie d'abord antérieure dans les lésions des trois premières vertébres cervicales. Neurochirurgie **12** (1966) 323–336.

[15] Seeger, W.: Microsurgery of the spinal cord and surrounding structures. Chapt 1, pp. 2–65. Springer, Wien–New York 1982.

[16] Stevenson, G. C., R. J. Stoney, R. K. Perkins, et al.: A transcervical transclival approach to the ventral surface of the brain stem for removal of a clivus chordoma. J. Neurosurg. **24** (1966) 544–551.

III Traumatic lesions

Double-threaded compression screws for osteosynthesis of acute fractures of the odontoid process

P. Knöringer

Introduction

Fractures of the odontoid process in most cases have been and continue to be treated conservatively. After closed reposition under image intensifier control with Crutchfield extension frame or halo ring, external immobilization is carried out with minerva plaster or halo vest. If the published results of conservative therapy are considered without taking into account the individual methods [4], it must be noted that stable bone healing of the injury did not occur in 32% (658 cases, 186 odontoid process pseudarthroses). Since the odontoid process pseudarthrosis is the only potentially fatal pseudarthrosis, it must be expected that about every third patient treated conservatively must undergo a stabilization

a

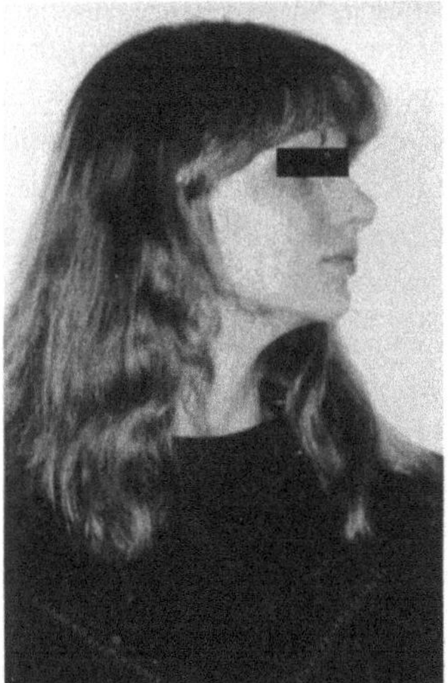

b

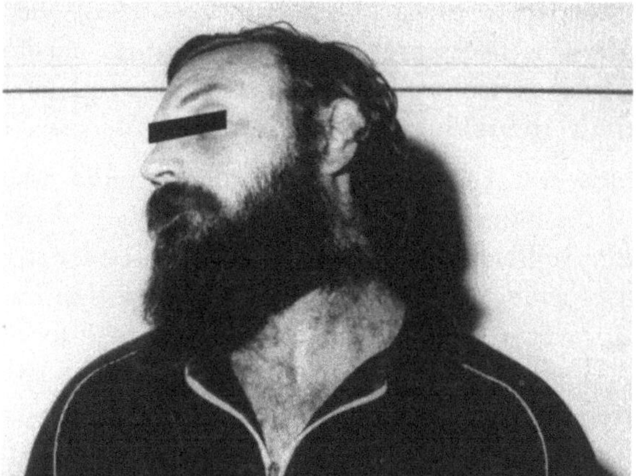

Fig. 1 a Condition after interarcuale spondylodesis C 1/2 from dorsal by cortico-spongious splints and plate osteosynthesis (Strehli plate). Due to elimination of the head rotation joint, marked restriction of rotation in glancing to the right. The rotation takes place in the joint C 2/3 – C 7/Th 1. The patient must carry out a dorsal flexion movement here in addition.

Fig. 1 b Condition after dens screwing two years after the operation. The rotatory movement is unrestricted and physiological.

operation. Jahna presents much better statistics of success with a pseudarthrosis rate of 8% (90 cases/7 pseudarthroses) in the largest number of individual cases. The publications stress that these results are achieved by consistent immobilization up to nine months [3].

In view of the relatively high rate of a pseudarthrosis following conservative treatment and the discomfort which must be accepted (in some circumstances over a long period of time) due to the immobilization of the injured neck with minerva plaster or halo vest, surgical alternatives to conservative therapy have been considered. During the dorsal (operation according to Brooks, Gallie, compression clamps, osteosynthesis with Strehli plate, transarticular screwing C 1/2) and lateral (atlanto-axial screw arthrodesis) fusion operations lead to restrictions of movement due to elimination of the head rotation joint (figs. 1 a and 1 b). The transoral operation must be reserved for special indications due to the raised danger of infection. However compression screw osteosynthesis of the axis from the anterolateral approach does not entail these disadvantages.

Method and material

Since 1982, we have been carrying out the odontoid screw fixation for treatment of acute fractures of the dens axis elaborated by Böhler [1, 2]. In the original method, two small-fragment spongiosa screws are used. At least one screw is intended to bring about compression of the fracture cleft whereas the second screw is necessary above all to attain a rotation-stable osteosynthesis. Böhler demands use of a disc washer to avoid penetration of the head of the screw into the vertebral body spongiosa (figs. 2 a – c).

However, these screws are not optimally adapted to the anatomical conditions of the injured vertebra. The thread part of these screws is relatively too long, so that individual threads may come to be located in the fracture cleft, thus causing a blocking action. The diameter of the screw thread is unfavourable (4.0 mm), since two screws have to be screwed into the odontoid process, which has a diameter of 8 to 12 mm. Too little reserve space remains and the screws project frequently through the lateral compact substance of the odontoid process. The screw heads almost regularly project so far downwards that they come into contact with C 3 in ventral flexion, and thus irritate the segment C 2/3 (fig. 2 c). This leads to bony reaction with osteophyt envelopment. Above all when working in a bent-over posture, a pain at the back of the head and neck can be felt. For these reason we omitted the disc washer in younger patients having a more solid compacta. Although we were able to obtain a stable bony healing of the injury, the disturbing action of the screw heads could not be eliminated (fig. 3).

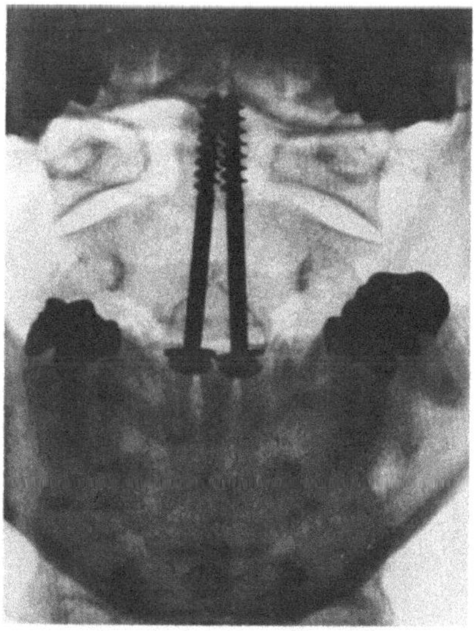

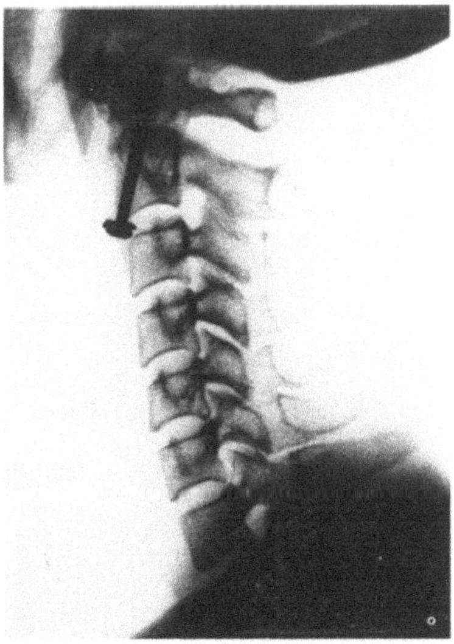

a b

Fig. 2 a Transoral X-ray after dens screwing for demonstration of the screw position.

Fig. 2 b Lateral middle section tomogram. The screws perforate the dorsal corticalis in the region of the dens tip. The disc underlays are intended to prevent impression of the screw heads into the spongiosa. Disc underlays and screw heads are situated caudal to the lower anterior axis region in the anterior upper region of C3.

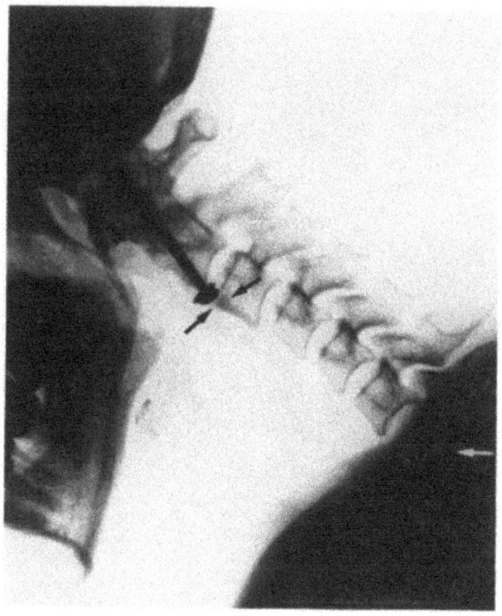

Fig. 2 c Functional X-ray one year after the operation. The screw heads lead to irritation in the anterior upper region C3 in ventral flexion. This is documented by the osteophytic apposition of the marginal edge (arrows). During and after forced holding of the head in ventral flexion, long-lasting headaches of the neck and the back of the head occur.

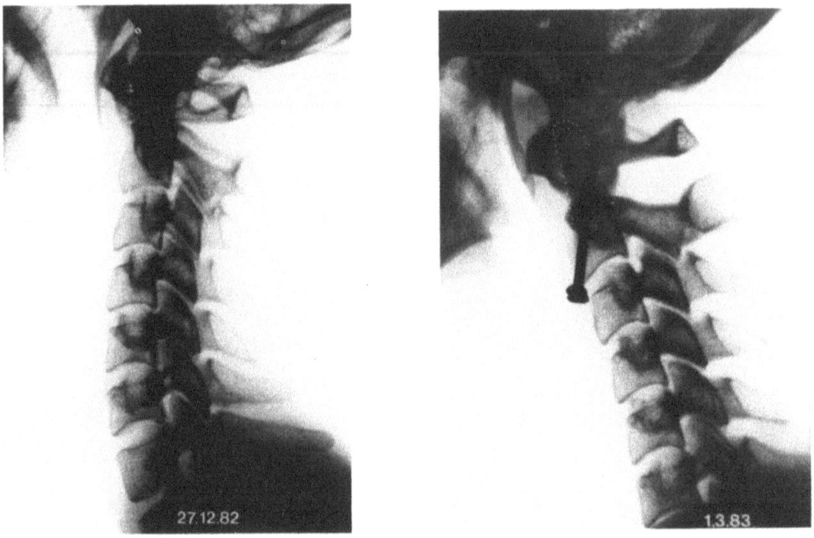

a b

Fig. 3 a Dens fracture with dislocation of the odontoid process to ventral. The fracture line runs horizontally.

Fig. 3 b Stable bony healing of the fracture in exact position. X-ray three months after operation. Two years after the operation: the screw heads have caused an irritation of the movement segment even without use of disc underlays. They are enveloped by osteophyte sheets.

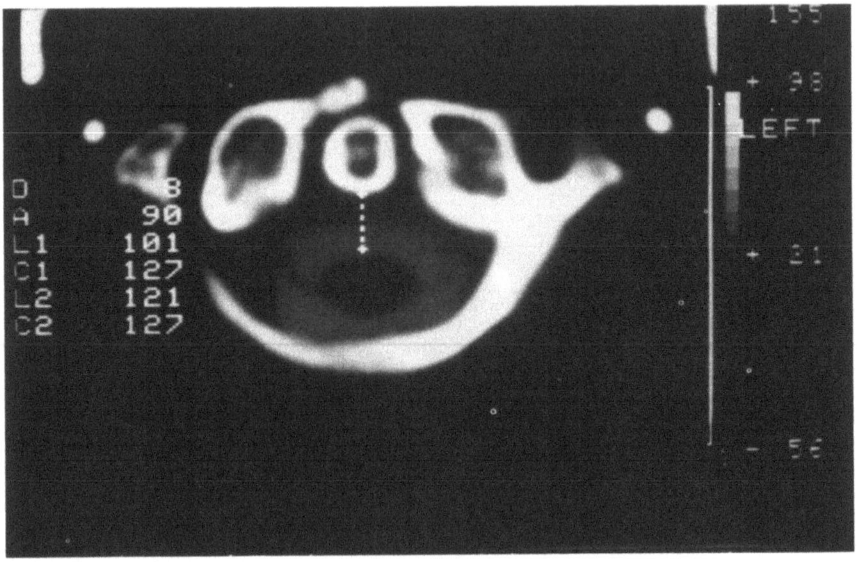

Fig. 4 Axial computer myelotomogram C 1 at the level of the odontoid process for demonstration of the spacial conditions. The distance of the dorsal corticalis of the dens axis from the dura is 4 mm, the distance of the dorsal dens axis corticalis to the spinal cord is 8 mm.

A further point requiring improvement are the commercially available Kirschner wires used. These have a tip which is too long and too sharp. Since the screws should grip the dorsal compacta, the compacta must be perforated with the Kirschner wire drills in predrill. The far too long and pointed Kirschner wires increase the danger of injury to the dura, to the vertebral and basal arteries and the medulla itself (figs. 4 and 5) forcing us to improve the instruments. In order to eliminate the irritating effect of the head of the screw, we have developed a screw with two terminal threads which are almost completely countersunk into the vertebra (fig. 6). The thread part at the anterior end of the screw is better adapted with regard to its diameter and length of the thread to the anatomical condition found in the most frequent fracture types than the usual spongiosa screw. The thread turns of the anterior part of the screw are steeper and are farther apart than on the posterior part. In tightening the screw, a compression is produced in the fracture cleft. The vertebral fragment gripped with the anterior screw thread must cover a greater distance than that associated with the posterior thread portion due to the arrangement of the threads.

The tip of the Kirschner drill wire which is too long and sharp was replaced by a chissel tip (fig. 5).

Fig. 5

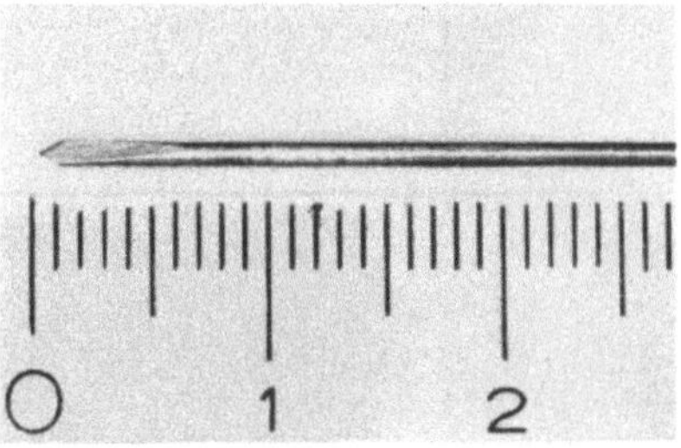

Fig. 6

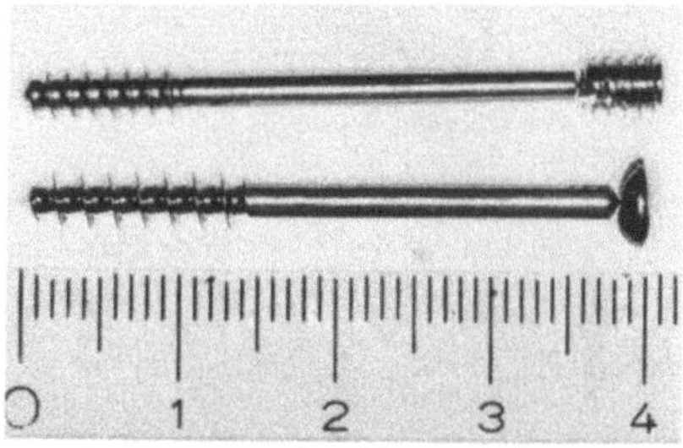

Fig. 5 Long sharp tip of a 1.8 mm Kirschner drill wire as compared to the chissle tip of a 1.2 mm drill wire for application of the double-threaded screw. Since the dorsal dens axis corticalis must be drilled through to screw the axis, there is a smaller danger of injury for the dura, spinal cord and vertebral artery in use of a chissle tip (spatula drill).

Fig. 6 On the left small fragment spongiosa screw, on the right double-threaded screw (length 40 mm in each case) for comparison of the nuclear and thread diameter and the length of the anterior part of the thread.

Surgical procedure

The preoperative diagnosis was made by scout X-rays (lateral and transoral) and axial computer tomography [1/2, 5]. The reposition is carried out with a Crutchfield extension frame modified according to Umbach (4 pins). The result is maintained by appropriate positioning and by extension on an average with

3.5 kg. The patient is orally intubated and strict attention is being paid to a location of the tube lateral to the middle (Fig. 6). Otherwise, the odontoid process is covered in the a. p. transillumination. The skin incision about 4 – 5 cm long, and runs in the tension lines in the region of the right side of the neck roughly at the level of the cricoid cartilage (C 5/6). This is important, as an exact procedure in the cleft spaces is possible without injuring important structures, and the level of the cutaneous incision exactly fits the later bore direction. The platysma is slit vertically. The cervical spine is reached at C 4/5 after looking for the upper edge of the omohyoid muscle as usual. From there, one proceeds retropharyngeally up to C 2/3 under control of the head light. By strict attention to this procedure, the submandibular space is not opened, so that the nerves and blood vessels (superior laryngeal nerve, hypoglossal nerve and the superior thyroid artery) passing through this space can be spared. If the level C 2/3 is reached and verified by lateral transillumination, two image intensifiers are placed in position. Under simultaneous transillumination in both planes, the fracture is bridged over with two bore wires which pass through the disc of C 2/3 at the anterior lower axis surface and just perforate the dorsal corticalis in the

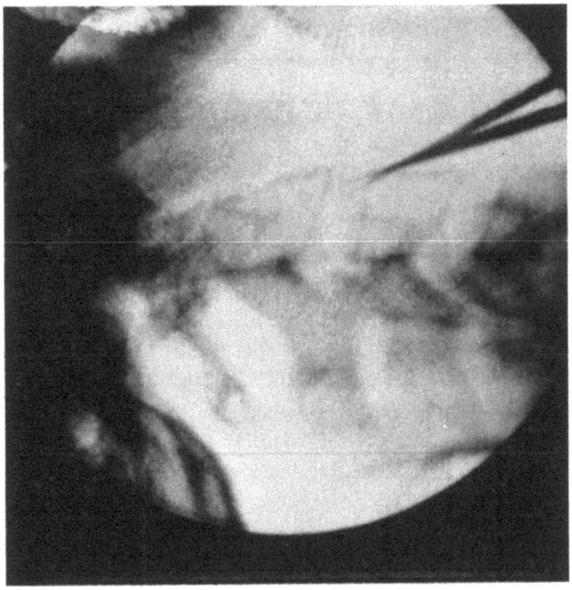

Fig. 7 X-ray negative retractor according to Knöringer for image converter-supported ventral operations on the upper cervical spine. In using a metal retractor, the entry point of the drill wires into the axis is made very much more difficult by the X-ray shadow of the retractor. Exact placing of the drill wires is rendered very much more difficult as well. When using the X-ray-negative retractor, free working is possible under image intensifier control.

region of the odontoid process tip. X-ray-negative retractors appreciably facilitate the operations supported by the image converter [6, 7] (fig. 7). Via the bore holes in postion, one predrills for the self-cutting wider posterior screw thread with a cannulated drill which has a depth stop. The predrilling by one of the wires in position for the anterior screw thread is likewise carried out with the cannulated instrument. After removal of this drill wire, the screw length is measured, the thread is cut for the anterior part of the screw and a suitably fitted screw is screwed in until it bridges over the fracture. The same process is carried out to introduce the second screw via the further drill wire. After ending the extension by unhinging the weights, the two screws are tightened (figs. 8, 9 a, b, 10 a, b). Afterwards, the stability can be checked under lateral transillumination. A prevertebral redondrainage is placed in position and the wound is closed by platysma and a subcutaneous and intracutaneous suture. Until the fracture has been firmly bridged by bone, we immobilize the neck for about six weeks with a plastic collar with chin support. This immobilization is indicated for the treatment of ligamentous instability at C 1/2, which is due to overstretching or rupture of the joint ligaments C 1/2 which is usually the case.

Results

From March 1982 to September 1985, 26 odontoid process fractures were treated surgically. Out of six dens pseudarthroses, four were stabilized from dorsal by interlaminar or interarcuale fusion with bone graft and Strehli plate, one by transarticular screwing C 1/2 and operation according to Brooks and a further case from ventral by plate osteosynthesis.

20 acute fractures were treated by compression screw osteosynthesis from the anterolateral approach in which the procedure according to Böhler was applied in eight cases and the method described by the author in 12 cases.

The oldest patient was 88 years old, the youngest patient 16 years old. Among these patients two deaths occured. One 71 year old patient who fell several times due to recurrent attacks of vertigo and who had contracted an odontoid process fracture died five days postoperatively from circulatory failure. An 81 year old patient (a doctor) was reanimated at the site of the accident successfully after odontoid process fracture with a high transverse lesion and respiratory paralysis, and regained full consciousness after reposition, chronic extension and artificial respiration. For the facilitation of nursing, the compression screw osteosynthesis was carried out. Postoperatively, the paraplegia syndrome transiently showed some sensory and motor improvement in the region of the proximal arms, whereas the respiratory paresis persisted. The tracheotomized and artificially ventilated colleague, who did not desire any continuation of the re-animation

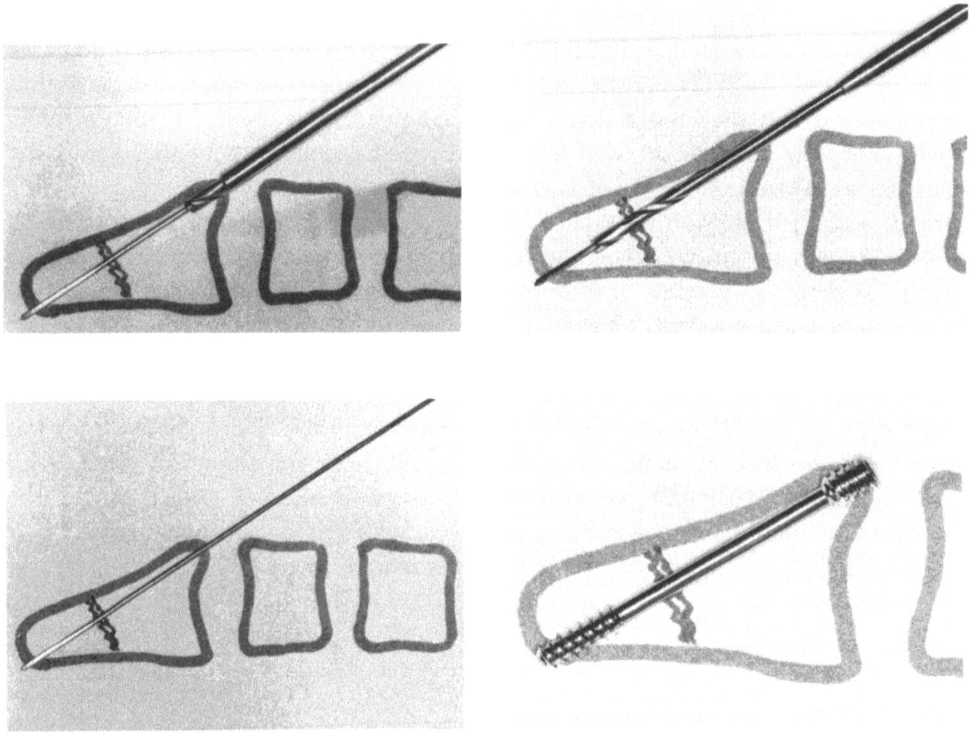

a c

b d

Fig. 8 a – d Schematic representation of the operation procedure for the application of a double-threaded screw.
a) The fracture is bridged by a drill wire which should just perforate the dorsal dens axis corticalis.
b) Via the bore wire in position, predrilling is carried out with the cannulated instrument with defined depth of penetration for the self-cutting posterior thread.
c) Predrilling is carried out via the bore wire in position with a thinner likewise cannulated drill for the anterior screw thread.
d) After removal of the drill wire, the screw length is measured, the anterior screw thread is cut and a matching two-threaded screw is screwed in which is almost completely countersunk into the vertebral body. The screw should penetrate the dorsal dens axis corticalis with 1 to 1.5 thread turns. The compression is brought about by the different parts of the thread. Since there are no screw heads, there is no irritation of the segment C 2/3.

measures, died 28 days after the operation, on the 32nd day after the accident. The remaining 18 injuries could be brought to stable healing without significant restriction of the mobility of the cervical spine, especially of the head rotation joint. However, the two latter cases cannot be finally evaluated as the period of follow-up observations is too short. Disorders of wound healing or other complications did not occur. Working patients could be reintegrated in their profession.

a b

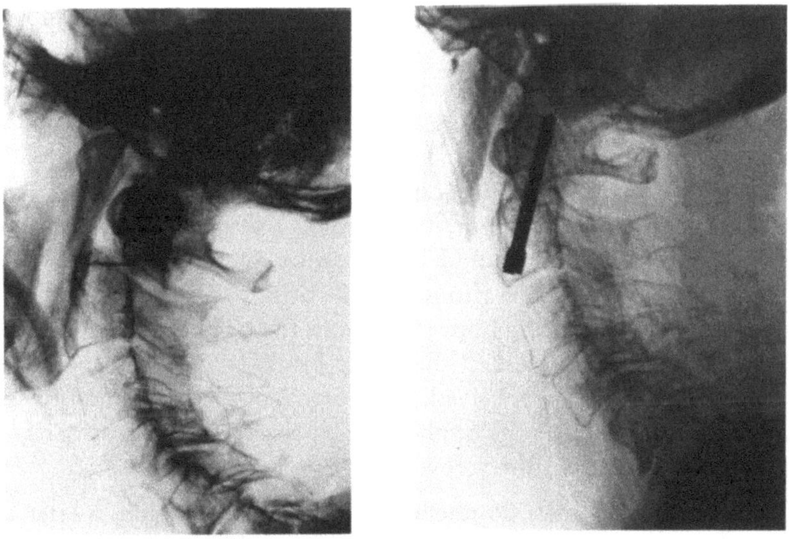

Fig. 9 a, b a) Odontoid process fracture with a dorsal displacement of the width of a vertebral body.
b) Condition after reposition and osteosynthesis with two double-thread compression screws. The anterior screw thread perforates the dens axis tip with 1.5 thread turns, the posterior is entirely countersunk in the vertebral body. An irriation of the moving segment C 2/3 is thus avoided and the fracture cleft is under compression and no longer visible.

b

a

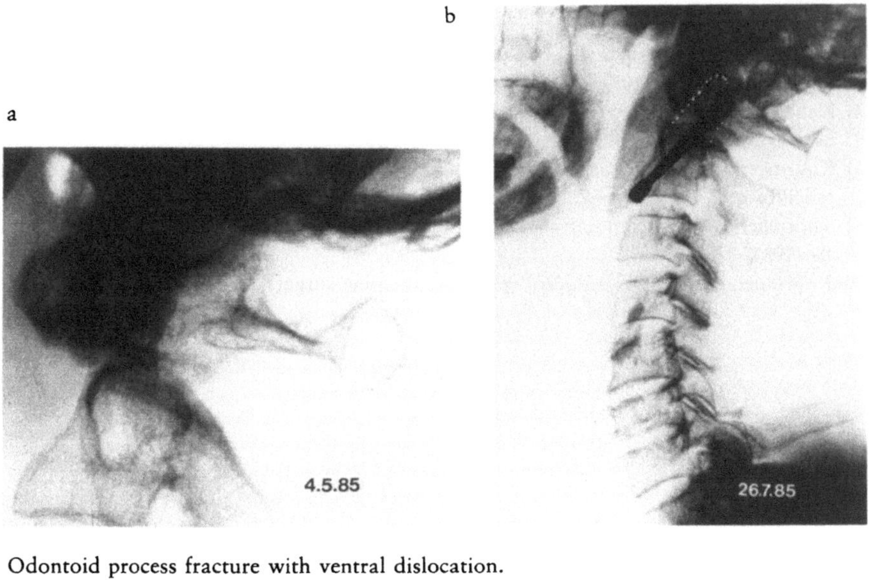

Fig. 10 a Odontoid process fracture with ventral dislocation.

Fig. 10 b Condition after reposition and osteosynthesis with double-threaded screws. Exact position of the fracture. The posterior screw threads are almost completely countersunk in the vertebral body. In ventral and dorsal flexion, the segment C 2/3 is not irritated.

Discussion and conclusion

Compression screw osteosynthesis of the axis in acute odontoid process fractures is a gentle and successful procedure. Among the surgical methods known at present, it is the method of choice in well trained hands since no functional disorders of the head rotation joint have to be accepted. Compared to the conservative method of treatment, it constitutes a safe procedure and the relatively small burden for the patient and the duration of his inability to work seems reasonable to bear. By alterations of the drill wires, on the application set (cannulated instruments) and above all due to the two-thread compression screw, in which the disturbing effect of the screw heads is lost, a further improvement of the technique could be achieved. At present, an experimental investigation is carried out to see whether the application of the screws can be safely simplified when the anterior part of the screw receives a self-cutting thread.

Since the implanted screws do not have an interfering action, a later removal of the metal is not necessary, and the patient can be definitively treated in one operation.

References

[1] Böhler, J.: Schraubenosteosynthese von Frakturen des Dens axis. Unfallheilkunde **84** (1981) 221–223.

[2] Böhler, J.: Anterior stabilization for acute fractures and non-unions of the dens. J. Bone Joint Surg. **64** A (1982) 18–27.

[3] Jahna, H.: Behandlung und Behandlungsergebnisse von 90 Densfrakturen und Luxationsfrakturen. H. Unfallheilkunde **108** (1971) 72–76.

[4] Knöringer, P.: Zur Behandlung frischer Frakturen des Dens axis durch Kompressionsschrauben-osteosynthese. Neurochirurgia 27 (1984) 68–72.

[5] Knöringer, P.: Diagnostischer Wert der Computertomographie bei spinalen Verletzungen. Unfallchirurg **88** (1985) 63–74.

[6] Knöringer, P.: Röntgennegative Retraktoren bei Osteosynthesen an der Wirbelsäule. Unfallchirurg **88** (1985) 373–376.

[7] Knöringer, P.: X-ray translucent retractors in spine surgery. J. Neurosurg. (in press).

Operative dorsal fusion in the region of the cranio-cervical junction after fracture of the odontoid process

A. Montazem

Introduction

A 17-year old male (fig. 1) was admitted to the Dept. of Accident Surgery with a traumatic dens fracture. An eight hour operation attempting to nail the odontoid process from ventral was unsuccessful, forcing us to carry out a dorsal fusion. It had become apparent intra-operatively that ligaments had been torn between the third and fourth cervical vertebra in the accident, rendering the fusion between the occipital bone up to and including C5 (fig. 2) necessary. After the operation, a halo ring with vest a was used for further immobilization. This external stabilization measure was removed after six weeks (fig. 3).

Fig. 1

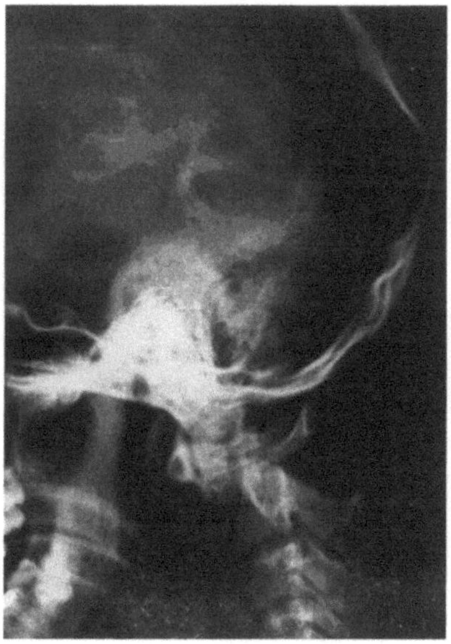

Fig. 2

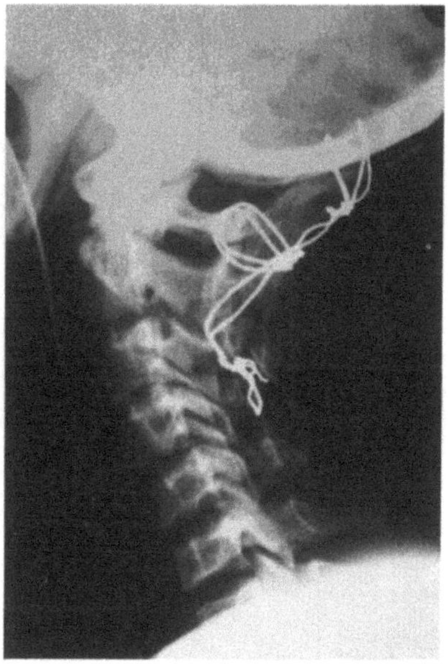

Fig. 1 Traumatic dens fracture with a 9 mm C1 – C2 dislocation.

Fig. 2 Reposition and fusion operation with bone graft and wiring between occiput and upper cervical vertebrae including C5.

After rehabilitation and a control examination after one year, we found very good ossification between the occipital bone and the upper cervical vertebrae including C 5 (fig. 4).

In X-rays the fusion area shows no pseudarthroses and head movements are carried out of necessity between C 5 and C 6.

Technique of operation [4, 7, 8, 9]

After exposure of the cranio-cervical transition area up to the necessary segment in the distal direction, a 0.6 mm thick wire was drawn through under the lamina on both sides. In the occiput, two boreholes were made on the right and on the left about one finger thickness apart beside the midline and wires drawn through these on the right and on the left. After roughening up of the entire bone area at the cranio-cervical transition up to the required level, bone was now removed from the iliac crest and modelled utilizing its natural curvature in such a way that it is wedged in the midline between the articular process of the desired

Fig. 3

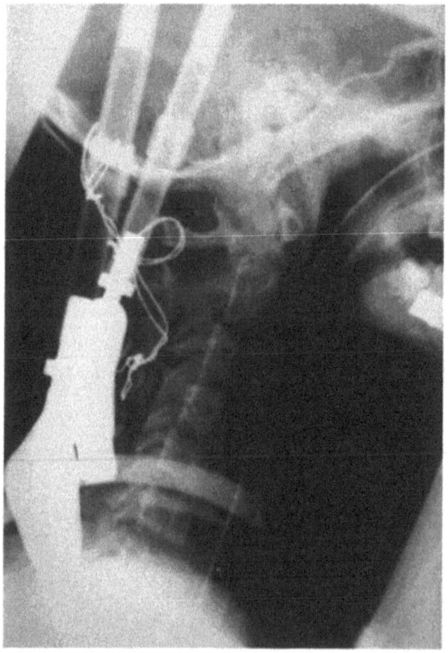

Fig. 4

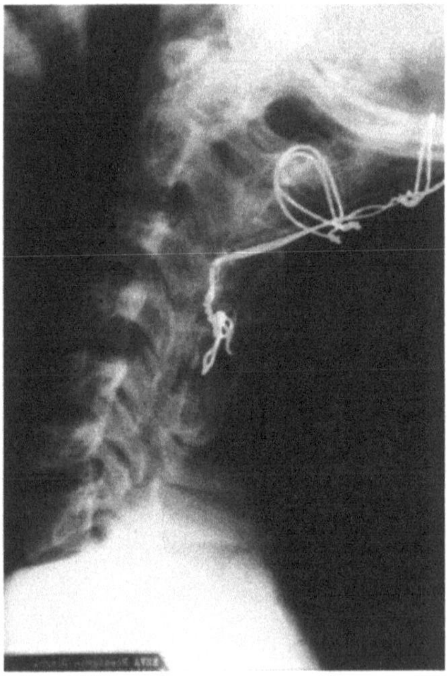

Fig. 3 After operation, a halo ring with vest was used for immobilisation.

Fig. 4 After one year: a very good ossification between The occipital bone and the upper cervical vertebrae including C 5.

segment and the occiput. The wiring over the interponate is now carried out both on the occiput and under C 1 so that this is fixed in a good position and in addition the C 1 arch is drawn up to this bone under image converter control until a satisfactory reposition of the displaced C 1 is attained. Further wires are likewise twisted and fixed over the bone interponate in the distal direction. Afterwards, the remaining gaps are filled with spongy bone which was taken at the same time from the iliac crest. This operation was carried out in the prone position and with a Codman support for the head. In the same anesthesia, the patient received a halo ring with a corresponding vest for complete immobilization for at least six weeks.

Discussion

In a dorsal fusion operation some severe, biomechanical alterations are caused which limit a nailing of the odontoid process from ventrally mainly in cases of dens axis fractures [3, 5, 10]. In cases in which multiple fractures are present in addition to the dens axis fracture with instability or if a primary nailing of the tooth of the axis from ventrally is not possible, a dorsal fusion operation is unavoidable [1, 2, 6].

The extent to which the fusion operation should be carried out further distally is determined by the relevant situation, especially the extent of simultaneous injuries to other vertebral bodies or to the postural apparatus are important considerations. Our case involved a fracture of the odontoid process which could not be nailed primarily from ventrally for technical reasons and in which a torn ligament at the level C 3/4 was revealed intra-operatively. For this reason, a fusion operation between the occipital bone was carried out up to and including C 5. By application of a halo ring and vest for six weeks, a sufficient immobilization was attained, and no formation of pseudarthroses occurred. After rehabilitation of the patient, he was followed up for one year. A native X-ray showed a solid ossification in the fused region, and head movements could be carried out at the level C 5/6 in the X-ray. In clinical testing, movement restriction of about 20% in all directions was present.

Summary

In fractures of the odontoid process, a primary nailing from ventrally should be aimed at. In individual cases in which the primary nailing from ventrally is not possible for technical reasons or due to a combination with other fractures of cervical vertebrae an instability has arisen, a dorsal fusion is indicated.

References

[1] Capen, D. A., M. D. Douglas, E. Garland, et al.: Surgical stabilization of the cervical spine. Clin. Orthop. **196** (1985) 229–237.

[2] Koop, S. E., M. D. St. Paul, R. B. Winter, et al.: The surgical treatment of instability of the upper part of the cervical spine in children and adolescents. J. Bone Joint Surg. **66 A** (1984) 403–411.

[3] Lee, P. C., S. Y. Chun, J. C. Y. Leong: Experience of posterior surgery in atlanto-axial instability. Spine **9** (1984) 231–239.

[4] Levine, A. M., C. C. Edwards: The management of traumatic spondylolisthesis of the axis. J. Bone Joint Surg. **67** (1985) 2–226.

[5] Lipson, S. J.: Cervical myelopathy and posterior atlanto-axial subluxation in patients with rheumatoid arthritis. J. Bone Joint Surg. **67 A** (1985) 593–597.

[6] Pepin, J. W., R. B. Bourne, R. J. Hawkins: Odontoid fractures, with special reference to the elderly patient. Clin. Orthop. **193** (1985) 178–182.

[7] Sadeghpour, E., H. R. Noer: Skull-C 2 fusion in rheumatoid patients with atlanto-axial subluxation. Orthopedics **4** (1981) 1369–1374.

[8] Trentz, O., P. Flory, V. Bühren: Verschiedene Techniken der occipito-cervicalen Fusion. Langenbeck Arch. Chirurg. **364** (1984) 347–350.

[9] Withe, A. A., M. M. Panjabi: The role of stabilization in the treatment of cervical spine injuries. Spine **9** (1984) 512–522.

[10] Whitehill, R., S. Reger, N. Weatherup: A biomechanical analysis of posterior cervical fusions using polymethylmethacrylate as an instantaneous fusion mass. Spine. **8** (1983) 368–372.

Operative treatment for traumatic arterio-venous fistulas of the vertebral artery

H. Friedrich, V. Seifert, H. Becker

Introduction

An arterio-venous fistula of the vertebral artery is uncommon and may be of either traumatic or congenital origin (tab. 1). Reviewing the literature most of the reported cases are caused by penetrating or blunt trauma to the head and/or cervical spine with consecutive injury of the vertebral artery [1, 3, 5, 23, 25]. Congenital or spontaneous occurrence of vertebral fistulas have been reported in very few cases [9, 10, 11, 15, 18, 20].

In this paper we present 3 relevant cases, their clinical picture (tab. 2), diagnostic procedures and operative treatment.

Table 1 Pathogenesis of traumatic arterio-venous vertebral fistula

1. Skull-base-fracture close to venous sinus
2. Hyperextension injury (whip lash) with interruption of intima and media of vertebral artery
3. Penetrating injury – traumatic (e.g. gun shot, stab wound) – iatrogenic (e.g. puncture of vertebral artery)

Case reports

Case 1: In October 1977 an 18 year old girl suffered a severe blunt trauma of the head and cervical spine with cerebral contusion and fracture of the pyramid of the right side with consecutive anosmia and persisting headache. In 1978 and 1980 she had two subarachnoid haemorrhages verified by lumbar puncture. Bilateral carotid angiography in an affiliated hospital did not reveal any arterio-venous malformation. Increasing tinnitus and an audible bruit behind the right ear led to vertebral angiography which demonstrated an arterio-venous fistula of the sigmoid sinus with the main feeders being the occipital artery and posterior auricular branches and muscular anastomoses from the vertebral artery (figs. 1 and 2). The basal dura was perforated by numerous dilated arterio-venous shunts

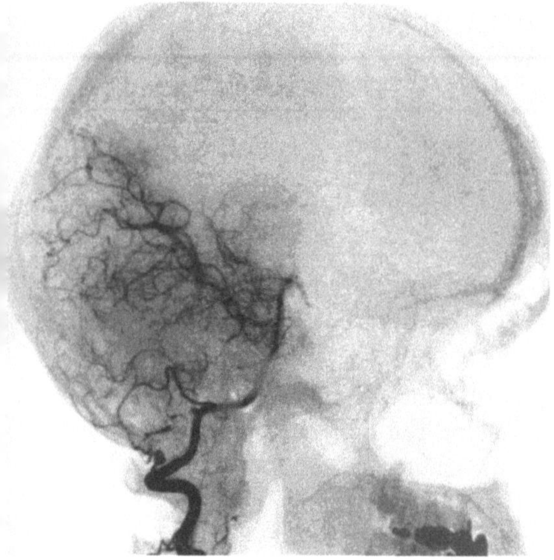

Fig. 1

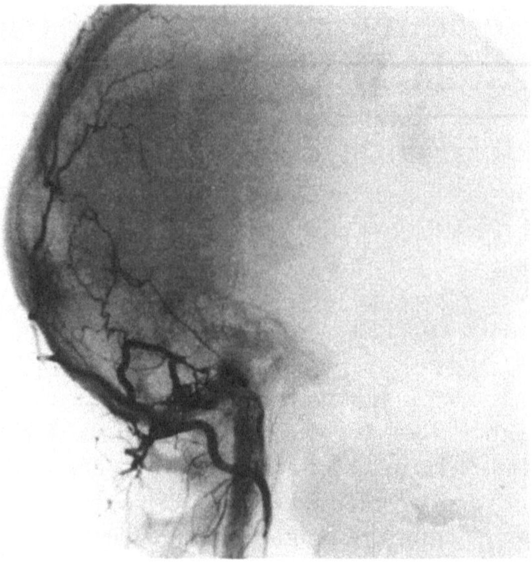

Fig. 2

Fig. 1, 2 Case 1: Pre-operative vertebral angiography.

reaching from the foramen magnum to the mastoid bone. Following a suboccipital craniotomy the angiomatous dilated vessels could be coagulated and occluded. The dura was excized and replaced by a dural graft. The postoperative course was uneventful. Angiography showed total obliteration of the fistulous vessels (fig. 3). The bruit had dissapeared. On examination three years later she was symptom-free and neurologically normal.

a b c

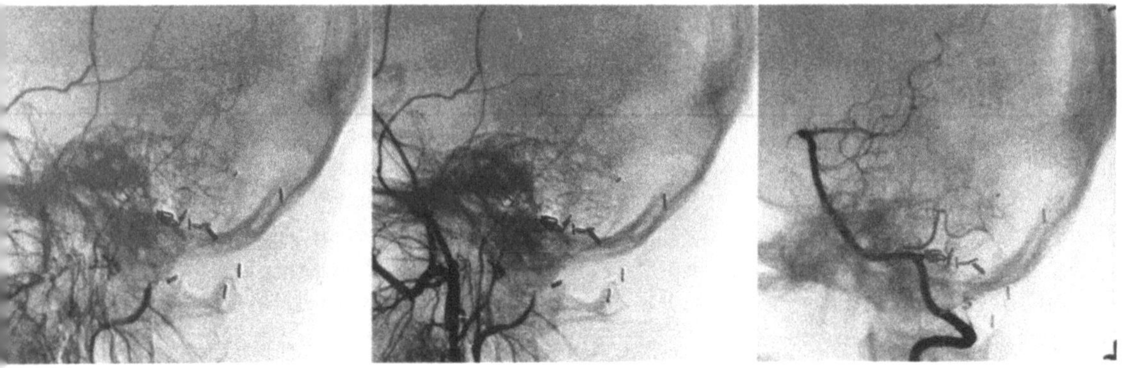

Fig. 3 Case 1: Post-operative vertebral angiography.

Case 2: In December 1983 this 64 year old woman suffered a whip lash injury of the cervical spine. From that time on she complained of increasing nuchal pain and occasional attacks of sudden unconsiousness. In June 1984 she noticed an audible bruit on the right occipital side of the head. On auscultation a machine-like murmur could be heard behind her right ear and in the upper neck. A digital subtraction angiography (DSA) performed in December 1984 revealed an arterio-venous fistula of the right vertebral artery (figs 4 and 5). Selective catheter angiography clearly demonstrated a fistula of the level of C 3 with communication of the vertebral artery and the vertebral venous plexus draining rapidly into deep paravertebral veins and into the internal jugular vein. Angiogra-

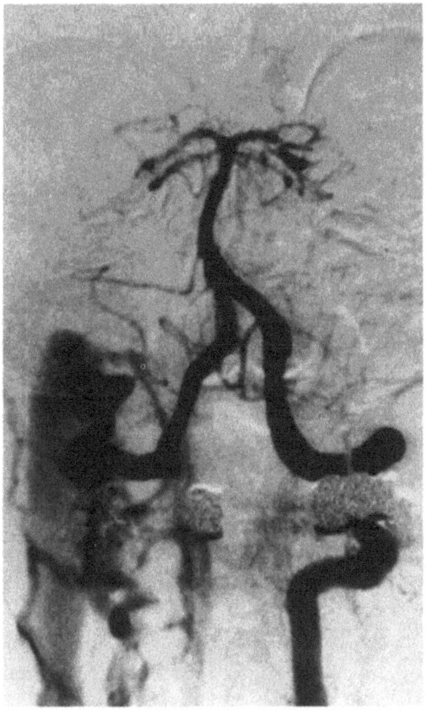

Fig. 4

Fig. 5

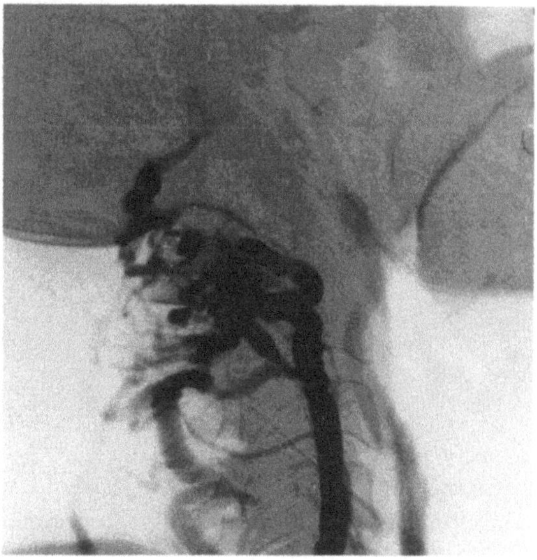

Fig. 4, 5 Case 2: Pre-operative digital subtraction angiography.

phy of the left vertebral artery showed a strong reflux with additional filling of the fistula and draining vein from that side with a considerable vertebro-vertebral steal effect. At operation a suboccipital craniotomy and a hemilaminectomy to the level of C 4 was performed. The vertebral artery was exposed at the C 2/3 level in the suboccipital region and intracranially. The vessel was occluded at the above mentioned levels with aneurysm clips and an additional embolisation of the artery within the occluded segments was performed using human fibrin glue. The patient's postoperative course was uneventful and no neurological deficits were present. The audible bruit had dissapeared and the patient remained symptom-free. Postoperative DSA showed complete obliteration of the arterio-venous fistulas (fig. 6).

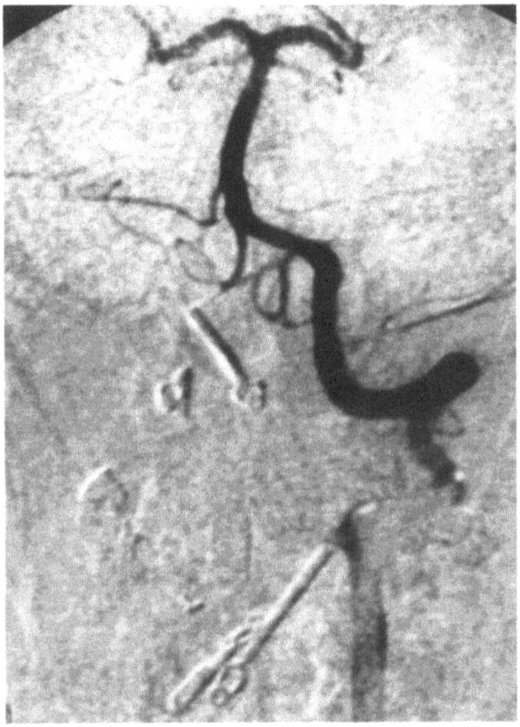

Fig. 6 Case 2: Post-operative digital subtraction angiography.

Case 3: In June 1984 this 62 year old woman had to undergo an exploratory abdominal operation. During the preoperative anesthesiological preparations an unsuccessful attempt was made to place an intravenous catheter in the left internal jugular vein. Postoperatively the patient complained about a swollen neck which lasted a couple of days. 4 weeks later she noticed an audible machinery type bruit which was localized behind the left ear and in the left side of the neck. From December 1984 on she developed an increasing number of transient ischaemic attacks with blurred vision and two events of sudden unconsiousness. A digital subtraction angiography revealed an arterio-venous fistula of the left vertebral artery. Selective vessel catheterization demonstrated a vertebral artery aneurysm at the C4 level and an arterio-venous fistula with filling of the venous complex around the vertebral artery and drainage into the deep para-vertebral veins and in the internal jugular vein (fig. 7). Using a ventro-lateral approach the

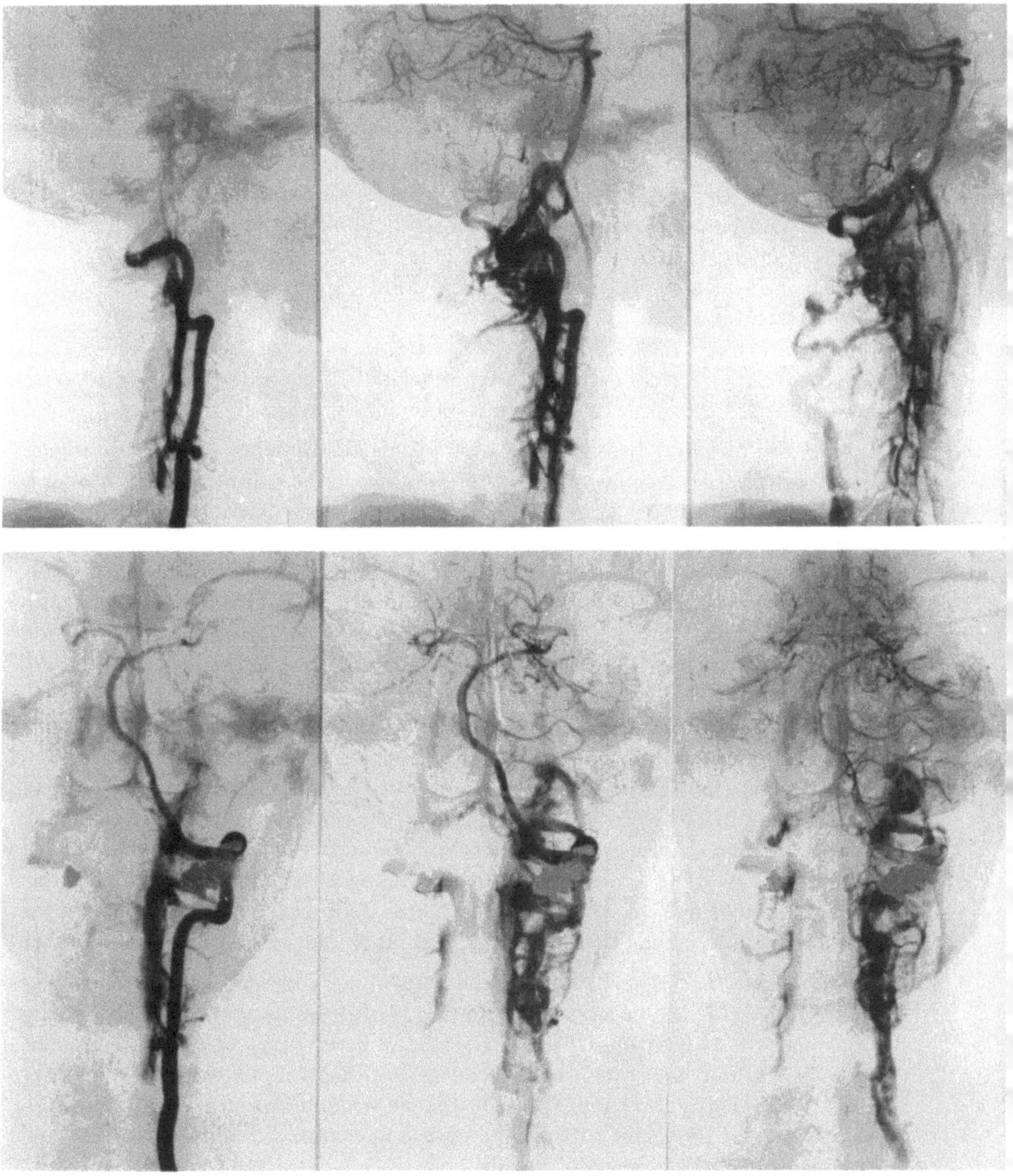

Fig. 7 Case 3: Pre-operative vertebral angiography.

region of the malformation at the C 3 to C 5 level was approached. The foramina transversaria of C 3 and C 4 were opened and the vertebral artery was dissected. After temporary occlusion of the vertebral artery the aneurysm was resected and the vascular wall was sutured. Thereafter the fistulous communications were occluded and divided. Although intraoperative Doppler flow examination had demonstrated good patency of the vertebral artery postoperative DSA showed occlusion of the vessel. Despite this fact the patient developed no neurological deficits and remained symptom-free on a follow-up examination.

Discussion

Arterio-venous vertebral fistulas may be classified according to their aetiology as traumatic, iatrogenic, spontaneous and congenital.

Traumatic vertebral fistulas have been reported following penetrating injuries from missiles or stab wounds or rarely after blunt trauma to the head and cervical spine [1, 3, 4, 5, 23, 25]. However, traumatic arterio-venous fistulas of the vertebral artery are thought to represent the rarest cases of all arterial injuries. Debrun [5] stressed the fact that not always a severe trauma is necessary to cause a vertebral fistula but that even very mild injury can induce the development of a fistula. Sudden [24] in 1962 was the first ro report an *iatrogenic* arterio-venous fistula following percutaneous vertebral angiography. Since then, a number of single cases have been reported throughout the literature [7, 12, 14, 16, 17]. Following the introduction of retrograde femoral catheterization by Seldinger [21] the risk of developing a postangiographic arterio-venous fistula has markedly decreased even if some cases remain unrecognized or unreported. Reviewing 11 000 femoral catheterizations Lang [13] in 1963 did not find any arterio-venous fistula as angiographic complications. Sudden and Pratt [25] in 1971 found only one single case of an arterio-venous fistula among 20 000 arteriograms of all types. To our knowledge no arterio-venous fistula following attempted percutanous catheterization of the internal jugular vein (as in our case 3) has been reported.

Spontaneous or *congenital* vertebral arterio-venous fistulas have only been reported on very rare occasions [9, 10, 11, 18, 20]. Some authors doubt the real incidence of these type of fistulas because in cases of so called "spontaneous" fistulas a minor injury months or years before the onset of symptoms may have been forgotten by the patient [5]. On the other hand obstetric injury during the direct pre- or postnatal period may escape detection although it is responsible for the so called "congenital" fistula.

There is a considerable variability concerning the time interval between the traumatic event and the onset of symptoms: it may range from a few days to several years because of the variety of clinical signs and symptoms. The difficulty of confirming the diagnosis of a vertebral arterio-venous fistula only by the clinical picture has been stressed by several authors [1, 3, 19, 25]. General symptoms are persisting headache mostly in the occipital and nuchal region, tinnitus in the affected ear, transient ischaemic attacks due to temporary vertebro-basilar insufficiency with vertigo, nausea, intermittent blurred vision, dysarthria and sometimes attacks of sudden unconsiousness (tab. 2). An almost always demonstrable symptom is the development of an audible machine-like bruit which can be demonstrated on auscultation. Normally plain X-rays of the skull and cervical spine, computerized tomography and carotid angiography do not reveal any abnormalities. The presence of an arterio-venous vertebral fistula can easily be demonstrated by the less invasive technique of digital subtraction angiography. Nevertheless a bilateral vertebral angiography is indispensible to clearly show the anatomical and pathological relationship of the vertebral artery and its surrounding fistulous vessels.

Table 2 Clinical symptoms of arterio-venous fistula of the vertebral artery

1. headache, occipital and nuchal pain
2. tinnitus
3. audible machine-like bruit
4. TIA's due to vertebro-basilar insufficiency
   - diplopia
   - blurred vision
   - nausea
   - vertigo
   - dysarthria
   - attacks of sudden unconcsiousness

The course of the vertebral artery can be divided into four anatomical segments (tab. 3) which can be affected by different traumatic mechanisms and which require different surgical approaches. *Segment 1* extends from the origin of the vertebral artery out of the subclavian artery to its entrance into the transverse foramen of C 6. Usually this segment can be reached using an anterior supraclavicular approach along the anterior border of the sternocleidomastoid muscle. If ligation of the vertebral artery is necessary, different forms of re-vascularisation of the vertebral artery may be used which have been described in detail elsewhere [6, 8, 22]. In the *2nd segment* the vessel runs in its bony canal from C 6 until it swings laterally to reach the arch of C 1. For the distal part of this segment also an anterior or antero-lateral approach may be used. The more proximal parts of segment 2 and the *segment 3* which extends from the level of C 1 to the entrance of the vertebral artery into the atlanto-occipital membrane should be approached according to the extension of the malformation by an anterior approach or by a submandibular-mastoid-suboccipital approach as described by Chou et al. [4] and modified by Senter et al. [22].

Table 3 Anatomic segments of the vertebral artery

Segment 1:	subclavian artery to level of C6
Segment 2:	transverse foramina of vertebrae C6 – C2
Segment 3:	arch of C1
Segment 4:	posterior fossa

Segment 4 which is situated in the posterior fossa is reached by a standard suboccipital retro-mastoid approach which should be extended far laterally. In most of the cases of arterio-venous fistulas of segment 2 and 3 the posterior fossa has to be opened in order to allow temporary occlusion of the vertebral artery proximal to the origin of the posterior inferior cerebellar artery.

Regardless of the location of the fistula it is of the utmost importance to expose the vertebral artery proximal and distal to the fistula in order to allow appropriate mobilisation and dissection of the artery and its surrounding fistulous vessels.

References

[1] Aronson, N. I.: Traumatic arteriovenous fistula of the vertebral vessels. Neurology **11** (1961) 817 – 823.

[2] Bergner, R., L. V. Andaya, R. B. Bauer: Vertebral artery bypass. Arch. Surg. **111** (1976) 976 – 979.

[3] Chou, S. N., L. A. French: Arteriovenous fistula of vertebral vessels in the neck. J. Neurosurg. **24** (1965) 77 – 80.

[4] Chou, S. H. N., J. L. Story, E. Seljeskog, et al.: Further experience with arteriovenous fistulas of the vertebral artery in the neck. Surgery **62** (1967) 779 – 788.

[5] Debrun, G.: Treatment of carotid cavernous and vertebral fistulas. In: Fein, J. M., Flamm, E. S. (eds.): Cerebrovascular surgery, pp. 1229 – 1257. Springer, Berlin – Heidelberg – New York 1985.

[6] Downing, E. F.: Surgical management of extracranial lesions of the vertebral artery. In: H. H. Schmidek, W. H. Sweet (eds.): Operative neurosurgical techniques, pp. 689 – 707. Grune and Stratton, New York 1983.

[7] Dutton, J., I. Isherwood: Iatrogenic vertebral arteriovenous fistula. Neurochirurgia **13** (1970) 49 – 60.

[8] Edwards, W. H., J. L. Mulherni: The surgical approach to significant stenosis of vertebral and subclavian arteries. Surgery **87** (1980) 20 – 28.

[9] Ehrlich, F. E., L. Carey, N. P. Kitrinos: Congenital arteriovenous fistula between the vertebral artery and vertebral vein. Case report. J. Neurosurg. **29** (1968) 629 – 630.

[10] Geraci, A. R., J. F. Upson, D. G. Greene: Congenital vertebral arteriovenous fistula. J. A. M. A. **210** (1969) 727 – 728.

[11] Goody, W., M. M. Scheckter: Spontaneous arterio-venous fistula of the vertebral artery. Br. J. Radiol. **33** (1960) 709 – 711.

[12] Jamieson, K. G.: Vertebral arterio-venous fistula caused by an angiography needle. Report of a case. J. Neurosurg. **23** (1965) 620 – 621.

[13] Lang, E. K.: A survey of the complications of percutaneous retrograde arteriography: Seldinger technique. Radiology **81** (1963) 257 – 263.

[14] Lester, J.: Arteriovenous fistula after percutaneous vertebral angiography. Acta radiol. Diag. **5** (1966) 337 – 340.

[15] Markham, J. W.: Spontaneous arterio-venous fistula of the vertebral artery and vein. J. Neurosurg. **31** (1969) 220 – 223.

[16] McDown, H. A.: Postarteriographic arteriovenous fistula of the cervical vertebral artery. South. Med. J. **64** (1971) 119 – 120.

[17] Newton, D. H., J. Darroch: Vertebral arteriovenous fistula complicating vertebral angiography. Acta radiol. Diag. **5** (1966) 428 – 440.

[18] Norman, J. A., K. W. Schmidt, J. B. Grow: Congenital arterio-venous fistula of the cervical vertebral vessels with heart failure in an infant. J. Pediat. **36** (1950) 598 – 604.

[19] Pritt, M. B., W. F. Chandler, G. W. Knidt: Vertebral artery disease: radiological evaluation, medical management and microsurgical treatment. Neurosurgery **9** (1981) 524 – 530.

[20] Robles, J.: Congenital arteriovenous malformation of the vertebral vessels in the neck. Case report. J. Neurosurg. **29** (1968) 206 – 208.

[21] Seldinger, S. I.: Catheter replacement of the needle in percutaneous angiography. A new technique. Acta radiol. **39** (1953) 368 – 376.

[22] Senter, H. J., S. M. Bittar, E. T. Long: Revascularization of the extracranial vertebral artery at any level without cross-clamping. J. Neurosurg. **62** (1985) 334 – 339.

[23] Shapiro, M., J. Polifrone: Traumatic vertebral arterio-venous fistula. J. Mt. Sinai Hosp. **36** (1969) 160 – 164.

[24] Sutton, D.: Angiography. Livingstone, Edinburgh 1962.

[25] Sutton, D., A. E. Pratt: Vertebral arterio-venous fistula. Clin. Radiol. **22** (1971) 289 – 295.

High quadriplegia combined with neurogenic respiratory insufficiency – Potentialities, limits and outlook

H. J. Gerner, P. Kluger, B. Meister

Respiratory insufficiency in paraplegia or quadriplegia can be caused by neurogenic loss of respiratory muscles, or by concomitant disturbances of pulmonary function [4, 9, 18].

When, depending on the level of a transverse lesion, a sudden failure of abdominal and intercostal muscles occurs, all symptoms of respiratory insufficiency may fully develop especially if obstructive or ventilatory disorders have been preexistent. We already have to expect primary dysfunctions at a level below D 6 and the problems increase with every higher spinal segments with C 4 the ultimate barrier is reached [12, 15, 22]. Since the origin of the phrenic nerves are the spinal segment C 3, 4 and 5, a functionally sufficient diaphragmatic respiration may be expected in cases of quadriplegia below C 4. Provided no severe pulmonary complications exist, an intubation should be avoided when the level lies below C 4, due to the high rate of future difficulties and complications during the transitional period between mechanical and spontaneous respiration. We also stress, that maintenance of articulation is of eminent importance during the early stage of spinal cord injury. In order to maintain spontaneous breathing, active breathing physiotherapy must start at once in regular day- and night rythm. In general, this can be guaranteed only in spinal cord injury centers or in hospitals with special units as the need for trained staff in great, this is an additional reason to insist upon immediate hospitalization in a specialized unit.

Respiratory insufficiency in transverse lesions between C 4 and D 6 is caused not so much by the reduction of minute volume, but by the incapability of expectoration. Inadequate expectoration leads to congestion in the respiratory tract, further restriction of ventilation leading to the development of atelectasis. Respiratory therapy has to achieve the following aims:

1. Conscious expectoration by supporting manual, rhythmical compression and decompression of the chest, in accordance with the patient's own efforts.
2. Support of patient's breathing during deep inspiration and expiration to compensate the neurogenic loss of intercostal muscles.
3. Stimulation of conscious diaphragmatic and auxiliary respiration (fig. 1).

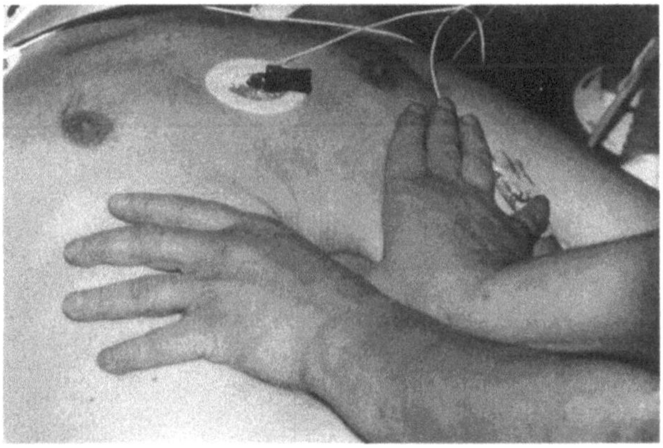

Fig. 1 Stimulation of respiration by stretching the diaphragm.

Further essential supportive treatments are humidifiers, secretolytic drugs, regular positional changes of the patient, standing training – even while in the intensive care ward, vibratory massage, manual percussion and the devices for augmentation of respiration dead-space. Other supportive apparatus such as Monoghan, Bird and other trigger machines (with C-PAP-respiration) too can help to avoid the intubation.

In the case of additional pulmonary disorders, of traumatic or non-traumatic nature, a temporary mechanical positive pressure breathing (PEEP) may be required. Indicative for this are the parameters of pulmonary function.

With sufficient physiotherapy the following limit values for an adult quadriplegia can be tolerated:

Tidal volume	> 300 ml
Vital capacity	> 800 ml
PO_2	> 60 mm Hg
PCO_2	< 60 mm Hg

We prefer nasotracheal intubation to the oral tube, because it simplifies oral hygiene, maintains the patient's verbal uttering by lip language and in most cases allows normal food intake over a time of prolonged mechanical respiration from two, at the most three weeks. Tracheotomy by quadriplegia below C 4 is the exception and is justified only by severe additional complications when artifical respiration for more than 14 days is to be expected. Weaning from the respirator by neurogenic respiratory insufficiency is exceedingly strenuous for the therapeutic team and weaning should start as early as possible, if no contraindications exist. The length of artificial respiration increases the difficulties of weaning, which must be done stepwise. The often troublesome procedure starts with first spontaneous breathing actions by which the patient (under controlled mechanical respiration) surmounts a trigger threshold by relative negative pressure or minimal inspiratory flow, so that the machine responds by an additional volume. A number of modern respirators offer further technical devices which intermittently support spontaneous breathing and facilitate the patient's inspiratory efforts.

At this stage medical date must be controlled frequently. Renal function as well as regular voiding of the bladder for reasons of neurogenic bladder dysfunction have to be observed. Regular defaecation is just as important, for flatulance and constipation may obstruct respiration considerably in this early and unstable stage. Whilst in hospital and at home when sufficient spontaneous breathing has been achieved, in order to improve pulmonary function, we use more and more breathing equipment – the so called C-PAP-breathing – so that there is a continuous positive airways pressure to minimize the tendency of alveolar collapse, the prevention of atelectasis, and to improve an maintain a better ventilation. To name a few: the Monoghan, Porta-Bird, and the Alveola II machines.

Up to September 1985, 46 quadriplegics with respiratory insufficiency had to be mechanically ventilated. Out of these patients 10 died, 3 suffered accompanying illnesses, 2 had cardiac problems, 1 a pulmonary embolism and another a massive tracheal hemorrhage, 3 had a severe pulmonary infection. Out of 36 patients 20 (80%) were able to be weaned from the ventilator. Special problems occur in paralyzed patient's with either a partial or total loss of diaphragmatic function, where a mechanical respiratory support must be calculated to be in use either for long periods, sometimes for ever.

Through modern emergency organization and rescue teams, sometimes also by helicopter transfer, it has been possible to admit a greater number of patients with total paralysis of the diaphragm to a medical unit.

The problems have been transfered from the place of accident into the clinic where some of these problems are thought to be insoluble.

The well-know problems occuring in high quadriplegia tend to multiply and are complicated by respiratory insufficiency. It is only through close teamwork between different medical disciplines that all the expectations can be met from the medical and non-medical staff. In 1982 we installed a respiratory unit with 5 beds for long term ventilation in high quadriplegia. This unit is run by the cooperation of the departments for anaesthesiology and intensive medicine at our spinal injuries center. These few beds are not thought to care for nursing-care to the end and under permanent artificial ventilation. These expensive wards are only justified when the outlook for the treatment such as the independance from the mechanical respirator and the ability to leave the intensive care ward are good. Without doubt, in specialiced centers under optimal conditions, many more paralyzed patients with a lesion above C4 can achieve spontaneous respiration than people presume nowadays. We have treated 22 quadriplegics with transverse lesions at C3/4 and above with neurogenic respiratory insufficiency, and have been able to achieve an independance from the mechanical ventilator in 11 of these patients.

Three possibilities have become apperent in weaning from the ventilator:
1. Spontaneous breathing with the auxiliary inspiratory muscles permanently.
2. Conscious breathing with the auxiliary inspiratory muscles for a few hours, and additional provision of transportable breathing appartus, which enables the discharge from hospital – also as a temporary compromise.
3. Diaphraghmatic pace-maker [17, 20].

A conscious breathing with cervical musculature is also possible when the lungs have not been damaged and the function of the accessory nerve remains.

The work of breathing is taken over by the auxiliary inspiratory muscles. They must be trained through intensive physiotherapy of each individual muscle group (fig. 2).

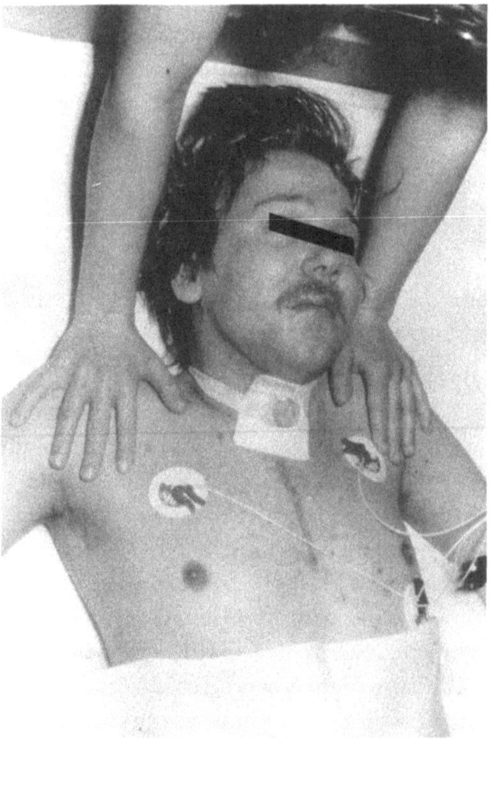

Fig. 2 Physiotherapy for strengthening the auxiliary muscles.

Available are the muscles in the neck, out of the upper cervical segments, especially in the region supplied by the accessory nerve, the hypoglossal muscles, an intact scalenus and above all the sternocleidomastoid.

They are able to elevate the chest, when at the same time the head and neck are fixed by the pre- and paravertebral muscles. The conscious use of the neck muscles can be trained, this training being supported and strenghtened at the same time through a tendency for the head to tip backwards.

Depending on the elasticity of the thorax and its own weight, it is found that the first conscious breaths are in the sitting position or lying down.

It is a long way from the first reaction, to inspiration by the patient for minutes, later hours, and can take a period of a year. This is a great strain both mentally and physically on the patients. If spontaneous breathing has been achieved over a period of hours, the quality of life is greatly improved. It is possible to insert an artifical larynx, and the patient will then be able to leave the intensive care ward in a chin-steered electrical wheelchair and is able to start occupational training at a mouth operated worktable. Sometimes cooperation fails in spite of good muscles, in young children and cranio-cerebral trauma cases.

During sleep problems arise because the auxiliary respiratory muscles are not stimulated from the respiratory center. The patient then "oversleeps" this breathing.

This problem can be solved by long training where a conscious and an unconscious arbitrary steered breathing is trained using the inspiratory muscles. Before reaching the stage where spontaneous respiration is achieved (also in the sleeping phase) and before removal of the tracheal cannula, we use an iron lung transitionally. In some cases it may be permanently necessary. In others a chest bell or "Kürass" may be sufficient.

The development in micro-electronics has opened a new possibility of functional stimulations of the diaphragmatic muscles through the phrenic nerve [1, 7, 10, 21]. Experiences of over 10 years has been gathered in the USA in the practical use of electronic stimulation of the phrenic nerves [2, 14, 16, 19]. This method demands that enough motory anterior horn cells must be left intact. Before the implantation of such a pacemaker a trial with a transcutaneous or open stimulus of the phrenic nerve is necessary. In the system used in the USA, both phrenic nerves and diaphragm halves were stimulated for 12 hours separately. After a time a certain amount of tiredness was noticed, which was traced back to the non-physiological stimulation of the nerve diameter through one electrode. A much improved pacemaker technique was developed by Thoma [20], Vienna, in which 4 electrodes are applied to each nerve, triggered by a processor and stimulated in constant rotation via a "carousel switch" [11]. The constant change in stimulation the different nerve sections allows for an extended recovery phase, and a possibility to stimulate the phrenic nerves spontaneously over a period of 24 hours. Two of our patients have been treated this way. In one of these patients data of the stimulations have been recorded for more than 2 years. This patient is now 23-year old and was discharged from hospital. He is only temporarily here for a check-up and to review the function of the system. In the spring of 1985 a subcutaneous re-implantation of the receiver was necessary and without problems. One disadvantage of this impressive technical possibility is its limited indication. A successful implantation of this method can only be promised when the anterior horn cells of the spinal column C3 – C5 are intact (fig. 3).

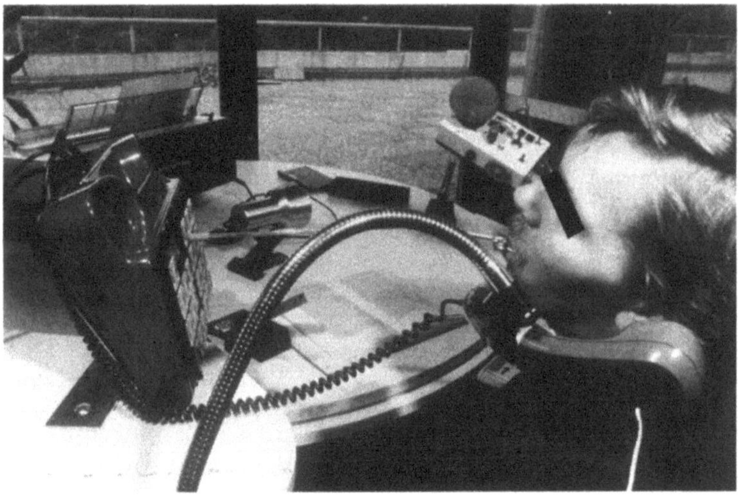

Fig. 3 Patient with electrophrenic respiration in OT.

In patients with insufficient functions of the auxiliary inspiratory muscles, and a phrenic nerve which cannot be stimulated, a temporary or permanent mechanical respiration is unavoidable [8, 13, 23]. Up to date this means in most cases a permanent stay in the intensive care ward, either in a spinal injuries centre or in another clinic.

Following Dutch experiences we are singularly trying to arrange a "home-care" unit for these patients, where it is possible to obtain a mechanical ventilation for overnight. Thus we see a possibility to free the paralysed patient from this dependancy on the hospital [3, 5, 6].

Summary

With this technique and at this time a very extensive and personnel-intensive therapy allows, patients with neurogenic failure after high spinal cord injuries, to survive longer than one expected.

We cannot foresee the expectation of life, and the quality of living in these high quadriplegic patients with a diaphragmatic paralysis. We, however, hold the point of view that these present methods of treatment have passed the experimental stage, and have given rise to improvement in the freedom and quality of life in those patients who are strongly attempting to maintain a normal life.

References

[1] Brancadoro, M., G. L. Guizzi, F. Ugolini: First experimental results on electrostimulated muscle energy output for total artificial heart. 1st Vienna Int. Work on Functional Electrostimulation. International Society for Artificial Organs 1983.

[2] Davis, J. N.: Phrenic Nerve conduction in man. Neurol. Neurosurg. Psych. **30** (1967) 420.

[3] Gerner, H. J., P. Kluger: Therapie et resultats du traitement de 82 tetraplégiques Reunion Euro-Mediterraneenne de la Paraplégie, Hyeres 1984.

[4] Gerner, H. J., P. Kluger: Ateminsuffizienz bei Querschnittlähmungen. In: Schirmer, M. (eds.): Querschnittlähmungen. Springer Verlag, Berlin – Heidelberg – New Xork – Tokio 1986.

[5] Gerner, H. J., M. Münz: Rollstuhlversorgung bei hoher Tetraplegie. Med.-Orthop.-Technik **101** (1981) 97 – 101.

[6] Gerner, H. J., D. W. Rauda, K. Witterstätter: Die soziale Situation von Querschnittgelähmten. Rehabilitation **18** (1979) 135 – 149.

[7] Glenn, W. W. L.: Diaphragm Pacing: Present status. Pace **1** (1978) 357 – 370.

[8] Glenn, W. W. L., J. F. Hogan, M. L. C. Phelps: Ventilatory support of the quadriplegic patient with respiratory paralysis by diaphragm pacing. Sur. Clin. N. A. **60** (1980) 1055 – 1078.

[9] Gürtner, Th.: Intensivmedizinische und anaesthesiologische Versorgung des frischverletzten Halsmark- und hoch-Brustmarkgelähmten. In: Die Rehabilitation traumatisch Querschnittgelähmter. Bibliomed **2** (1983) 37 – 64.

[10] Holle, J., E. Moritz, H. Thoma: Die Wirkung der Electrophrenic-Respiration auf den Lungen-Kreislauf. Anaesthesist **20** (1971) 102 – 106.

[11] Holle, J., E. Moritz, H. Thoma, et al.: Die Karusselstimulation, eine neue Methode zur elektrophrenischen Langzeitbeatmung. Wien. Klin. Wschr. **86** (1974) 23.

[12] Kelley, W. O.: Phrenic nerve paralysis, special consideration of the accessory phrenic nerve. F. Thoracic Surg. **19** (1950) 923.

[13] Mletzko, M.: Krankengymnastische Maßnahmen zur Normalisierung der alveolären Ventilation. In: R. H. Borst (ed.): Anästhesie und Intensivmedizin **3**. pp. 67 – 70 (1981).

[14] Moritz, E., J. Holle, H. Thoma, et al.: Further experiences with electrophrenic respiration. 1st Vienna Int. Work on Functional Electrostimulation. International Society for Artificial Organs (1983).

[15] Pernkopf, E.: Atlas der topographischen und angewandten Anatomie des Menschen. H. Ferner (ed.). Verlag Urban & Schwarzenberg, München, Berlin 1963.

[16] Sato, G., W. W. L. Glenn, W. G. Holcomb, et al.: Further experience with electrical stimulation of the phrenic nerve: electrically induced fatigue. Surg. **68** (1970) 817.

[17] Shaw, R. K., W. W. L. Glenn, J. F. Hogan, et al.: Electrophysiological evaluation of phrenic nerve function in candidates for diaphragm pacing. J. Neurosurg. **53** (1980) 345.

[18] Suter, P. M.: Übergang zur Spontanatmung nach Langzeitbeatmung. In: P. Lawin, M. Wendt: Aktuelle Probleme der Intensivbehandlung II, Intensivmedizin, Notfallmedizin, Anaesthesie 17 (1980) 174 – 180.

[19] Thoma, H.: Phrenicusstimulation. Jahrestagung der Deutschen Gesellschaft für Anaesthesiologie, Würzburg 1978.

[20] Thoma, H.: Vorrichtung zur örtlich und zeitlich variablen elektrischen Reizstrom-Langzeitstimulation eines Reizobjektes, wie Nerven und Muskeln. Österreichische Patentschrift Nr. 330342, 1970.

[21] Ugolini, F.: Multipolar non invasive electrode for partial, direct cyclic skeletal muscle nerve stimulation. 1st Vienna Int. Work. on Functional Electrostimulation. International Society for Artificial Organs, 1983.

[22] Waldeyer, A.: Anatomie des Menschen, Bd. II, 4. u. 5. Auflage. Verlag Walter de Gruyter, Berlin – New York 1967.

[23] Walter, W.: Intensivmedizin und Beatmungstechnik bei Querschnittlähmung. Manuskript zum Deutsch-Griechischen Symposium "Querschnittlähmung". Bad Wildungen, 6. 9. – 9. 9. 1984.

Occipital condyle fractures – Pathophysiology, clinical signs, and diagnosis

H.-G. Höllerhage, R. R. Renella, S. Hussein

Introduction

The occipital condyle fracture is one of the rarest fractures at all [15). Whereas fractures of the cervical spine in general and even fractures of the atlas and the odontoid process are routine cases in major neurosurgical and traumatological departments occipital condyle fractures occur only sporadically. This fact is also reflected by the literature. We found only 22 cases of which 14 are well documented regarding to the nature of accident and the clinical course. 4 of the 14 cases were necroptic findings. In 10 patients who survived the fracture was diagnosed radiologically. Guided by the literature and one personal observation the pathophysiology, clinical signs, and diagnostic procedures of this rare fracture are to be discussed.

Pathophysiology

The majority of occipital condyle fractures ocurred after motor-vehicle accidents and only two reporting other circumstances. The first description of Bell [3] reports the case of a young man who fell on his head. Kissinger [11] reports a fatal railway accident. We observed an occipital condyle fracture in an 18 year old man who rode against a wall with a motor-cycle. These different pathophysiological mechanisms can cause in an occipital condyle fracture.

1. an impact to the skull causes a linear fracture extending down to the occipital condyle. This mechanism was seen in one case [14].

2. a massive impact to the craniocervical junction causes a complete rupture of all ligaments except the atlanto-occipital membrane and the alar ligaments leading to an avulsion fracture of the attachment of the alar ligament to the occipital condyle. This mechanism was observed in 3 primarily fatal injuries [5, 11].

3. the most important mechanism, however, is the compression between the occipital condyle and the lateral mass of the atlas. This compression can be due to the transmission of force from the vertex through the occipital condyles to the vertebral column or to an extreme flexion of the head as will be outlined

below. Jefferson [10] gave an excellent explanation of the pathophysiology of atlas fractures which is helpful for the understanding of occipital condyle fractures, too: the net result of the compression between the occipital condyle and the atlas is a horizontal force because of the wedge-shaped figure of the lateral masses in the anterior-posterior view and the oblique articular facets. This force usually results in a lateral spread, a separation of the two lateral masses from each other and a consequent tension fracture of the atlas ring (Jefferson-fracture). It is on the other hand not impossible that the same force which in one case splits the lateral masses asunder in the other case leads to a fracture of the occipital condyle driving the fragment medially to the foramen magnum. Schliack [13] cites a case of bilateral hypoglossal nerve palsy in a man who had been struck upon the head by a falling object of 30 kg of weight. He presumes that this palsy was due to an occipital condyle fracture. However, such a fracture could not be proved in this case nor is there another case in the literature with such a pathophysiological mechanism. Whereas axial force to the vertex more likely leads to an atlas ring fracture there is evidence that compression between atlas and occiput due to extreme flexion of the head sometimes results in an occipital condyle fracture. This extreme flexion is in fact present in all reported cases in which the course of events is mentioned except the primarily fatal injuries with complete disruption of the ligamental junction of the head with the vertebral column [5, 11]. This flexion may come about by a sudden fall on the occiput like in Bell's case [3]. In all other cases it was due to a craniocervical whiplash injury. As Bucholz and Burkhead outlined in their analysis of atlanto-occipital dislocations on primarily fatal motor-vehicle accidents [5] the posterior atlanto-occipital membrane is not liable to be torn even by severe violence. This means that an extreme flexion of the head in the atlanto-occipital joint necessarily leads to a compression between the occipital condyles and the lateral masses as soon as the atlanto-occipital membrane is maximally strained. As the tension of the posterior atlanto-occipital membrane on the other hand prevents the lateral masses from drifting apart (in contrast to compression due to mere vertical force) a fracture of the occipital condyle with medial dislocation can occur. We suggest that this is the main pathophysiological mechanism at least in cases in which the patients survive the injury.

Clinical signs

The clinical course of 11 patients who survived the occipital condyle fracture including our own observation was analysed. In 7 patients [1, 2, 4, 9, 13, 14] the clinical presentation on admission was dominated by unconsciousness. In 3 cases [4, 14] there was even a severe head injury. Our patient was drowsy and had a multiple trauma. 2 patients [7, 12] who were conscious on admission complained

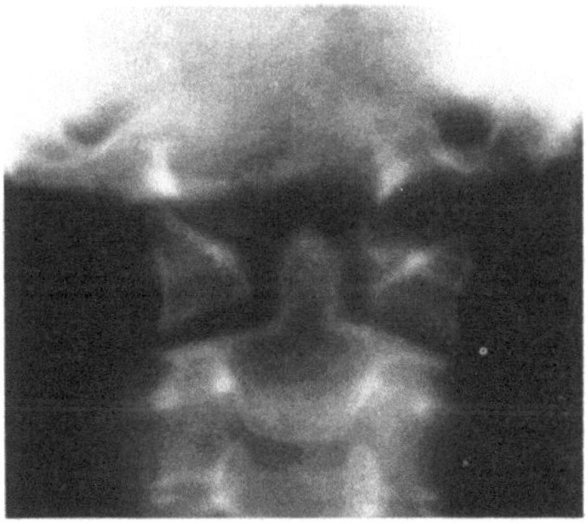

Fig. 1 Tomogram of the craniocervical junction in anterior-posterior view showing a right occipital condyle fracture in our patient.

of pain in the neck without any other clinical signs. Neck pain was present in other 5 patients including our patient after regaining of consciousness [2, 2, 6, 13]. 2 of the primarily unconscious patients [9, 14] did not show any clincical signs pointing to an injury of the craniovertebral junction. 4 patients including our case had cranial nerve palsies which were diagnosed, however, not before recovery of consciousness [4, 13]. There were 3 cases of multiple cranial nerve palsies [4, 13] including 1 case of bilateral [4] and 2 cases of ipsilateral [4, 13] involvement. We observed a palsy of the contralateral hypoglossal nerve. Including our patient we had 3 cases of hypoglossal nerve palsy [4, 13]. This means that it was rarer than it might have been expected because of the neighbourhood of the hypoglossal canal to the occipital condyle. Besides palsies of the abducens [2 cases; 4, 13], facial [1 case; 4]; glossopharyngeal [1 case; 4], vagus [2 cases; 4], and accessory nerves [1 case; 4] occurred.

Diagnosis

The diagnosis of the occipital condyle fracture is a radiological one. However, x-rays of the skull and the cervical spine in 2 planes as usually carried out at admission could in no case confirm and in only 1 case [9] point to an injury of the craniocervical junction. The anterior-posterior view with open mouth could in all cases in which when made point to the diagnosis [1, 12] or even confirm it [2]. The diagnosis could be proved by tomography (fig. 1) in all cases [1, 2, 4, 6, 7, 9, 13], in 1 case, however, not before the 2nd attempt [13]. The paramount diagnostic procedure is unequivocally the computed tomography (fig. 2). It gives the best impression of the fracture (fig. 3), the extent of dislocation, and thus the possibility of injury to neighbouring structures [4, 6, 8, 12, 14].

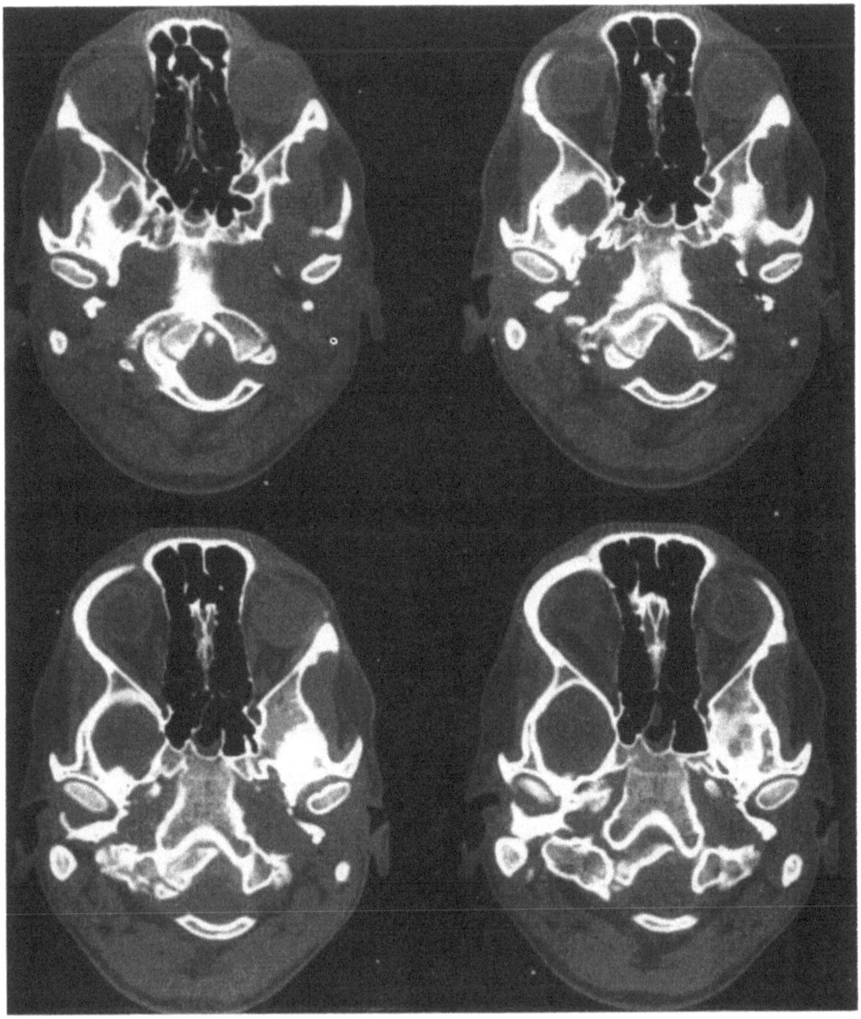

Fig. 2 The computed tomogram of the same patient showing the fracture and giving a good impression of the extent of the dislocation of the fragment.

Clinical course

All patients who had survived the initial injury recovered by simple immobilisation of the head without any or with only minor deficits. Our patient still shows a complete left hypoglossal nerve palsy (fig. 4) 2 years after the accident but feels only little disabled by it. This means that occipital condyle fractures have generally a rather good prognosis once the patient has survived the initial trauma. An exception is Bell's case [3]. His patient was already so well that he was to

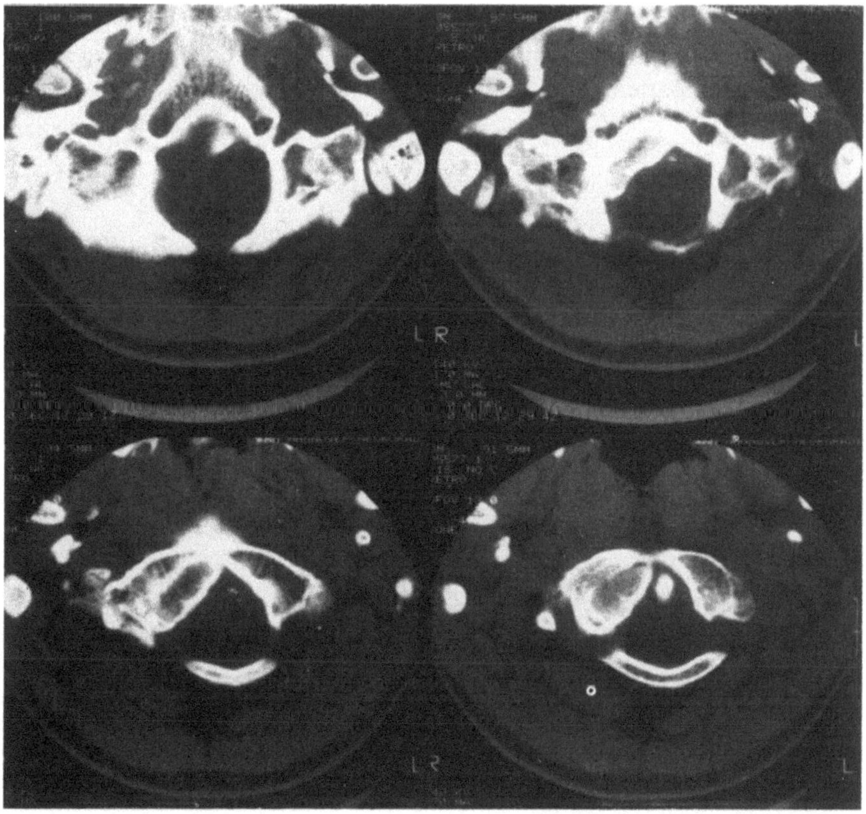

Fig. 3 The same fracture as in figures 1 and 2. The computed tomogram shows the consolidated fracture 2 years after the injury.

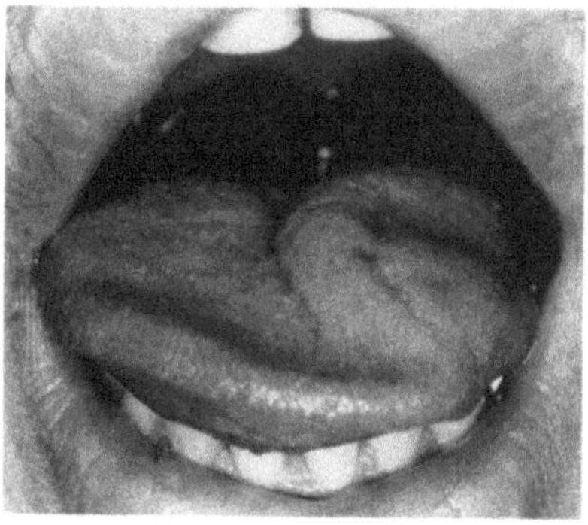

Fig. 4 Typical left hypoglossal nerve palsy observed in our patient.

be discharged when he suddenly died after rotation of his head. Of course Bell could not prove the diagnosis in 1817. His case shows, however, that it is important to the patient to diagnose the fracture, if there is one.

Conclusions

The main pathophysiological mechanism in occipital condyle fractures is the hyperflexion injury. The main clinical sign is neck pain. Cranial nerve deficits are less frequent. It is important to confirm the diagnosis radiologically in order to avoid sudden death by the dislocation of the fragment into the medulla oblongata. Therefore neck pain following "whiplash injury" should not be underestimated as only functional. In unconscious patients with adequate trauma the computed tomography should be extended to the craniocervical junction.

References

[1] Ahlgren, P., T. Mygind, B. Wilhjelm: Eine selten vorkommende Fractura Basis cranii. Fortschr. Röntgenstr. **97** (1962) 388–391.

[2] Ahlgren, P., J. V. Dahlerup: Fractura Condylus occipitalis. Ein neuer Fall von isolierter Fraktur. Fortschr. Röntgenstr. **101** (1964) 202–204.

[3] Bell, C.: Surgical observations. Middlesex Hospital J. **4** (1817) 469–470.

[4] Bolender, N., L. D. Cromwell, L. Wendling: Fracture of the occipital condyle. Am. J. Roentgenol. **131** (1978) 729–731.

[5] Bucholz, R. W., W. Z. Burkhead: The pathological anatomy of fatal atlanto-occipital dislocations. J. Bone Joint Surg. **61** (1979) 248–250.

[6] Camssa, N. W., C. Casavola, M. Castelli, et al.: Frattura del condilo occipitale. Radiol. Med. **69** (1983) 154–155.

[7] Goldstein, S. J., J. H. Woodring, A. B. Young: Occipital condyle fracture associated with cervical spine injury. Surg. Neurol. **17** (1982) 350–352.

[8] Handel, S. F., Y. Y. Lee: Computed tomography of spinal fractures. Radiol. Clin. North Am. **19** (1981) 69–89.

[9] Harding-Smith, J., P. K. MacIntosh, K. J. Sherbon: Fracture of the occipital condyle. A case report and review of the literature. J. Bone Joint Surg. **63** (1981) 1170–1171.

[10] Jefferson, G.: Fracture of the atlas vertebra. Brit. J. Surg. 7 (1920) 407–422.

[11] Kissinger, P.: Luxationsfraktur im Atlantooccipitalgelenke. Centralbl. Chir. **37** (1900) 933–934.

[12] Peeters, F., B. Verbeeten: Evaluation of occipital condyle fracture and atlantic fracture, two uncommon complications of cranio-vertebral trauma. Fortschr. Röntgenstr. **138** (1983) 631–633.

[13] Schliack, H., P. Schaefer: Hypoglossus- und Accessoriuslähmung bei einer Fraktur des Condylus occipitalis. Nervenarzt **36** (1965) 362–364.

[14] Spencer, J. A., J. W. Yeakley, H. H. Kaufman: Fracture of the occipital condyle. Neurosurgery **15** (1984) 101–103.

[15] Wackenheim, A.: Roentgen Diagnosis of the cranio-vertebral Region. Springer Verlag, Berlin–Heidelberg–New York 1974.

IV Malformations, system diseases and functional disturbances

A review and classification of malformations of the cranio-cervical region

H. P. Schmitt

The development of the central nervous system (CNS) and its osseous coverings are closely interrelated. Thus, malformations of one compartment are frequently accompanied by maldevelopment of the other and vice versa. However, in some complex malformation syndromes involving both the CNS and the cranium it may be difficult to decide which malformation was primary and which was secondary. In other cases, it seems obvious that both the CNS and the osseous structures must have been simultaneously affected by the teratogenic agents.

The changing interpretation of the pathogenesis of the Arnold-Chiari malformation may serve to illustrate the difficulty of establishing priority, brain or bone. The classical hypotheses emphasize various pathogenetic mechanisms of cerebral origin [2, 10, 12, 30, 31, 33, 42]. Others favour those of thc osscous compartment as primary causes of the syndrome since developmental abnormalities of the cranio-cervical structures are as a rule associated with the malformations of the hindbrain structures in the Arnold-Chiari syndrome. In addition, recent observations in animal experiments [37] seem to indicate that developmental defects in the formation of the posterior fossa may be the primary cause for the abnormal development of the related nervous structures in this syndrome, and will be discussed later.

Doran and Guthkelch [16] defined the "encephalo-cranial dysproportion" as a fundamental feature of well-known malformation syndromes of the infratentorial space. This also underscores the significance of the involvement of osseous malformations in the developmental defects of the CNS.

Contrary to the common usage, the developmental abnormalities of the osseous parts of the cranio-cervical region will accordingly serve as a systematic guide for the discussion of the malformations of the anatomically related brain structures in the following survey.

Malformations of the cranio-cervical bones and the related brain structures

The malformations of the cranio-cervical region subsumed under the term *"occipital dysplasia"* [45] may be best understood by considering the complex development of the posterior fossa and the adjacent parts of the spinal column. The posterior skull base is phylogenetically derived from the primordial chondrocranium. The latter is probably formed from of the anlage of primordial vertebrae by the process of somite reduction, which is repeated in ontogenesis (Goethe's *vertebral theory* of skull base development). From this theory (pp. 6–8 of this volume) it becomes clear that overshoot somite reduction should result either in an abnormal fusion of single cervical vertebrae with each other or with the occiput (atlanto-occipital fusion, atlanto-axial fusion etc.), or, in severe cases, in the total absence of cervical vertebrae or of the entire cervical spine (e.g. iniencephaly, Klippel-Feil syndrome).

Up to the fossa hypophyseos, the posterior skull base corresponds to the chordal part of the cranial anlage while the anterior part is derived from the prechordal plate. The rostral part of the posterior skull base is formed by the basio-occipitale, while its lateral parts comprise the paired exoccipitalia and its posterior part is formed by the chondral supraoccipitale. The latter fuses with the desmal interparietale to form the occiput. In rare instances, the supraoccipitale and the interparietale may remain separated throughout life by a persistent *sutura mendosa* [cf. 46]. The four chondral bones mentioned embrace the foramen occipitale magnum and are connected with each other and with the sphenoidal bone by synchondroses. These normally ossify in early childhood or in the case of the synchondrosis spheno-occipitalis (tribasilaris) as early as at the end of the second decade.

Premature closure of these synchondroses will cause disturbances of the formation of the posterior fossa and may be regarded as one important, if not the most common cause of a hypoplastic posterior fossa with narrowing of the foramen magnum. In particular, the "tribasilar synostosis", for example, has already been considered by Virchow as the basic mechanism responsible for the dysproportionate development of the posterior skull base in achondroplastic cretinism. Premature synostosis of the sphenoidal synchondroses causes shortening of the skull base. The most severe type of malformation in this context is the *"cloverleaf skull"* which occurs in achondroplasia or thanatophoric dwarfism [27]. The basic defect in this syndrome is a severe maldevelopment of the posterior skull base and narrowing of the foramen magnum due to premature synostosis of the basal synchondroses. The other striking abnormalities of the skull shape in the cloverleaf syndrome are likely to be secondary to the disturbance of the skull base formation. It is easy to imagine that developmental defects of osseous structures which cause a narrowing of the posterior fossa and the foramen magnum will have a significant influence on the development of the infratentorial brain structures and on the intracranial pressure conditions, since they interfere directly with an important junction of the CSF pathways.

A systematic survey of the most important osseous malformations of the cranio-cervical region and the related brain structures is presented in table 1.

Table 1 Malformations of the cranio-cervical region

I. Osseous compartment and related CNS structures
- A) Occipital bone
  - 1. Occipital Hypoplasia
    - a) proportionate o. h.
      special form: *Platybasia*
    - b) dysproportionate o. h.
      (with osseous dysoplasia, e. g.:
      Cloverleaf Skull)
      special form: *Basilar Impression*
      - anterior type
      - lateral type
      - posterior type
      - classical type
      [cf. 26, 45]

      related CNS: *Chiari Type 1*
      Chiari Type 2
      "Inverse Chiari Type 2"
      (cf. 47)
  - 2. Cranio-spinal Dysraphism
    Cranioschisis occipitalis
    related CNS: *Occipital Encephalocele*
    "Inverse Cerebellum" [cf. 41]
- B) Cervical Spine
  - 1. *Atlanto-Occipital Fusion*
  - 2. *Manifestation of Occipital Vertebra*
  - 3. *Hypo- and Aplasia of Cervical Vertebrae*
    (e. g. Klippel-Feil Syndrome)
  - 4. *Vertebral Fusion*
  - 5. *Spinal Dysraphism*
    Defective arch of Atlas
    Rachischisis cervicalis dorsalis
    - ventralis
    - lateralis

    related CNS: *Cervical Meningomyelocele*
- C) Combinations of A and B
  - 1. *Basilar Impression* with *Platybasia*
  - 2. *Basilar Impression* with *Atlanto-Occipital Fusion*
    related CNS:
    Basilar Impression with *Hydrosyringomyelia*

continuous page 170

3. *Cranio-Rachischisis occipito-cervicalis*
   related CNS: *Suboccipital Encephalocele*
   Chiari Type 3
   (with associated anomalies of cervical vertebrae:)
   Iniencephaly
4. *Cranio-rachischisis totalis*
   related CNS: *Platyneuria* or
   Aneuria
   Anencephaly
   (with defective cervical spine:)
   Iniencephalic Anencephaly

II. Infratentorial Brain Structures with Secondary Changes of the Posterior Fossa
1. *Dandy-Walker Syndrome*
   (enlargement of posterior fossa)
2. *Cerebellar Hypoplasia and Agenesis*
   (hypoplastic posterior fossa)
   - *paleocerebellar (vermal) A.*
     - sporadic
     - familial: *Joubert Syndrome* [cf. 22]
   - *neocerebellar (hemispheric) A.*
   - *complete A.*
3. *Rhombencephalosynapsis* [cf. 40]

Many of the classical malformation syndromes of the hindbrain and less well-known ones are as a rule accompanied by a mostly proportionate *hypoplasia of the posterior fossa*. Therefore, this will not be stressed separately with the delineation of each of these syndromes in the following. The designation "encephalo-cranial dysproportion" [16] mentioned above characterizes this situation.

In addition to hypoplasia of the posterior fossa, further osseous malformations or abnormalities, such as listed in table 1 B are frequently associated with cerebral malformations.

Apart from premature ossification of the synchondroses proportionate hypoplasia of the posterior fossa may be also due to primary disturbances of bone formation (e.g. osteoblastic insufficiency) and to "chondral" as well as "vascular" factors [27].

A special form of hypoplasia of the posterior fossa occurs in the *platybasia* [15, 45, 57]. The latter is characterized by a flattened kyphosis of the skull base with an elevation of the floor of the posterior fossa. This results in a narrowing of the infratentorial space (fig. 1). The average value of Welcker's sphenoidal angle of the skull base is normally 134° in Caucasian males and 138° in females. In platybasia, the angle may be increased up to 180°, the plane of the clivus being in a horizontal position, while the plane of the foramen magnum remains unaltered in mere platybasia (fig. 1 C, D).

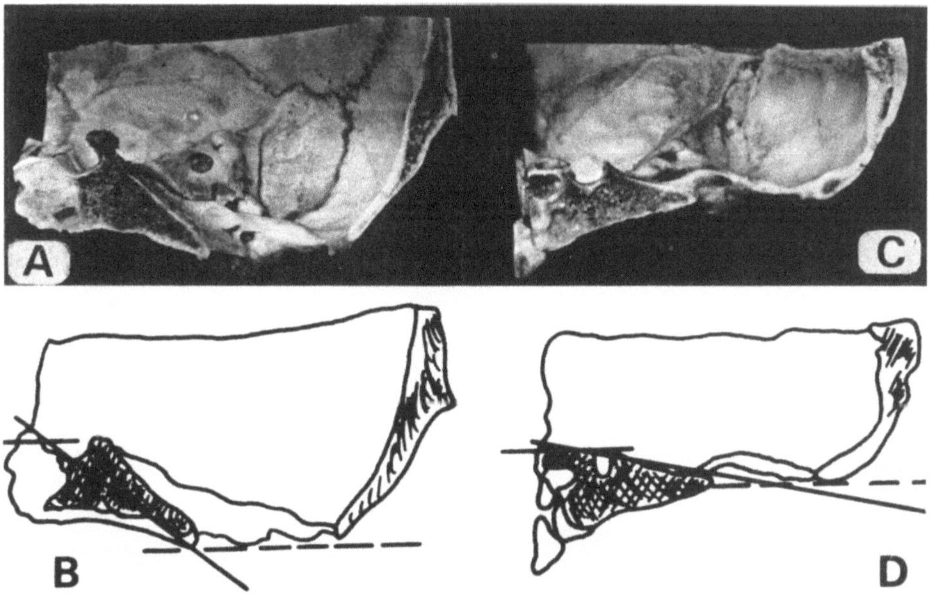

Fig. 1 Platybasia. A, B: Median-sagittal section of a normal skull base with a regular sphenoid angle. B, C: Median-sagittal section of a skull base in platybasia showing an enlarged sphenoid angle with an elevation of the clivus.

Although mere platybasia has only slight clinical significance, the associated narrowing of the posterior fossa may result in an infratentorial encephalo-cranial dysproportion. This may turn out to be an additional unfortunate genetic factor stigma when acute space occupation occurs in the posterior fossa [51].

Basilar impression (BI) [15, 20, 26, 45, 57], which should not be confused with platybasia (although it is often combined with a flattening of the skull base angle) is characterized by a funnelshaped impression of the floor of the posterior fossa with an alteration of the plane of the foramen magnum. The latter may be found in an inclined or even perpendicular position. In the "classic form" of BI [26], the impression is symmetrical while in other variations of the BI spectrum either the anterior, the lateral or the posterior circumference of the foramen magnum may be involved asymmetrically. The most typical radiologic feature of BI is an elevated position of the dens epistropheus which appears in the plane of the foramen magnum or may even project beyond it (fig. 2 A, B). This results in a narrowing of the foramen often leaving only little space for the passage of the cervical spinal cord. In the observation delineated in figure 2, the latter was reduced to the caliber of a knitting-needle at its transition to the medulla oblongata. Nevertheless, throughout his life the patient had exhibited very few clinical symptoms, which may be different in other cases of BI. The symptoms

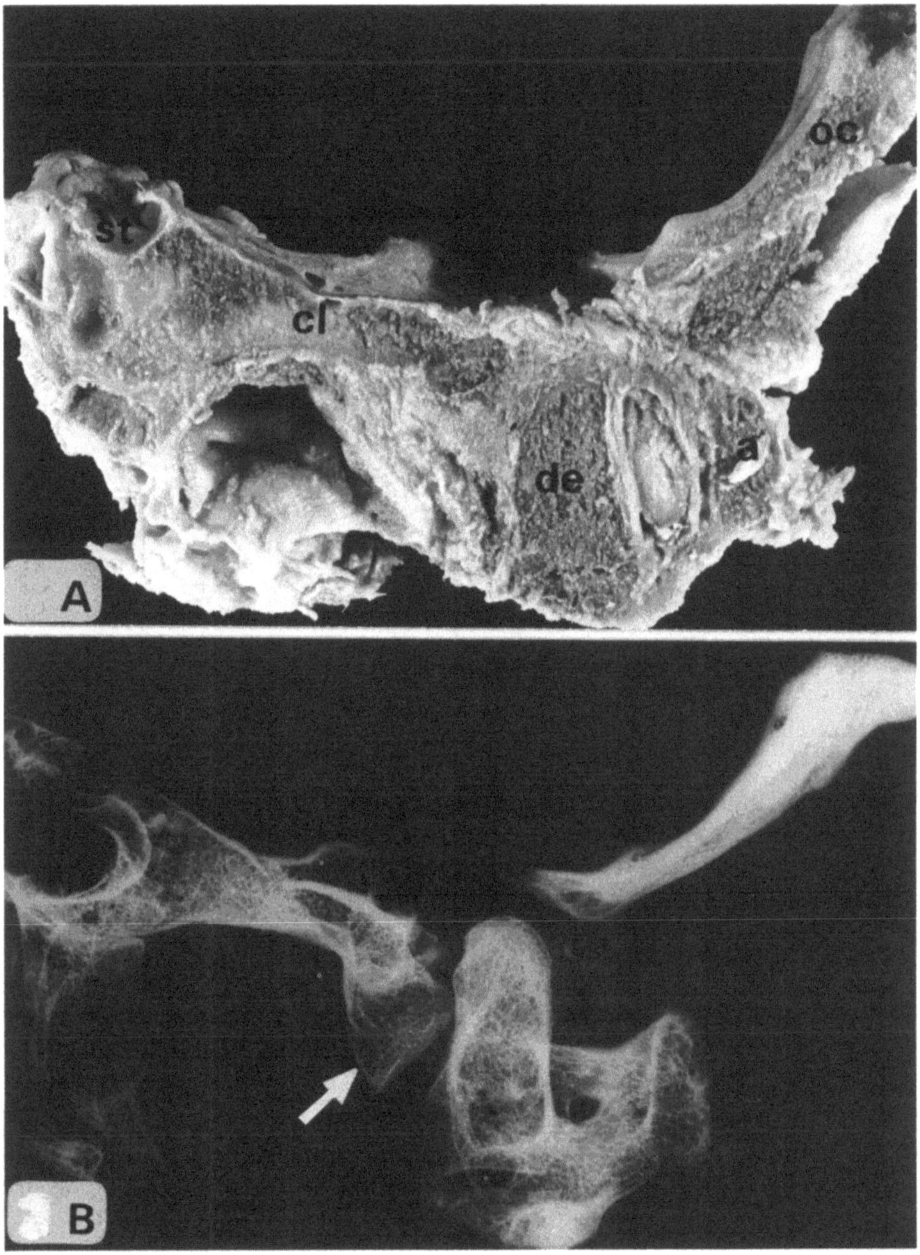

Fig. 2 Basilar impression. A: Median-sagittal section of a skull base in basilar impression. Note that the plane of the clivus in this case is also elevated (combination with platybasia). (a = atlas, cl = clivus, de = dens epistropheus, st = sella turcica). B: X-radiograph of the section in A demonstrating the elevated position of the dens and an inclined plane of the foramen magnum. The osseous structure ventral to the dens (arrow) is supposed to be a condylus tertius.

in BI are variable and may first occur only in advanced age, or earlier but occasionally with certain movements of the head. The spectrum of symptoms may include disturbances of the cochleo-vestibular system, the long tracts of the spinal cord, the cranial and cervical nerve roots, the cerebellum, and bulbar and vegetative signs [15, 54]. *Atlanto-occipital fusion*, the *manifestation of occipital vertebrae* and *fused vertebrae* are frequently associated with BI [15, 20, 45].

Secondary impressions of the floor of the posterior fossa, which may occur due to systemic disorders of bone development (e. g. osteogenesis imperfecta etc.), metastases of malignant tumors and fractures of the posterior skull base may not be included in the spectrum of BI, which is a primary developmental abnormality.

Here, the malformation described by Chiari [11, 12] and Arnold [1], the *Arnold-Chiari syndrome* or *Chiari type 2* malformation may be stressed since it is frequently associated with osseous abnormalities such as described above. From recent findings with induction of the Arnold-Chiari malformation by vitamin A application in pregnant hamsters, the authors [37] concluded that maldevelopment of the osseous parts of the posterior fossa may be the primary cause of this syndrome which is mainly characterized by a downward displacement through the foramen magnum of the inferior cerebellar vermis with elongation of the rhomboid fossa [3, 9, 10, 12, 16, 18, 24, 30, 37]. The earliest and most striking finding in these animal experiments was an underdevelopment of the basioccipitale resulting in a shortening of the posterior skull base and hypoplastic posterior fossa due to a "primary para-axial mesodermal insufficiency" [37]. In addition, the floor of the posterior fossa was elevated and showed changes which the authors parallelled with the human basilar impression. The authors concluded that the significant narrowing of the infratentorial space was the reason for the maldevelopment of the hindbrain structures in the Arnold-Chiari syndrome.

The same is true for observations in the *Chiari type 1* malformation or *"chronic tonsillar herniation"* [21] of the cerebellum. Here too, the posterior fossa can be shown to be hypoplastic [39] and suboccipital craniotomy yielded good results in symptomatic Chiari type 1 patients.

Finally, the mechanism of a narrowed infratentorial space may be employed in interpreting the pathogenesis of the *syndrome of transtentorial upward displacement of the cerebellum* (TUDC) or *"inverse Chiari type 2 syndrome"* [17, 42, 47, 52], although underdevelopment of the posterior skull base and the occiput cannot be clearly demonstrated craniometrically in all of these observations [57]. Nevertheless, as a rule there is a low insertion of the hypoplastic tentorium cerebelli [13, 42] so that the infratentorial space is always definitely narrowed in TUDC. The syndrome, which is closely related to the Arnold-Chiari malformation, as can be demonstrated by transitional forms between the two [48, 49], is

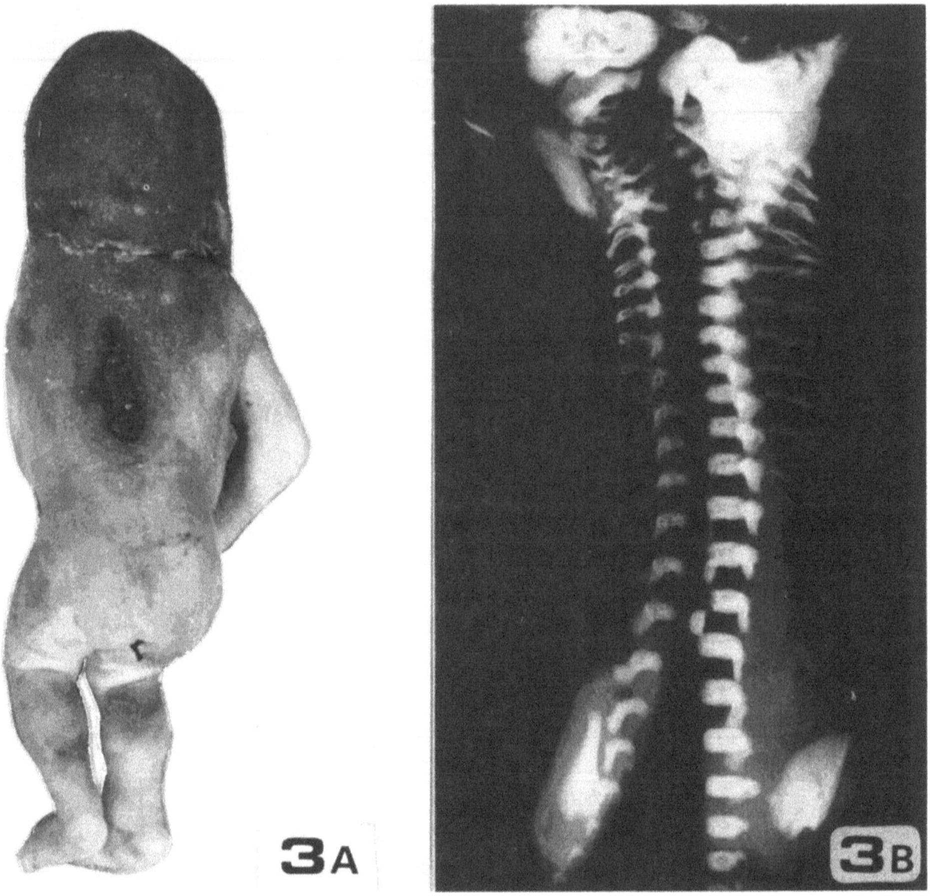

Fig. 3 Klippel-Feil syndrome. A: male fetus of the 26th week of gestation. Absence of the neck and a thoracic bifid spine. B: X-radiograph of the spine and skull base (obtained postmortally after sagittal sectioning of the spine). Note that, except for some small rudiments, there are no cervical vertebrae.

chiefly characterized by a displacement of the superior cerebellar vermis and adjacent parts of the lobuli quadrangulares into the supratentorial space. There they cause a deep-bowl-shaped impression of the posterior base of the forebrain [52].

The clinically most important malformations of the cranio-cervical region are the different forms of *cranio-spinal dysraphism.*

In *cranioschisis occipitalis*, brain structures and/or their coverings are displaced extracranially into an *occipital encephalocele* (fig. 4). Even in those cases with a low insertion of the cele, the latter mostly contains parts of the forebrain *(telencephalic encephalocele)*. In single cases of this kind, the brainstem and the cerebellum may be found in an abnormal retroflexion, the brainstem being at the top and the cerebellum in a caudal position *("hindbrain upside-down")* [50]. In other observations, the cerebellum was absent or severely hypoplastic [34].

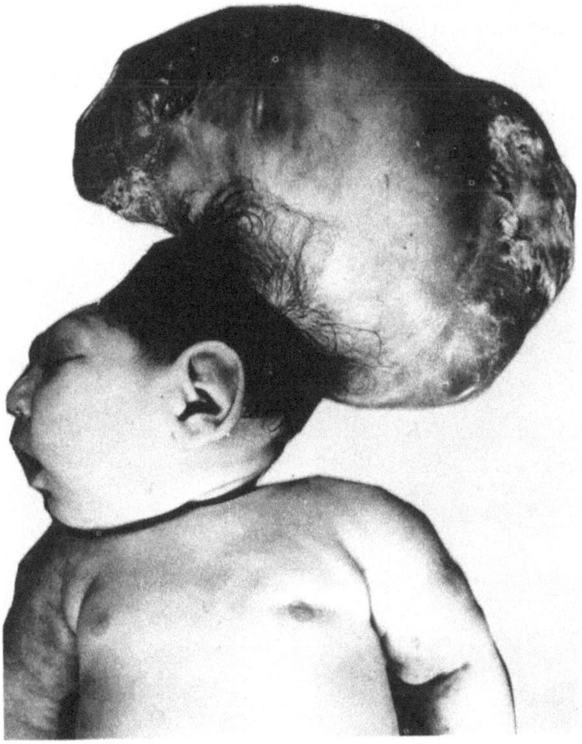

Fig. 4 New-born infant delivered at term with a huge highly inserting occipital encephalocele which contained the major parts of the forebrain.

Rachischisis of the cervical spine is associated with dysraphic changes of the spinal cord and/or its coverings subsumed in the *"meningomyelocele"* spectrum. The most moderate change without formation of a cele is the *defective dorsal arch of the atlas*. In more severe occipito-cervical dysraphism *(cranio-rachischisis occipito-cervicalis)*, the entire cerebellum may be displaced into a *suboccipital encephalocele (rhombencephalic encephalocele)* which is consistent with the very infrequent *Chiari type 3 malformation* [11, 12].

In rare events, a deeply inserting occipital encephalocele may harbor the cystic roof of the fourth ventricle in a cerebellum with agenesis of the vermis and ventrally dislocated ("inverse") cerebellar hemispheres [41, 53]. This *inverse cerebellum with occipital encephalocele* [53] or the *syndrome of Padget and Lindenberg* [41] is related to both the Arnold-Chiari and the Dandy-Walker spectrum as a kind of an intermediate form between them [53].

In *inciencephaly* [36], an occipito-cervical cranio-rachischisis with occipital encephalocele is combined with fused or defective vertebrae resulting in a shortening of the neck and abnormal retroflexion of the head.

In the most severe *iniencephalic anencephaly* [35], a subtotal or total dysraphism of the cranium and the spine with platyneuria or aneuria is associated with absence and fusion of cervical vertebrae, short neck and retroflexion of the head (fig. 5). These *arrhaphic anencephalics* are not viable.

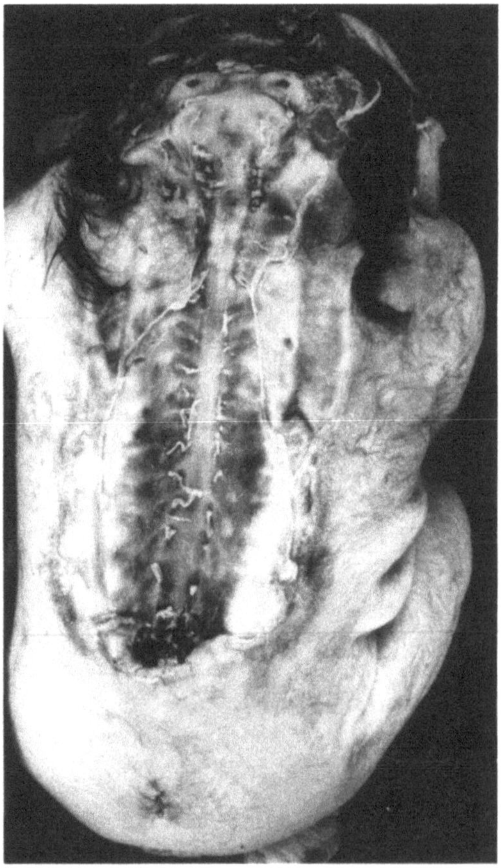

Fig. 5 Arrhaphic anencephalus with platyneuria and shortening of the neck ("iniencephalic anencephalus").

Conversely, the *Klippel-Feil syndrome* represents the more moderate, mostly viable type in the teratologic spectrum of deficient cranial vertebrae with shortening of the neck. In the observation delineated in fig. 3, the cervical spine is almost completely absent except some poor rudimentary cervical vertebrae. The posterior fossa is hypoplastic and Chiari type 1 or type 2 malformations are frequently associated. The same is true for spinal dysraphism. As in other malformation syndromes, the changes of the cranio-spinal region and the related hindbrain structures are frequently part of a more comprehensive malformation complex with involvement of other organs or body regions.

Finally, some malformation syndromes of the hindbrain will have to be mentioned in this context in which the associated abnormalities of the cranio-cervical region, in particular the posterior fossa, have to be regarded as definitely secondary to the changes of the CNS structures.

The first one is the *Dandy-Walker syndrome* (DWS) [4, 14, 44, 55, 56] in which a large ventriculocele in place of the defective cerebellar vermis constitutes the roof of the fourth ventricle and results in a severe enlargement of the posterior fossa. The torcular is elevated and the plane of the tentorium cerebelli is inclined. A present, disturbances in the formation of the foramen anterius, which occurs as a transitory opening in the primitive roof of the rhomboid fossa during early embryonic development, are chiefly discussed as the cause of the DWS [7, 23, 25]. The classical hypothesis relating the DWS to an atresia of the apertures of the fourth ventricle has been invalidated by the demonstration of patent foramina in several observations [19, 29).

Paleocerebellar agenesis, i.e. a defective cerebellar vermis without formation of a rhombencephalic ventriculocele, may occur sporadically or as an inherited disorder termed the *Joubert syndrome* (JS) [5, 6, 22, 32]. Episodic hyperpnea, abnormal eye movements, ataxia and other symptoms have been outlined as typical clinical signs of the JS. Together with the DWS the JS belongs to the spectrum of cerebellar dysraphism.

The same is true for the very infrequent *rhombencephalosynapsis* of Obersteiner [40] although in this syndrome the absence of the cerebellar vermis does not result in a median defect of the cerebellum but in a fusion of the cerebellar hemispheres and the dentate nuclei [28, 38, 40].

Neocerebellar (hemispheric) agenesis or *hypoplasia* and *complete agenesis of the cerebellum* may also occur either sporadically or as inherited defects. Their occurrence with telencephalic encephalocele has already been mentioned above. Moreover, they may be associated with malformational posterior fossa cysts which may sometimes cause difficulties in the clinical differentiation from true Dandy-Walker cysts [25].

Summary

The main objective of the foregoing survey was to emphasized that the malformations and abnormalities of the osseous parts of the cranio-cervical region and those of the neighbouring cerebral structures are interactively related to each other and may not be considered independently if one wishes to gain a more complete concept of their pathogenesis and the developmental mechanisms involved.

References

[1] Arnold, J.: Myelocyste, Transposition von Gewebskeimen und Sympodie. Path. Anat. **16** (1894) 1 – 28.

[2] Barry, A., B. M. Patten, B. H. Steward: Possible factors in the development of the Arnold-Chiari malformation. J. Neurosurg. **14** (1957) 285 – 301.

[3] Bell, J. E., A. Gordon, A. F. Y. Maloney: The association of hydrocephalus and Arnold-Chiari malformation with spina bifida in the fetus. Neuropath. Appl. Neurobiol. **6** (1980) 29 – 40.

[4] Benda, C. E.: The Dandy-Walker syndrome or the so-called atresia of the foramen of Magendie. J. Neuropath. Exp. Neurol. **13** (1954) 14 – 29.

[5] Boltshauser, E., W. Isler: Joubert syncrome: episodic hyperpnea, abnormal eye movements, retardation and ataxia, associated with dysplasia of the cerebellar vermis. Neuropediatrie **8** (1977) 57 – 66.

[6] Boltshauser, E., M. Herdan, G. Dumermuth, et al.: Joubert syndrome: Clinical and polygraphic observations in a further case. Neuropediatrics **12** (1981) 181 – 191.

[7] Brodal, A., E. Hauglie-Hanssen: Congenital hydrocephalus with defective development of the cerebellar vermis (Dandy-Walker syndrome): clinical and anatomical findings in two cases with particular reference to the so-called atresia of the foramina of Magendie and Luschka. J. Neurol. Neurosurg. Psychiat. **22** (1959) 99 – 108.

[8] Burkhardt, L., H. Fischer: Pathologische Anatomie des Schädels. In: O. Lubarsch, F. Henke, R. Rössle (eds.): Handbuch der speziellen pathologischen Anatomie und Histologie, Bd. IX, Teil 7. Springer, Berlin – Heidelberg – New York 1970.

[9] Case, M. E. S., H. B. Sarnat, P. Monteleine: Type II Arnold-Chiari malformation with normal spine in trisomy 18. Acta neuropath. (Berl.) **37** (1976) 259 – 262.

[10] Caviness, V. S. jr.: The Chiari malformations of the posterior fossa and their relation to hydrocephalus. Dev. Med. Child Neurol. **18** (1976) 103 – 116.

[11] Chiari, H.: Ueber Veränderungen des Kleinhirns infolge Hydrocephalie des Großhirns. Dtsch. Med. Wochenschr. **17** (1891) 1172 – 1175.

[12] Chiari, H.: Ueber Veränderungen des Kleinhirns, des Pons und der Medulla oblongata infolge von kongenitaler Hydrocephalie des Großhirns. Denkschr. kaiserl. Akad. Wissensch., Wien, Math.-Naturw. Kl. **63** (1896) 71 – 116.

[13] Daniel, P. M., S. J. Strich: Some observations on the congenital deformity of the central nervous system known as the Arnold-Chiari malformation. J. Neuropath. Exp. Neurol. **17** (1958) 255 – 266.

[14] Dandy, W. E., K. D. Blackfan: Internal hydrocephalus, an experimental, clinical and pathological study. Amer. J. Dis. Child **8** (1914) 406 – 482.

[15] Dieckmann, H.: Basilare Impression, Atlasassimilation und andere Skelettfehlbildungen der Zervico-okzipital-Region. Klinische Untersuchungen und angiographische Studien der Arteria vertebralis. In: H. Junghanns (ed.): Die Wirbelsäule in Forschung und Praxis, Bd. 32. Hippokrates, Stuttgart 1966.

[16] Doran, P. A., A. N. Guthkelch: Studies in the spina bifida cystica. I. General survey and reassessment of the problem. J. Neurol. Neurosurg. Psychiat. **24** (1961) 331 – 345.

[17] Emery, J. L.: Intracranial effects of longstanding decompression of the brain in children with hydrocephalus and meningomyelocele. Dev. Med. Child Neurol. 7 (1965) 302 – 309.

[18] Emery, J. L., R. K. Levick: The movement of the brain stem and vessels around the brain stem in children with hydrocephalus and the Arnold-Chiari deformity. Dev. Med. Child Neurol. Suppl. **11** (1966) 49 – 60.

[19] Finizio, F. S.: Dandy-Walker syndrome with patency of the foramina of Luschka and Magendie. J. Neurosurg. Sci. **23** (1979) 77 – 80.

[20] Frank, P., P. J. Prager, V. Menges, et al.: Klinik und Röntgendiagnostik der Fehlbildungen des craniocervikalen Überganges. Radiologe **17** (1977) 296 – 304.

[21] Friede, R. L.: Developmental neuropathology. Springer, Wien – New York 1975.

[22] Friede, R. L., E. Boltshauser: Uncommon syndromes of cerebellar vermis aplasia. I: Joubert syndrome. Dev. Med. Child Neurol. **20** (1978) 758 – 763.

[23] Gardner, E., R. O'Rahiley, D. Prolo: The Dandy-Walker and Arnold-Chiari malformations. Clinical, developmental, and teratological observations. Arch. Neurol. (Chic.) **32** (1975) 393 – 407.

[24] Gardner, W. J.: The dysraphic states from syringomyelia to anencephaly. Excerpta Medica (Amsterdam), pp. 1 – 35 1973.

[25] Gardner, W. J.: Hydrodynamic factors in Dandy-Walker and Arnold-Chiari malformations. Child's Brain 3 (1977) 200 – 212.

[26] Gátai, G.: Über die Veränderungen des Schädels und der Wirbelsäule bei basaler Impression. Z. menschl. Vererb.-Konst.-Lehre **35** (1959) 77 – 92.

[27] Gathmann, H. A., R. D. Meyer: Der Kleeblattschädel. In: W. Doerr (ed.): Veröffentlichungen aus der Forschungsstelle für theoretische Pathologie der Heidelberger Akad. d. Wiss., Suppl. 2 1977.

[28] Gross, H.: Die Rhombencephalosynapsis, eine systematische Kleinhirnfehlbildung. Arch. Psychiat. Nervenkrh. **199** (1959) 537 – 552.

[29] Hart, M. N., N. Malamud, W. G. Ellis: The Dandy-Walker syndrome. A clinicopathological study based on 28 cases. Neurology **22** (1972) 771 – 780.

[30] Hoytema, G. J. van, R. van den Beg: Embryological studies of the posterior fossa in connection with Arnold-Chiari malformation. Dev. Med. Child Neurol., Suppl. **11** (1966) 61 – 76.

[31] Ingraham, F. D., H. W. Scott: Spina bifida and cranium bifidum: Arnold-Chiari malformation. N. Engl. J. Med. **229** (1943) 108 – 114.

[32] Joubert, M., J. J. Eisenring, J. P. Robb, et al.: Familial agenesis of the cerebellar vermis: A syndrome of episodic hyperpnea, abnormal eye movements, ataxia, and mental retardation. Neurology **19** (1969) 813 – 825.

[33] Kapsenberg, J. G., J. A. VanLookeren: A case of spina bifida combined with diastematomyelia, the anomaly of Chiari and hydrocephalus. Acta Anat. (Basel) **7** (1949) 366 – 388.

[34] Karch, S. B., H. Urich: Occipital encephalocele: a morphological study. J. Neurol. Sci. **15** (1972) 89 – 112.

[35] Lemire, R. J., J. B. Beckwith, J. Warkany: Anencephaly. Raven Press, New York 1978.

[36] Lewis, H. F.: Iniencephalus. Amer. J. Obstet. Gynaecol. **35** (1897) 11 – 53.

[37] Marin-Padilla, M., T. M. Marin-Padilla: Morphogenesis of experimentally induced Arnold-Chiari malformation. J. Neurol. Sci. **50** (1981) 29 – 55.

[38] Noetzel, H.: Rhombenzephalosynapsis (Kleinhirn ohne Wurm). In: W. Doerr, G. Seifert, E. Uehlinger (eds.): Spezielle pathologische Anatomie, Bd. 13/II; G. Ule (ed.): Pathologie des Nervensystems, p. 189. Springer, Berlin – Heidelberg – New York 1983.

[39] Nyland, H., K. G. Krogness: Size of posterior fossa in Chiari type 1 malformation in adults. Acta Neurochir. (Wien) **40** (1978) 233 – 242.

[40] Obersteiner, H.: Ein Kleinhirn ohne Wurm. Arb. a. d. Neurol. Inst. (Wien) **21** (1916) 124 – 136.

[41] Padget, D. H., R. Lindenberg: Inverse cerebellum morphogenetically related to Dandy-Walker and Arnold-Chiari syndromes: Bizarre malformed brain with occipital encephalocele. Johns Hopkins Med. J. **131** (1972) 228 – 246.

[42] Peach, B.: The Arnold-Chiari malformation. Arch. Neurol. (Chic.) **12** (1965) 527 – 535, 613 – 621.

[43] Penfield, W., D. F. Coburn: Arnold-Chiari malformation and its operative treatment. Arch. Neurol. Psychiat. **40** (1938) 328 – 336.

[44] Sawaya, R., R. L. McLaurin: Dandy-Walker syndrome. Clinical analysis of 23 cases. J. Neurosurg. **55** (1981) 89 – 98.

[45] Schmidt, H., E. Fischer: Die okzipitale Dysplasie. In: W. Bargmann, W. Doerr (eds.): Zwanglose Abhandlungen aus dem Gebiete der normalen und pathologischen Anatomie, Heft 9. Thieme, Stuttgart 1960.

[46] Schmitt, H. P.: Ein Beitrag zum Problem der Sutura frontalis und Sutura mendosa persistens. Virch. Arch. A Path. Anat. **368** (1975) 213 – 227.

[47] Schmitt, H. P.: Syndrome of primary transtentorial cerebellar displacement – "inverse Chiari type II" syndrome. Neuropädiatrie **9** (1978) 268 – 276.

[48] Schmitt, H. P.: "Inverse Chiari Type II syndrome" in untreated hydrocephalus and its relationship to typical Arnold-Chiari syndrome. Brain Dev. (Tokyo) **3** (1981) 271 – 275.

[49] Schmitt, H. P.: Der Hydrozephalus bei Mißbildungen der hinteren Schädelgrube im Umfelde des dysraphischen Formenkreises. Morphologie und Überlegungen zur Pathogenese. In: D. Voth, P. Gutjahr, P. Glees (eds.): Hydrocephalus im frühen Kindesalter, pp. 79 – 88. F. Enke, Stuttgart 1983.

[50] Schmitt, H. P.: "Hindbrain upside-down" with occipital encephalocele. Alternative to the syndrom of Padget and Lindberg. In: D. Voth, P. Glees, J. Lorber (eds.): Spida bifida-neural tube defects, pp. 61 – 66. Walter de Gruyter, Berlin – New York 1986.

[51] Schmitt, H. P., L. Tamaska: Die Bedeutung occipito-cervikaler Mißbildungen für die forensische Pathologie. Z. Rechtsmed. **72** (1973) 140 – 150.

[52] Schmitt, H. P., W. Waidelich, E. Harms, et al.: Partial transtentorial displacement of the cerebellum and the brain stem in hydrocephalus – A primary condition or a result of treatment? Acta Neurochir. (Wien) **33** (1976) 151 – 165.

[53] Smith, M. T., H. W. Huntington: Inverse cerebellum and occipital encephalocele. A dorsal fusion defect uniting the Arnold-Chiari and Dandy-Walker spectrum. Neurology **27** (1977) 246 – 251.

[54] Sollmann, A. H.: Die basiläre Impression. Med. Klin. **58** (1963) 1301 – 1304.

[55] Taggart, J. K., A. E. Walker: Congenital atresia of the foramens of Luschka and Magendie. Arch. Neurol. Psychiat. **48** (1942) 583 – 612.

[56] Tal, Y., B. Freigang, H. G. Dunn, et al.: Dandy-Walker syndrome: analysis of 21 cases. Dev. Med. Child Neurol. **22** (1980) 189 – 201.

[57] Wackenheim, A.: Roentgendiagnosis of the craniovertebral region. Springer, Berlin – Heidelberg – New York 1974.

Neurological diagnosis of malformations at the cranio-cervical junction

R. W. Heckl, J. Harms

The discussion of the malformations of the cranio-cervical junction has been limited to the more prevalent bony malformations. These include
- basilar impression
- atlanto-axial dislocation
- os odontoideum

Cerebellar tonsil ectopia (Arnold Chiari I) must be included as it does not occur only in isolation but can be combined with bone malformation.

The complaints of the patients vary and include a combination of the following symptoms:
- headache
- vertigo
- paralysis
- disturbance of equilibrium
- sensory disturbances.

Headache is one of the most constant complaints and the following types can be observed:
- neck and occipital headache (dull)
- occipital neuralgia
- pain in the forehead and temporal regions
- more frequently onesided
- press headache ("cough headache").

The dull neck and occipital pain is by far the most frequent sign. Not quite as frequently occur pains refered to as occipital neuralgia and also pains in the forehead and temple regions which chiefly are an extension of the neck and occipital pain. The press headache ("cough headache") will be dealt with below.

The other symptoms like vertigo, paralysis, disturbance of equilibrium and sensory disturbances are not very characteristic because they can be caused by other neurological ailments. Even the *course of the disease* can develop in different forms. The following forms can be differentiated:
- slowly progressing
- primarily slowly progressing/rapidly progressing

- slowly progressing – with inhibition
- acute exacerbation (after trauma)
- intermittent recidivation symptoms.

Most prevelant is the slowly progressing form which can develop into the rapidly progressing type before one is able to establish the cause for the symptoms. We also experienced patients which develop the slowly progressing form of the disease but the symptoms came to a standstill. It often occurs that patients who previously showed no symptoms suddenly develop grave deficiencies after a trauma with no correlation to the severity of the trauma. Not well known is the fact that intermittent signs and symptoms can also occur (see later). Frequently the radilogist discovers a cranio-cervical junction disability, whereby the patient is not at all impeded by any discomfort. There is no specific sign or symptom characteristic to the course of development of the various forms described. Every neurological disease can run a course with exactly the same symptoms as one of these types. Multiple sclerosis is the only disease which can show a course of development with so many different forms. There is no clinical grouping of symptoms, which is characteristic of any of the deformities described. The diverse symptoms can be made more complicated not only through cerebellar ectopia but also often through a syringomyelia combined with bony cranio-cervical junction malformation.

During the course of the investigation the seat of the lesion is usually located in the cervical medulla and to be exact at the cranio-cervical junction. Without extra x-ray examinations the aetiology can not be determined. However there are often outward signs and symptoms which are suggestive of a process located at the cranio-cervical junction. We found that in basilar impression patients often have a conspicuously short neck (fig. 1).

The congenital basilar impression is a dysplasia and has to be included in the group of the so called "status dysraphicus". It is therefore not a surprise that syringomyelia which also belongs to the "status dysraphicus" is often associated with this bone malformation. Sometimes one finds other signs of dysplasia such as hypertrichosis at the lumbo-sacral junction as an expression of a spina bifida or accessory nipples. It is not uncommon to find an asymmetry of the face in cranio-cervical malformations.

Dysfunctions of the cranial nerves are not very common. We found one case of paralysis of the hypoglossal nerve and often a paralysis of the accessory nerve.

The most conspicious sign among the clinical findings is usually a *lesion of the pyramidal tract* with a spastic paralysis confined to the legs.

After a recurrence of the disease due to trauma a distinctive paralysis of the arms can sometimes be found. This type of paralysis is called "Bell's cruciate paralysis"

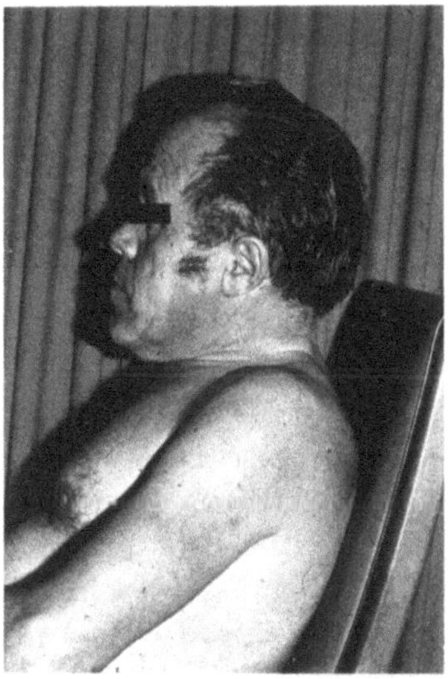

Fig. 1 Basilar impression. Note conspicuously short neck.

caused by the tip of the dens injuring the crossing of the pyramidal tracts ventrally of the medulla oblongata.

Intermittent vestibulo-cerebellar signs are found but usually occur simultaneously in connection with an existing cerebellar tonsillar ectopia.

Similarly as frequently as the pyramidal tract disturbances are *posterior tract lesions* of various degrees. As with other high spinal cord signs or disease processes at the spino-medullary junction it is very common to see a deficiency more pronounced in the arm.

Sensory disturbances on the body surface are common but are not very distinct. A dissociated sensory disturbance even when not very marked, should remind the examiner of a accompanying syringomyelia.

Disturbances of the urinary bladder are not common. In case these develop, other symptoms such as paralysis are already present in an advanced degree. The diagnosis can be very difficult when the course of the disease is not of the usual slowly progressive, but when intermittent signs and symptoms develop or the slowly progressive course is interrupted with exacerbations.

In 12 patients suffering from cranio-cervical junction disturbances (including some with secondary forms such as rheumatic cases) the following intermittent signs and symptoms were observed:

press headache ("cough headache")	3 cases
sudden transient paralysis	3 cases
Lhermitte's sign	3 cases
drop attacks	2 cases
transient blindness	1 case
transient global amnesia	1 case
thermparesthesia	1 case

Press headache can be defined as a headache which occurs when the abdominal pressure is raised for instance by sneezing, by pressing during defecation or by coughing ("cough headache"). Tonsillar ectopia was always present in our three cases [1]. It has to be assumed that when the abdominal pressure rises an increase of the intracranial pressure through which the ectopic cerebellar tonsil is pressed into the foramen magnum. A compensation for the raised pressure is not achieved in the spinal canal. In some patients *transient paralysis* developed from neck movements which are still in physiological limits (for instance trampoline springing, slight whip lash trauma). The *Lhermitte's sign* is also very common and indicates sensory disturbances of an electric shock character mostly in the arms or along the vertebral column caused by certain movements of the head and neck. In two patients there were *drop attacks* whereby it could not be determined whether a direct lesion of the medulla was present or was there a vertebro-basilar insufficiency. In one patient *episodes of amnesia* occured, which might have been coincidental. However, some authors have reported that episodes of amnesia do occur in cranio-cervical junctions disturbances [3].

Thermparesthesia developed in one patient. By this we mean sensory disturbances to cold and heat sensation in the legs, and has been observed in patients with tumours at the cranio-cervical junction [2].

The complaints, signs and symptoms and the outcome in patients with malformations in the cranio-cervical region are so varied that clinically the presumed diagnosis can only seldom be established and additional investigations are needed. Even when a cranio-cervical junction disturbance is identified by x-ray, the entire differential diagnostic spectrum must be considered. We know that a variety of patients with cranio-cervical junction defects show no clinical symptoms. Even when a cranio-cervical junction disturbance is diagnosed there is no typical set of related clinical symptoms. In case of a cranio-cervical junction symptom, a detailed differential diagnosis must still be carried out to exclude multiple sclerosis, tumours of the spinal cord or a funicular myelosis.

References

[1] Heckl, R. W.: Der Preßkopfschmerz ("Hustenkopfschmerz"). Begriffsbestimmung und Überlegungen zur Ätiologie. Fortschr. Neurol. Psychiat. 1986 (in press).

[2] Haymaker, W.: Bing's local diagnosis in neurological diseases, 15th ed. Mosby Co., St. Louis, Mo. 1969.

[3] Jones, M. W., J. G. E. Kaufmann: Vertebro-basilar insufficiency in rheumatoid atlanto-axial subluxation. J. Neurol. Neurosurg. Psychiat. **31** (1969) 15 – 20.

Clinical findings in syringomyelia in contrast to the lesions seen in NMR imaging

G. Hertel, W. Schörner, D. Köhler, B. Trempenau

Introduction

Syringomyelia is a congenital disease of the spinal cord that can progress throughout the patient's lifetime. The primary symptoms of this disorder are: pain in the neck and in the upper limbs, dissociated sensory loss, vegetative symptoms, weakness and wasting in one or more limbs, and in severe cases, spastic paraparesis.

In cases having several of these symptoms the diagnosis of syringomyelia is easy to establish; however, this is rarely the case in the early stages of this illness. There are few flagrant cases that develop rapid muscle wasting within a few years. In most cases (2/3rds of our patients) the illness progresses very slowly and can remain stable for decades. It is not surprising that in a previous study of 323 patients (which included the necessary long period of time for follow-up) an average of six years had passed before symptoms led to hospitalization. Nearly a quarter of the patients had some symptoms for more than ten years prior to their first neurologic examination [7].

Prior to the development of computer tomography, myelographic studies with contrast medium or with air (collapsing cord sign) were used to confirm the diagnosis of syringomyelia. Due to the limitations of this type of myelography one could only suspect a diagnosis of syringomyelia although the patient had been followed up for more than 20 years. Once computed tomography became available, it could be used in combination with metrizamide-myelography, and cystic lesions in the spinal cord could be more easily visualized [1, 2, 4].

However, a superior method for the diagnosis of syringomyelic cavities in the spinal cord is now available: NMR-imaging is, at present, the safest and most elegant method of examination. It is not invasive and the entire brain stem and cervical cord can be shown on one picture. The caudal spinal cord can also be examined. Other diseases, such as, meningioma and glioma, can be excluded and one can assess the possibility whether a Arnold-Chiari Malformation may be present [3, 9, 12].

Cases (General data)

In the past 1 1/2 years we were able to establish the diagnosis of syringomyelia with NMR-imaging in 12 cases. The group of patients is extremely heterogenous. Ages of patients at the time of NMR-examination varied between 19 and 73 years and the duration of the disease was between one and 35 years. The neurologic symptoms were highly variable. 8 representative cases will be discussed.

Case reports

1. A 27 year old turk presented initially complaints of brief episodes of pain and weakness (fig. 1) in both arms. His initial neurologic examination was normal. His cervical spine X-rays revealed widening of the anteroposterior diameter of the canal and despite the paucity of findings syringomyelia was suspected. NMR-imaging showed a large cystic spinal cord lesion extending from the level of C_2 to C_7. A subsequent neurologic examination 6 months after the NMR examination was normal.

2. A 19 year old Turk developed wasting and weakness in both arms, a dissociated sensory loss, and spastic paraparesis over approximately 12 months. The possibility of syringomyelia was considered and NMR-imaging revealed a large intramedullary cyst extending from the level of C_1 into the thoracic region.

3. In 1983 a 41 year old woman (figs. 2, 3) complained of pain in the right arm and a few months later pain also appeared in the left arm. The attacks of pain

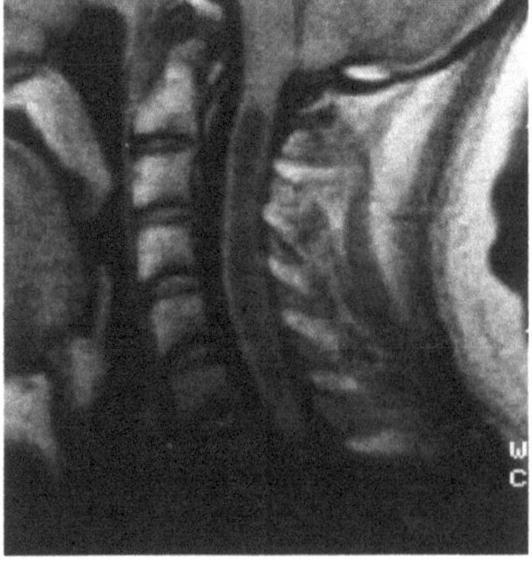

Fig. 1 Patient 1. Short case history with attacks of pain and some weakness without other symptoms. Neurological examination was normal.

were initially associated with coughing and bending forward, but later on laughing and even mild physical exertion also caused the pain. Computed tomography with myelography were performed and the diagnosis of syringomyelia was made. The patients symptoms remained unchanged for one year. At this time she developed the additional complaint of intermittent right sided dysaesthesia that first appeared in the arm, then in the breast, ear, lips and finally in the legs. In 1985 she developed proximal, asymmetric, weakness of the legs. Throughout her clinical course she has had no dissociated sensory loss. The EMG evaluation was normal. NMR-imaging revealed a cyst in the spinal cord extending from the level of C_2 to C_6. The cavity was greatly enlarged in the cranial region. There was an associated severe Arnold-Chiari malformation.

Fig. 2

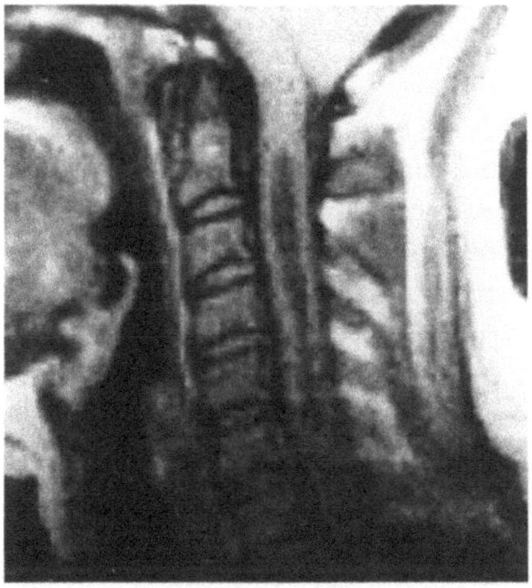

Fig. 3

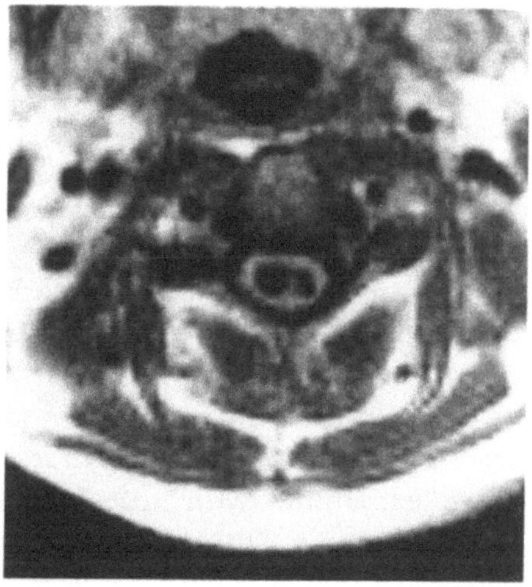

Fig. 2, 3 Patient 3. Short case history, very few symptoms.

4. A 49 year old Turkish woman came for a neurologic evaluation having a two year history of progressive weakness in both legs. This was accompanied by pain in the neck and shoulders. On neurological examination she had a left Horner's syndrome, proximal muscle wasting more pronounced on the right, spastic paraparesis and absent tendon jerks in the upper extremities. There was severe atrophy in the right arm and the patient was unable to use her right hand. The patient recently indicated that these right arm symptoms had been present for 20 years (after trauma to the right shoulder!). She had no dissociated sensory loss. The X-rays of the cervical spine demonstrated an increased sagittal diameter. On NMR-imaging there was a very large cyst in the spinal cord from the level of C 1/C 2 and terminating in the thoracic cord at approximately T 6. An Arnold-Chiari malformation was also present.

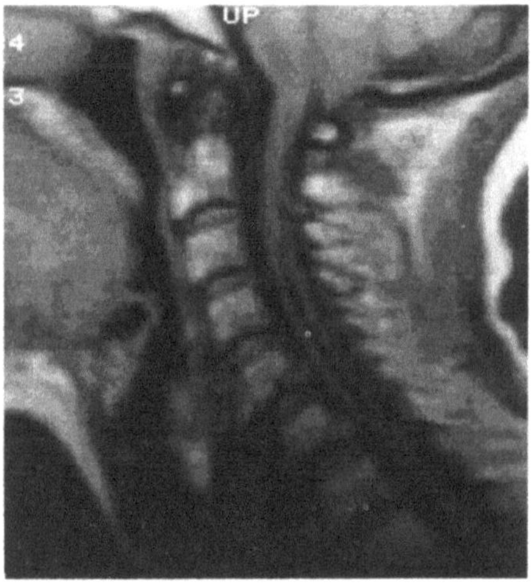

Fig. 4 Patient 5. Case history of about 36 years, very severe symptoms.

5. A 60 year old woman (fig. 4) presented with a long history starting when she was 24 years old when she developed pain, weakness, and paresthesias. At this time she began to suffer from repeated accidental burns. At 35 years of age the patient was believed to have a glioma of the spinal cord and she received X-ray treatment. Two years later the diagnosis of syringomyelia was considered in her case. Over the ensuing years this patient had very slow progression of weakness in the right arm and a slight spastic paraparesis. By 1984 she had developed a severe scoliosis, a Horner's syndrome on the left, and severe weakness of both upper extremities with little function in her left hand. The slight paraparesis remained stable. Dissociated sensory loss was detected in the upper extremities and severe numbness in both legs. On NMR-imaging a very thin intramedullary cyst extending from the level of C2 to C7 could be demonstrated.

6. A 62 year old woman had her first neurologic symptoms at 28 years of age. She experienced progressive weakness in the left arm followed by dysesthesia in both upper extremities. In order to exclude the presence of an angioma, numerous clinical and laboratory examinations were performed, included three myelograms and two angiograms. In 1985 she developed typical signs of syringomyelia and dissociated sensory loss, severe weakness of the shoulder girdle muscles was noted in addition to a virtually useless right hand. The radiograph of the cervical spine showed an increased sagittal diameter. Computed tomography was inconclusive although there was suspicion of a small cyst in the spinal cord. NMR-imaging revealed a very thin cyst which extended from C2 to C6.

7. A 59 year old woman became ill when 18 years old. The diagnosis syringomyelia was made early in the clinical course and confirmed several times. On examination in 1985 she was found to have severe weakness throughout the

proximal and distal portions of both upper extremities, and she had little functional use in her hands. There was a dissociated sensory loss, but no signs of spastic paraparesis were present. NMR-imaging showed a large cyst in the spinal cord from C 1 and to the thoracic region but severe scoliosis prevented an exact determination of the caudal end of the cavity.

8. A 73 year old woman presented with a 30 year history of peculiar pains in the arms, dysesthesias, and fluctuating weakness which was felt to be atypical for syringomyelia. At present her neurological examination is without diagnostic abnormalities. The tentative diagnoses made previously were multiple sclerosis, tumor, angioma, and disc herniation. In 1984 NMR imaging was performed on the patient and a small intramedullary cyst extending from C 3 to C 7 was detected. In the throracic region additional cysts were detected.

Conclusions

Syringomyelia is nowadays a very rare disease (at least in Germany). While making the plans for an epidemiological multicentre study, we stated that in the past 30 years, the number of cases had diminished considerably. In Würzburg, where one of the 12 hospitals was involved, we had 15 cases between 1950 and 1959. Between 1960 and 1969 we had only 8, and from 1980 to the present about 1 – 2 new patients per year [8].

Over the past 1 1/2 years we were able to make the diagnosis of syringomyelia 12 times with NMR-Imaging in Berlin. Five out of the 8 patients in the present report had a unequivocal case history of syringomyelia of at last 20 years. Among the three patients with short history (less than two years) there were two Turks and only one German, who was living in Hannover. We did not see a single new patient in Berlin. It is obvious that during the next years many "old patients" with long case history and diffuse symptoms as well as those patients with symptoms typical for syringomyelia over many years, will have NMR-imaging. This will lead to an apparent increasing number of cases.

NMR-imaging [3, 9, 12] permits an immediate diagnosis of syringomyelia, but the immediate therapeutic significance of the finding is less certain. The rate of progression of the disease can be very varied (from rapid progression with severe weakness and spastic paraparesis within a few years to microsymptoms for decades) [7]. In our opinion impressive findings on NMR-imaging should not lead to hasty surgery. It seems that the suboccipital craniotomy as proposed by Gardner [5, 6] is nowadays more rarely used than in the past. The results of our carefully controlled studies with 20 operated patients were disappointing similar to those reported by Cahan and Bentson [2]. With the introduction of new catheters and the use of microsurgery the myelotomy and syringostomy with drainage of cysts is now reappearing. However, well documented follow-up studies are not yet available [11].

Already in the 60's we noticed that in two patients who had died after suboccipital craniotomy, the size of the cysts did not correlate with the severity of the clinical symptoms. One patient had a very short case history with little symptoms, the other had already had a very severe syringomyelia for many years. In both cases the cyst was extremely large.

The experience with NMR-imaging confirms our view that the severity of the symptoms and the extent of spinal cord pathology seen on NMR-imaging may differ radically. In patients with severe symptoms the cysts are often but not always large. In patients with microsymptoms the cysts can be very large. It is remarkable that the cysts in our three younger patients (19, 28 and 41 years of age) with short case history (less than two years) are much bigger than in several of the older patients (60, 62 and 73 years old) with a long case history (more than 20 years). It is not clear if this cyst, which probably already existed at birth, became measurably bigger during lifetime of the patient and whether the increase in size correlated with the appearance of new symptoms and signs.

We assume that a spinal cyst can remain without symptoms for decades until it, for whatever reason, becomes manifest. This agrees well with Staemmler's oppinion. In 1942 he examined systematically the spinal cord in 1200 unselected autopsies and found in ten cases (0,8%), a pathological cyst (syringomyelia). In 14 further cases he described a very large central canal (hydromyelia) or a gliosis [10]. These results support Karge's thesis who assumes only one out of every 100 persons with an congenital cyst will develop syringomyelia-symptoms during life. This correlation between the frequency of symptoms and signs with the actual presence of a cystic cavity in the spinal cord may have increasing importance in the future. With the increased use of NMR-imaging in spinal cord diagnostic it is likely that we will observe cysts but find that they have little clinical relevance.

References

[1] Bonafé, A., C. Manelfe, J. Espagno, et al.: Evaluation of syringomyelia with Metrizamide Computed Tomographic Myelography. J. Comput. Assist. Tomogr. 4 (1980) 797 – 802.

[2] Cahan, L. D., J. R. Bentson: Considerations in the diagnosis and treatment of syringomyelia and the Chiari-malformation. J. Neurosurg. 57 (1982) 24 – 31.

[31] De La Paz, R. L., T. J. Brady, F. S. Buonanno, et al.: Nuclear Magnetic Resonance (NMR) Imaging of Arnold-Chiari Type I Malformation with Hydromyelia. J. Comput. Assist. Tomogr. 7 (1983) 126 – 129.

[4] Di Chiro, G., D. Schellinger: Computed Tomography of spinal cord after lumbar intrathecal introduction of Metrizamide. Radiology **120** (1976) 101 – 104.

[5] Gardner, W. J., J. Angel: The mechanism of syringomyelia and its surgical correction. Clin. Neurosurg. 6 (1958) 131 – 138.

[6] Gardner, W. J.: Hydrodynamic mechanism of syringomyelia: its relationship to myelocele. J. Neurol. Neurosurg. Psychiat. **28** (1965) 247 – 259.

[7] Hertel, G., S. Kramer, E. Placzek: Die Syringomyelie. Klinische Verlaufsbeobachtungen bei 323 Patienten. Nervenarzt **44** (1973) 1 – 13.

[8] Hertel, G., K. Ricker: A geomedical study on the distribution of syringomyelia in Germany. Excerpta Medica International Congress series **434** Neurology (Amsterdam) (1977) 353 – 365.

[9] Pojunas, K., A. L. Williams, D. L. Daniels, et al.: Syringomyelia and hydromyelia: Magnetic Resonance evaluation. Radiology **153** (1984) 679 – 683.

[10] Staemmler, M.: Hydromyelie, Syringomyelie und Gliose. Monogr. Gesamtgeb. Psychiatr. Springer, Berlin 1942.

[11] Tator, Ch. H., K. Meguro, D. W. Rowed: Favorable results with syringosubarachnoid shunts for treatment of syringomyelia. J. Neurosurg. **56** (1982) 517 – 523.

[12] Yeates, A., M. B. Zawadski, D. Norman, et al.: Nuclear Magnetic Resonance Imaging of syringomyelia. J. J. N. R. **4** (1983) 234 – 237.

A historical review of syringomyelia in the cranio-cervical region and new aspects for operative treatment possible after NMR examination

N. Hüwel, J. Schumacher

Introduction

Since the introduction of Nuclear Magnetic Resonance Technique (NMR) and after radiologists and neuroradiologists have learned to plan and apply the technical details of nuclear magnetic resonance efficiently, a considerable change in operative procedures can be observed [1, 2, 11, 13, 18, 22, 23, 33, 38, 51]. To start with a brief review will be given of the previous treatment of syringomyelia and the extent of how far NMR has superseded former neuroradiological examination techniques for the diagnosis of syringomyelia. The term 'syringomyelia' was first mentioned in 1827 by Olivier [3] in a French article describing longitudinal cavities in the spinal medullary grey matter. The French author could already demonstrate that the underlying changes and their characteristic localisation were closely connected with morphological changes and neurological symptoms. Neither in those early days nor today has a clear view concerning the pathogenetic causes been found and it seems that a number of pathogenetic factors are responsible for the clinical syndrome [34]. At the time of Olivier's publication syringomyelia is equated with terms like 'glia pin' or spinal gliosis and we know now that this only characterizes a special form of the disease by its predominant morphological character.

Syringomyelia can be divided into a communicating and non-communicating form [42, 45] which has different consequences for the operative treatment. The communicating form is characterised by a communication between the 4th ventricle and the dilated central canal of the spinal cord. This is caused by a stenosis of the normal outlets of the 4th ventricle due to developmental abnormalities of the skull base, inflammatory changes or space occupying lesions [3–5, 9, 11]. The disturbance in CSF dynamic leads to a permanent connection between the 4th ventricle and the central canal causing a gradual dilation and finally hydromyelia. Such a connection however does not exist in the non-communicating type and other causes must be responsible for the syrinx. In the communicating form the essential disturbance in CSF circulation is caused by the fact that the central canal is not yet or incompletely obliterated and a dilatation of the central canal results which is a part of the ventricular system [36]. In the literature a so-called idiopathic syringomyelia is mentioned. From a morphological point of view this resembles a spinal gliosis but must be separated from a gliomatous tumor in a differential diagnosis [31]. These three different pathogenic assumptions demand different operative techniques. The communicating form was treated after a laminectomy in the upper region of the cervical vertebral column, an exposure of the skull base by enlarging the foramen magnum, by removal of blocking membranes in the region of the outlet foraminae, and furthermore by draining the cavity in the cervical cord into the subarachnoid space. In some cases the operatively induced obliteration of the obex was sealed by muscle grafting [19].

The non-communicating form has been mostly treated by draining into the subarachnoid space after a laminectomy at the maximal level of the syrinx. The treatment of the idiopathic syringomyelia is similar to the operative procedure used for a removal of a glioma [47, 48, 50].

Overview of theories, diagnostics and operative procedure

A paper of von Leyden as early as 1876 is based on the assumption that the syringomyelia develops as consequence of a developmental error in the formation of the central canal and is combined with a hydromyelia and a myelocele [30].

In 1883 Hoffmann described a malformation of the central canal as sequela of an insufficient occlusion of the central canal and assumed that embryonic cells persist in the surrounding of the central canal which later proliferate and result in a gliosis [13]. Due to a secondary softening it comes to the formation of a cavity in the central gliosis.

Gardner et al. [22] published the first interpretation of syringomyelia representing a combination with other clinical syndromes. These authors consider malformations in the region of skull base related to either a Arnold-Chiari-malformation, a Dandy-Walker-syndrome or a cerebellar cyst. Gardner et al. assume that all these changes have a common pathogenetic factor. During embryonic development the foramina connecting the 4th ventricle and the subarachnoid space fail to develop. As the CSF production starts in the 6th embryonic week an incomplete development of the Foramina Magendii and Luschkae prevents a sufficient drainage between the ventricular system and the subarachnoid space. The result is the development of a hydrocephalus with displacement of the cerebellar tonsils into the upper cervical canal. In this developmental anomaly the 4th ventricle and the central canal remain connected and a hydromyelia develops acting as a compensation for the hydrocephalus. In most cases we find here a normal-pressure-hydrocephalus [43].

In 1965 Gardner completed his work in evolving a hydrodynamic theory leading to the formation of a cavity in the spinal cord. Gardner's work is based on the fact that a combination of disturbed CSF production in the 4th ventricle into the cisterna magna occurs leading to a connection between 4th ventricle and the central canal. The missing foramina of Luschkae and Magendii cause a flow disturbance from the ventricular system to the cisterna magna. When a sudden CSF production takes place due to the increase of arterial pulsation in the plexus chorioideus the CSF pushes into the central canal. This "water hammer"-effect leads, according to Gardner, to the development of a hydro- and syringomyelia.

Williams [50] assumed that during increase in the pressure within the spinal space by coughing, sneezing and physical exercises CSF is pushed into the cisterna magna and unable to return into the spinal subarachnoid space as the foramen magnum is displaced. In this instance CSF flows into the 4th ventricle and through the open connection between this ventricle and central canal into the cavity of the cord. Foster et al. (1969) published a paper on patients with syringomyelia and state that after physical strain patients suffer from pain and disturbed sensory functions [19, 20].

Other authors advanced the hypothesis that the cavity develops by CSF forces which come from the subarachnoid space through Virchow-Robin-spaces into the spinal cord. This mechanism becomes effective when an increase in pressure in the spinal canal occurs and obstructed liquor flows into the cisterna magna.

Foster et al. (1980) in a further paper on communicating syringomyelia conclude that an intramedullary tumor, arachnitis or a spinal cord contusion could be the case. After this historical review of the etiology of syringomyelia we proceed discussing the operative treatment preceeded by a short historical introduction.

Before the clinical picture of syringomyelia was subdivided into a communicating and a non-communcating form, two therapeutic procedures were generally used. One was the conventional treatment with X-ray and the other the surgical treatment which, however, was subject to numerous modifications in finding a combination of treatment between changes occuring in the basis of the skull and syringomyelia [14, 24]. At first the surgeon was mainly concerned reducing the patient's disease progress by a fluid drainage of the cyst [47]. However, the post-operative results were not successful, and a change in procedure was necessary.

Other surgeons recommended the drainage of a cyst into the subarachnoid space [17, 35]. This resulted in a better prognosis and gave a longer period of arrest in the disease progress. The X-ray-treatment and the follow-up control of patients for a period of about 20 years does not justify radiotherapy which causes extensive gliosis. In the majority of patients no difference in the disease process of treated and untreated cases could be observed. However, a reduction of pain was noticeable, although the risk of an ensueing leucosis and myelin degeneration cannot be overlooked. Various pathogenic causes for the filling of the syrinx resulted in different operative procedures [6, 10]. A great change in the operative procedure came only in 1965 initiated by Gardner, who realised the combination of syringomyelia with other malformations in the area of the base of the skull connected with alteration of the CSF circulation. Due to this new methods for treatment which correct CSF flow aroses. Gardner suggested a decompression at the base of the skull to alleviate a stenosis of the foramen magnum caused by ectopic cerebellar tonsils. This cause – he believed – should be responsible for the disease progression [21].

The *operative procedure* starts with an exposure of the base of the skull and a laminectomy of the upper cervical vertebral column. After opening of the dura ectopic cerebellar tonsils are resected, allowing a view of the 4th ventricle. In a number of patients the outlet of the 4th ventricle, the Foramen Magendii, occluded by a membrane of embryonic origin, was perforated [9]. In other patients the CSF flow was found to be arrested by cerebellar tonsils in front of the 4th ventricle. Gardner recommended a closure in case a connection between the 4th ventricle and the central canal was present. In most cases a muscle graft is used inserted below the obex. However, this procedure is more effective in the communicating form, when a decompression of the base has been performed instead of only blocking the connection between the 4th ventricle and the central canal. In some cases even the reclosure of the dura was omitted in order to support the effect of decompressing the base.

Postoperative rigidity of neck, muscles, headaches and fever were frequently observed due to an unavoidable contamination of CSF with blood and tissue fluid. This surgical procedure produced some positive results completely independent of the duration of the disease. Some surgeons carried out a ventriculo-atrial shunt even in cases where a hydrocephalus internus could not be proved. An indication for the application of a ventriculo-atrial and peritoneal shunt was seen necessary when arachnitis, hydrocephalus and syringomyelia were present and in cases where no decompression was performed. When the ventriculo-atrial shunt was occluded, a second operation involving an exposure of the foramen occipitale magnum and a high cervical laminectomy became necessary.

Gardner et al. recommended in 1977 terminal ventriculostomy. However, a satisfactory operational result was only possible if the cavity covered the whole cervical spine. The methods myelotomy, terminal ventriculostomy and high myelotomy carry only few complications, i. e. they have distinctly less complications than the exposure of the base, but it is not the method of first choice. A disadvantage lies in the fact that this approach could not treat an existing hydrocephalus or correct CSF flow. We reached the conclusion that the decompression by exposure of the base and the dilatation of diverted liquor passages are the methods of choice. In case this should not be sufficient in treating

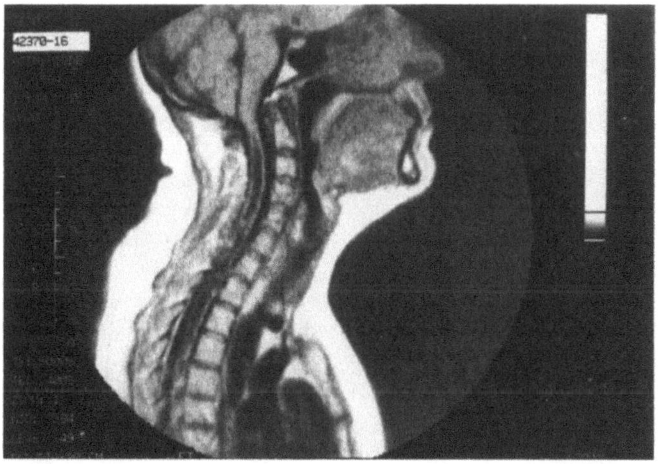

Fig. 1 NMR-findings of a thirty years old woman with syringomyelia in the cervical-thoracal spinal cord (preoperative state).

syringomyelia with hydrocephalus, an additional application of a shunt is necessary. Of course a dilated syrinx is of advantage when a myelotomy is planned and the intervention gives a better result also when the drainage of the cyst can be channeled into a zone of lower pressure, like the subarachnoid space or the peritoneum. Williams' publication in 1983 stated that decompression is not the right procedure if signs of a basal arachnitis or hydrocephalus exist. On the other hand, extopic cerebellar tonsils and craniospinal pressure dissociation justify decompression. However, it seems of great importance to us to point out that the pressure dissociation is responsible for the progression of disease and can only be treated by decompression. These pressure dissociations originate from a displacement of the cisterna magna because of ectopic cerebellar tonsils. A pressure compensation into the external subarachnoid space can be avoided and CSF which is under pressure reaches the slowly dilating central canal via the 4th ventricle, transmitting the pressure wave in a caudal direction. At the non-communicating form the syringo-subarachnoid shunt is the method of choice and we use this procedure since nuclear magnet resonance imaging allows a high rate of correctly assessing extension and maximal distinction of syringomyelia [37, 41].

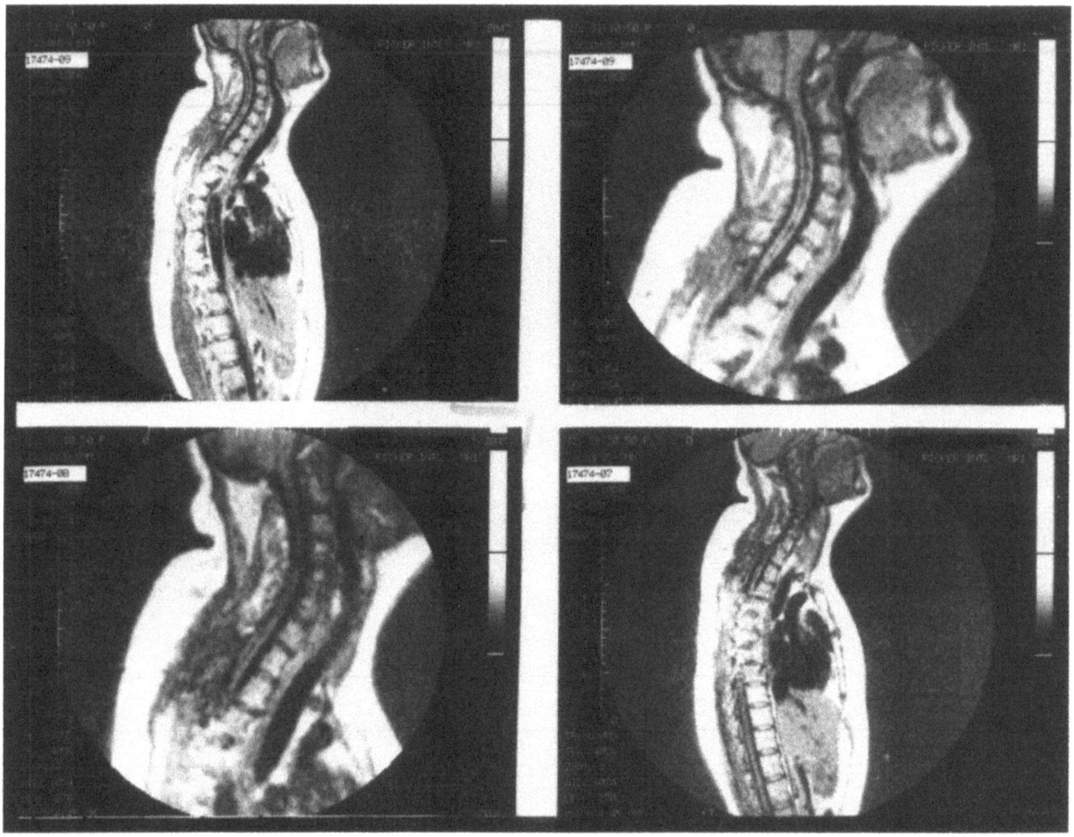

Fig. 2 The same patient: postoperative state.

Case reports

A 30 year old woman had developed a progressive spinal ataxia, a dissociated paralgesia and finally a paraparesis of the legs (fig. 1, 2). During surgical treatment of this non-communicating syringomyelia, a small laminectomy of 1 1/2 vertebrae was made and a microsurgical approach to the syrinx, which was shunted to subarachnoidal space. The spinal ataxia receded almost completely and the paraparesis of the legs as well as the dissociated paralgesia of the upper extremities was minimal and the pain disappeared completely. About four months after the decompression similar complaints as preoperatively were stated and the NMR clearly showed a considerable regression of the spread of the syrinx into the cervical suggesting a shunt failure which will have to be excluded. But if a definite stenosis of the shunt had occurred the syrinx should have again reached the preoperative size and further surgery was excluded.

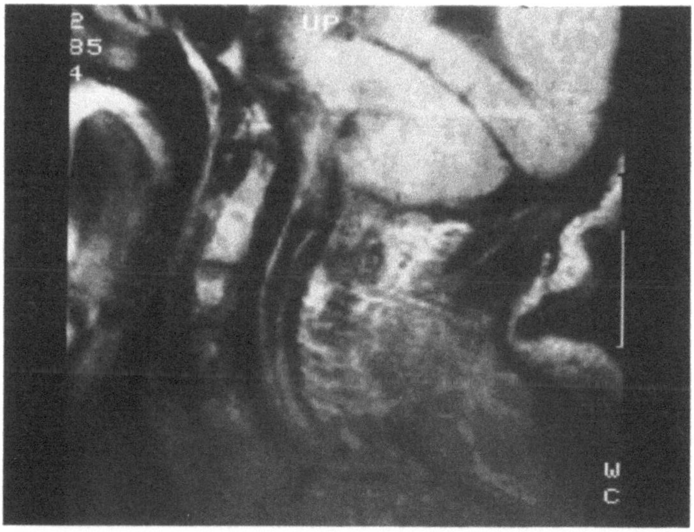

Fig. 3 NMR of a twenty-three years old man with syringobulbia, syringomyelia, Arnold-Chiari-Syndrome.

For discussing the second form of syringomyelia (a communicating syringomyelia with malformation of the base) we describe the case of a 23 year old patient suffering from a syringobulbi, a syringomyelia as well as an Arnold-Chiari-Syndrome, beside a serious kyphoscoliosis requiring a number of orthopedic interventions. It is of interest to note that the patient already suffered as child from a nystagmus, a facial paresis and from a spinal ataxia [25]. The malformation caused extreme kyphoscoliosis, but only the NMR-examination allowed the exact diagnosis and the extent of the malformation (figs. 3, 4). Here we would like to point out that at the age of 10 the boy had all current neuroradiological examinations procedures but no clear diagnosis was possible. We exposed the base, dilated the Foramen magnum, resected the arch of the atlas and fenestrated the outlet of the 4th ventricle. In this way a wide communication of the internal CSF passages with the subarachnoid space was achieved. In addition we performed a longitudinal splitting of the lower medulla and the upper cervical cord, voiding the cyst and shunting it into the subarachnoid space.

Summary

Radiotherapy of syringomyelia is obsolete and the necessary operational choice should be made according to the etiopathogenesis. This is essentially determined by the exact diagnosis bases on NMR imaging which is clearly superior to any other neuroradiological procedures [7, 8, 12, 15, 16, 26–28, 32, 39, 40, 44, 46].

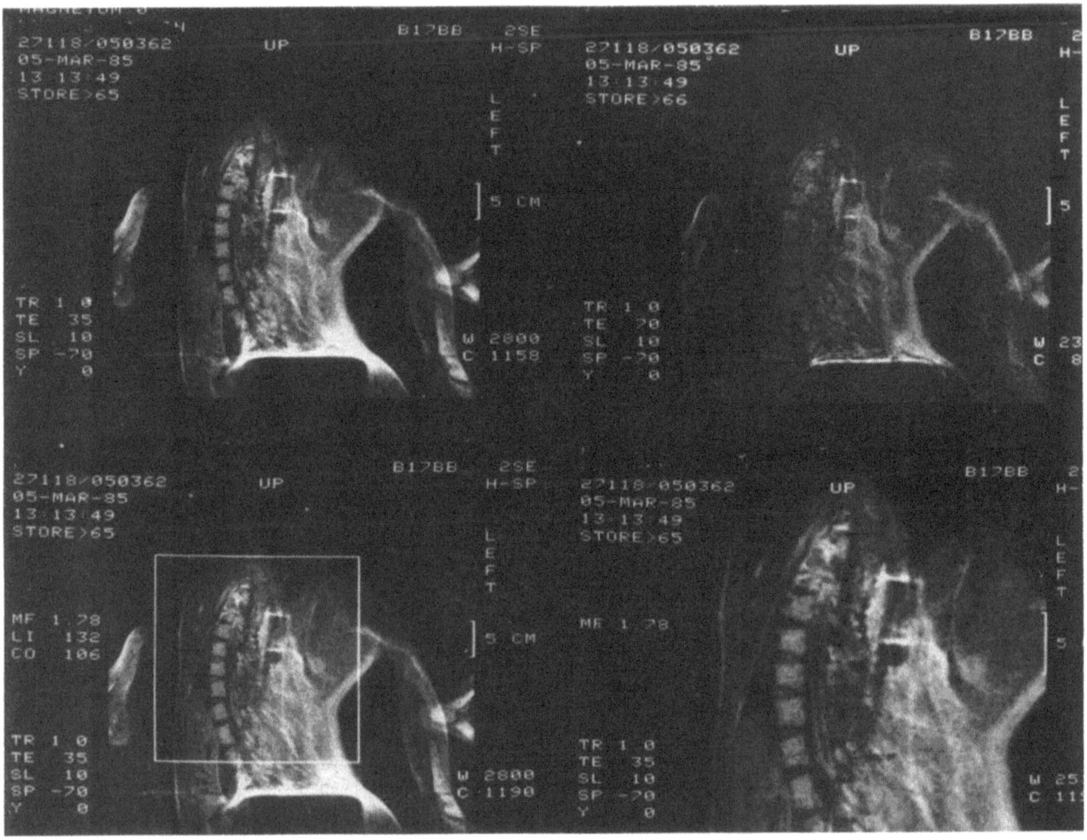

Fig. 4 NMR-findings by the same patient as figure 3 (thoracal spinal cord and extreme kyphoscoliosis).

References

[1] Aichner, F., F. Gerstenbrand, W. Huk, et al.: NMR-tomographie in der Diagnostik der Syringohydromyelie. Nervenarzt **55** (1984) 324 – 327.

[2] Aubin, M. L., J. Vignaud, D. Bar, et al.: Apport de la Scannographie a l'étude des Syringomyélies. Rev. Neurol. (Paris) **136/3** (1980) 271 – 277.

[3] Ballantine, H. T., R. G. Ojemann, J. H. Drew: Syringohydromyelia. Progr. Neurol. Surg. **4** (1971) 227 – 245.

[4] Barraro, N. M., Ch. B. Wilson, Ph. Gutin, et al.: Surgical treatment of syringomyelia. J. Neurosurg. **61** (1984) 531 – 538.

[5] Benini, A., H. Krayenbuehl: Ein neuer chirurgischer Weg zur Behandlung der Hydro- und Syringomyelie. Schweiz. Med. Wochenschr. **99** (1969) 1137 – 1142.

[6] Boman, K., M. Iivanainez: Prognosis of Syringomyelia. Acta Neurol. Scand. **43** (1967) 61 – 68.

[7] Boncaf, A., C. Manelfe, J. Espagno, et al.: Evaluation of syringomyelia with metrizamide computed tomographic myelography. J. Comp. Ass. Tomogr. **4** (1980) 797 – 802.

[8] Brain, R., M. Wilkinson: Cervical arthropathy in syringomyelia, Tabes Dorsalis and Diabetes. Brain **81**, Teil 3 (1958) 275 – 289.

[9] Cahan, L. D., J. Bentson: Considerations in the diagnosis and treatment of syringomyelia and the Chiari malformation. J. Neurosurg. **57** (1982) 24–31.

[10] Conway, L. W.: Radiographic studies of syringomyelia. Trans. Amer. neurol. Ass. XG (1961) 205–209.

[11] Conway, L. W.: Hydrodynamic studies in syringomyelia. J. Neurosurg. **27** (1967) 501–514.

[12] Crolla, D., L. Hens, G. Wilms, et al.: Metrizamide enhanced CT in hydrosyringomyelia. Neurorad. **19** (1980) 39–41.

[13] Crooks, L. E., D. A. Ortendahl, L. Kaufman, et al.: Clinical efficiency of nuclear magnetic resonance imaging. Radiol. **146** (1983) 123–128.

[14] Decker, K.: Über die Roentgenstrahlenbehandlung der Syringomyelie. Strahlenther. **80** (1965) 265–270.

[15] Di Chiro, G., S. P. Axelbaum, D. Schellinger, et al.: Computerized axial tomography in syringomyelia. N. Engl. J. Med. **2** (1975) 13–16.

[16] Di Chiro, G., D. Schellinger: Computed tomography of the spinal cord after lumbar intrathecal introduction of metrizamide (Computer-Assisted Myelography). Radiol. **120** (1976) 101–104.

[17] Dietemann, J. L., E. Babin, A. Wackenheim, et al.: Percutaneous puncture of spinal cysts in the diagnosis and therapy of syringomyelia and cystic tumors. Neurorad. **24** (1982) 59–63.

[18] Droege, R. T., S. N. Wiener, M. S. Rzeszotarski, et al.: Nuclear magnetic resonance: A gray scale model for head images. Radiology **148** (1983) 763–771.

[19] Foster, J. B., P. Hudgson, G. W. Pearce: The association of syringomyelia and congenital cervico-medullary anomalies. Pathological Evidence Brain **92** (1969) 25–34.

[20] Foster, N. L., S. D. Wing, P. F. Bray: Metrizamide ventriculography in syringomyelia. Neurology **30** (1980) 1323–1326.

[21] Garcia-Uria, J., G. Leundia, R. Carillo, et al.: Syringomyelia: long-term results after posterior fossa decompression. J. Neurosurg. **54** (1981) 380–383.

[22] Gardner, W. J., L. J. Karnosch: Syringomyelia, 144–145, Cleveland, Ohio.

[23] Hall, P., M. Turner, S. Aichinger, et al.: Experimental syringomyelia. J. Neurosurg. **52** (1980) 812–817.

[24] Hertel, G.: The width of the cervical spinal cord and the size of the vertebral bodies in Syringomyelia. Eur. Neurol. **9** (1973) 168–182.

[25] Hopf, H. C., H.-J. Hufschmidt, G. Schaltenbrand: Elektromyographische Untersuchungen bei Syringomyelie und amyotrophischer Lateralsklerose. Dtsch. Z. Nervenheilkd. **168** (1965) 529–540.

[26] Hutchins, W. W., R. L. Vogelzang, H. L. Neinan, et al.: Differentation of tumor from syringohydromyelia: Intraoperative neurosonography of the spinal cord. Radiology **151** (1984) 171–174.

[27] Jenkins, J. P. R., D. S. Hickey, X. P. Zhu, et al.: MR-Imaging of the intervertebral disc: a quantitative study. Br. J. Radiol. **58** (1985) 705–709.

[28] Kan, S., A. J. Fox, F. Vinuela, et al.: Spinal cord size in syringomyelia: Change with position of metrizamide myelography. Radiology **146** (1983) 409–414.

[29] Kempe, L. G.: Cervical Laminectomy. Neurosurgery **2** (1970) 98–107.

[30] Love, A. G., R. Olafson: Syringomyelia: A look at surgical therapy. J. Neurosurg. **24** (1966) 714–718.

[31] Maeder, R. P., M. Mumenthaler, H. Markwalder: Symptomatische zervikale Syringomyelie. Dtsch. Med. Wochenschr. **95** (1970) 164–168.

[32] Marin, G.: Matters arising. J. Neurol. Neurosurg. Psychiatry **36** (1983) 365–367.

[33] Modic, M. T., M. A. Weinstein, W. Pavlicek, et al.: Nuclear Magnetic Resonance-imaging of the spine. Radiology **148** (1983) 757–762.

[34] Newman, Terenty, Foster: Some observations on the pathogenesis of syringomyelia. J. Neurol. Neurosurg. Psychiatry **44** (1981) 964–969.

[35] Pearce, J. M. S.: Surgical management of syringomyelia. Br. Med. J. **283** (1981) 1204–1205.

[36] Perot, P., R. Musella: Observations on the pathogenesis and surgical treatment of syringomyelia. Neurochirurgia **8** (1965) 90 – 97.

[37] Pitts, W. F., R. A. Groff: Syringomyelia: Current status of surgical therapy. Surgery (1964) 806 – 809.

[38] Pojunas, K., A. L. Williams, D. L. Daniels, et al.: Syringomyelia and hydromyelia: Magnetic resonance evaluation. Radiology **153** (1984) 679 – 683.

[39] Pullicino, P., B. E. Kendall: Computed tomography of "cystic" intramedullary lesions. Neuroradiology **23** (1982) 117 – 121.

[40] Resjoe, M., D. C. Harwood-Nash, C. R. Fitz, et al.: Computed tomographic metrizamide Myelography in Syringohydromyelia. Radiology **131** (1979) 405 – 407.

[41] Scheid, W.: Die Syringomyelie. In: Lehrbuch der Neurologie und Psychiatrie. 5. Aufl. Thieme Stuttgart 1983.

[42] Schielp, G.: Probleme der Syringomyelie. Fortschr. Neurol. Psych. **47** (1979) 557 – 608.

[43] Schürmann, K., M. Brock, H. J. Reulen, D. Voth: Cerebello Pontine Angle Tumors. Adv. in Neurosurg. 1, Springer, Berlin – Heidelberg 1973.

[44] Sotaniemi, K. A., J. Pyktinen, V. V. Myllylá: Computed tomography in the diagnosis of syringomyelia. Acta Neurol. Scand. **68** (1983) 121 – 127.

[45] Tator, Ch., K. Meguor, D. Rowed: Favorable results with syringosubarachnoid shunts for treatment of syringomyelia. J. Neurosurg. **56** (1982) 517 – 523.

[46] Thomas, A., P. G. Morris: The effects of NMR exposure on living organisms. I. A. microbial assay. Br. J. Radiol. (1980) 615 – 621.

[47] Toennis, W., H. Olivecrona: Syringomyelie und Hydromyelie, pp. 335 – 338. In: Handbuch der Neurochirurgie 7, 1. Teil, IV. Springer, 1969.

[48] Van der Bergh, R., I. Dehaene: New concepts in the neurosurgical treatment of syringomyelia. Acta Neurochir. **26** (1972) 352.

[49] West, R. j., B. Williams: Radiographic studies of the ventricles in syringomyelia. Neuroradiology **20** (1980) 5 – 16.

[50] Williams, B., G. Fahy: A critical appraisal of "terminal ventriculostomy" for the treatment of syringomyelia. J. Neurosurg. **58** (1983) 188 – 197.

[51] Yeates, A., M. Brant-Zawadzki, D. Norman, et al.: Nuclear Magnetic Resonance imaging of syringomyelia. AJNR **4** (1983) 234 – 237.

Bilateral microsurgical accessoriolysis for the treatment of spasmodic torticollis

N. Freckmann, H.-D. Herrmann

Introduction

Since 1980 the bilateral microsurgical accessoriolysis (BMA) has been performed on 33 patients for treatment of spasmodic torticollis (ST) [4, 5].

In our opinion a peripheral cause is usually present in the aetiology of ST, especially if it is of the purely horizontal type. Findings which point towards a central cause of the disease are not available. In contrast to our previous view however, we now assume that the development of ST is based on a pathology in the afferent, but not in the efferent part of head control. It cannot be verified, that neurovascular relation of the spinal accessory nerve roots (SRAN) might be causal as in other cranial nerve dysfunction syndromes. Against this view are recent findings of Lang who showed that the oligodendral segment of the accessory nerve (AN) is extremely short [9].

On the other hand the assumption of a pathogenic factor in the *afferent* part of head control is supported by the results of this follow up study.

Patients and methods

All patients (22 male, 11 female) suffered from a severe ST with involuntary spastic movements of the head towards one side. They had been selected from more than 200 outpatients. Conservative treatment had been unsuccessfull and 24 patients were incapable of working. Signs of torsion dystonia were not present in any of the patients prior to surgery.

The mean age of the patients at the onset of the disease was 37.7 years. The average duration of the disease until surgical intervention was 3.8 years. The average length of postsurgical evaluation is 3.1 years. In 22 patients the torticollis was predominantly horizontal (12 to the right, 10 to the left). Two patients suffered from a rotatory torticollis with inclination of the head towards the right. 9 patients showed combined symptoms with involvement of deep neck muscles. A rotatory-horizontal torticollis was found in 5 patients, a retrocollis with a horizontal component in 3 patients and an antecollis with rotatory component in 1 patient (tab. 1). Of these 9 patients 4 suffered additionally from pain syndroms in the neck and arm. 11 patients could influence their symptoms by the "Counterpressure Sign".

Table 1 Torticollis-patients treated by BMA

Case	Sex	Age	Symptoms	Dir.	Type of A N.-Cl-Anastomosis right	Type of A N.-Cl-Anastomosis left	Fol-low-up (ms)	Assessment of Results Physicians	Assessment of Results Patients	Dys-tonic
1	m	37	horizontal	r	I	–	64	excellent	excellent	
2	m	21	horizontal	l	–	III	63	good	–	
3	m	47	horizontal	r	III	IV	59	improved	improved	
4	f	46	horizontal	r	IV	III	56	good	good	
5	m	52	horizontal	l	IV	I	46	unchanged	⊞	
6	m	22	horizontal	r	II	III	52	good	good	
7	m	36	horizontal	l	IV	IV	52	good	improved	
8	m	26	horizontal	l	IV	IV	49	excellent	excellent	
9	m	42	horizontal	l	IV	IV	47	excellent	excellent	
10	f	25	horizontal	r	IV	IV	40	improved	–	
11	m	41	horizontal	l	IV	III	39	good	good	
12	m	51	horizontal	l	IV	III	39	good	good	
13	m	47	horizontal	r	IV	IV	38	improved	unchanged	
14	m	39	horizontal	r	IV	III	37	improved	improved	
15	f	38	horizontal	r	II	III	34	excellent	excellent	
16	f	47	horizontal	r	III	III	28	good	good	
17	m	45	horizontal	r	III	IV	26	excellent	excellent	
18	m	57	horizontal	l	I	I	15	good	good	
19	m	41	horizontal	r	IV	III	13	improved	improved	
20	f	50	horizontal	l	IV	III	9	improved	improved	
21	f	24	horizontal	r	III	III	8			
22	m	54	horizontal	r	IV	IV	3	improved	improved	
23	f	49	rotatory	r	IV	IV	57	good	improved	
24	m	41	rotatory	r	IV	IV	41	improved	⊞	
25	f	48	rot/hor	r	IV	I	42	unchanged	unchanged	×
26	f	54	rot/hor	l	IV	I	31	improved	unchanged	
27	m	41	rot/hor	l	IV	I	28	unchanged	unchanged	
28	m	30	rot/hor	l	III	IV	22	worsened	worsened	×
29	m	51	rot/hor	l	IV	III	20	improved	unchanged	
30	f	40	rot/ante	r	IV	IV	26	worsened	unchanged	×
31	m	37	retro/hor	r	–	III	64	improved	improved	×
32	f	55	retro/hor	r	IV	IV	56	improved	unchanged	
33	m	42	retro/hor	r	III	IV	13	improved	unchanged	
	m	43	retro/hor	r	III	IV	2	⊞	⊞	

Preoperative evaluations

Besides the clinical investigation the patients received EMG, computed tomography (CT) and angiography. In 11 out of 25 patients the angiography of the vertebral arteries revealed a low origin of the PICA with a caudally loop, sometimes extending below the foramen magnum. Because there were no additional anomalies, we no longer perform angiography. CT did not give any clues which could have been helpful in establishing a morphological correlation for the disease.

Operative technique

The operations were performed in prone position under general anaesthesia. A small suboccipital craniotomy as well as a laminectomy of C1 was carried out. After longitudinal incision of the dura, the spinal as well as the cranial roots of the AN can be inspected on both sides as far down as C2. Under the operating microscope we especially look for anastomoses between SRAN and the dorsal roots of the first and second cervical nerve (DRC 1/2). These anastomoses are cut while preserving the radicular arteries. If present, DRC 1 was cut bilaterally and sometimes removed. In addition SRAN was freed on both sides from all adhesions and vascular contacts. In some cases the SRAN was protected from vascular contacts by inserting a small teflon-sponge.

Operative findings

In analogy to a previous anatomical study on non selected postmortem specimens [7], our torticollis patients showed a high variety of anatomical relationships in the cranio-cervical region. Especially remarkable were numerous relationships of DRC 1 and to a lesser extent also of DRC 2 with the SRAN. According to Quaknine 4 types can be destinguished [11]:

Type I: Lack of DRC 1 (fig. 1),
Type II: Normal course of DRC 1,
Type III: DRC 1 has an anastomosis with SRAN,
Type IV: DRC 1 anastomoses with SRAN without direct connection to the spinal cord (fig. 2).

Following incidences were noted, Type I 7 times, Type II 2 times, Type III 19 times, Type IV 35 times on 63 sides (3 cases were not inspected bilaterally). In many cases we found a small ganglion next to the anastomosis, sometimes on the SRAN, more often on DRC 1. In Type IV SRAN frequently was pulled into the intervertebral foramen of C1 with tight adhesion to the vertebral artery.

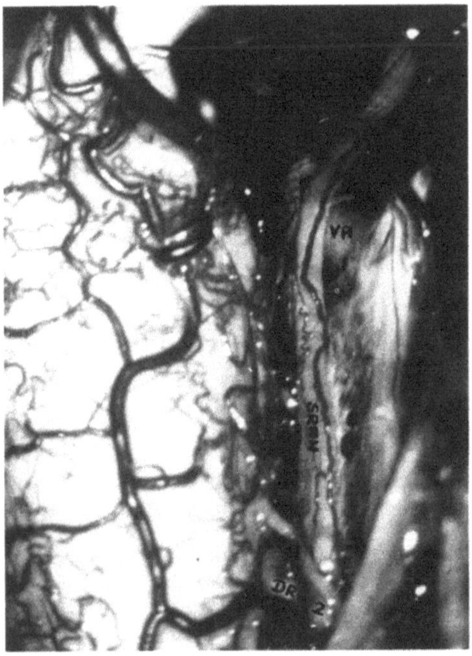

Fig. 1

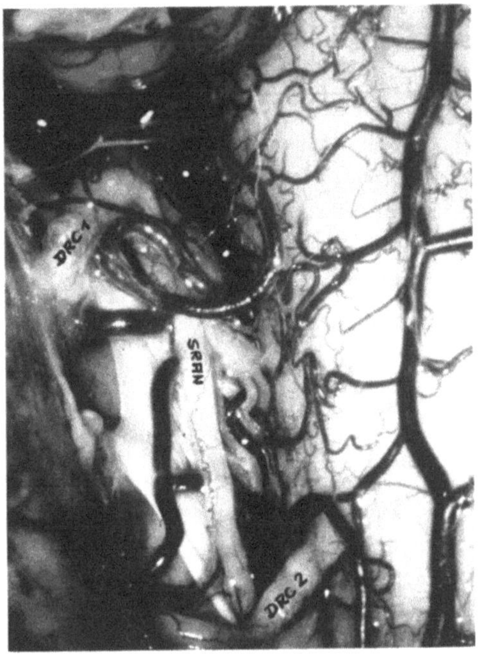

Fig. 2

Fig. 1 Relationship of the SRAN to DRC 1. Right side: Type I (Lack of DRC 1). VA: Vertebral artery.

Fig. 2 Relationship of the SRAN to DRC 1. Left side: Type IV (DRC 1 anastomoses with SRAN without direct connection to the spinal cord).

Postoperative evaluation

After surgery all patients were re-examined at regular intervals. In most cases surgical treatment was followed by an extensive physical therapy and if necessary by medical treatment with Dartalan or Xylotocan. Ambulatory controls were done 6, 9 and 12 months post surgery. In June 1985 we sent out questionaires for self-evaluating the effectiveness of the surgical intervention. Simultaneously all patients were asked to show up for a follow up study.

Results

Three of our patients have died. One patient underwent a second operation 13 months after the first intervention because the symptoms had little improved. Two weeks after surgery this patient developed medullary symptoms with severe respiratory insufficiency of which he died. The other patients died 3 1/2 and 4 years respectively after surgery from unrelated causes (asthma attack/intoxication). 28 patients returned their questionnaires. Two patients had moved and no address is available. Of these patients only those results from the first year follow up are included.

Evaluation of the questionaires showed that in 5 cases the result was "excellent". 7 patients rated the surgical result as "good", 8 patients described their status as "improved". In 7 patients no improvement of the symptoms was noted and one patient noted a deterioration.

We marked as an „excellent" result if the patient has no residual symptoms or pain, as "good" if the patient can keep his head voluntary straight without pain for a longer duration and is able to move it in all directions. We consider as "improved" if the patient still experiences some involuntary movements of the head in particular if attention is distracted by other activities. Compared to the pre-operative state these symptoms have to be markedly reduced and should be voluntarly suppressable.

Side effects related to the surgical procedure were described by 4 patients. In all cases there were unilateral pareses of the AN of varying degree.

The outpatient follow up revealed the following results: together with our own rating of the last reports of those two patients who could not be traced and those two who died from an unrelated cause, 5 results were rated as "excellent", 7 as "good", 12 as "improved". In three patients the symptoms were regarded as "unchanged", in two patients a deterioration was noted, one patient died due to the treatment. 19 patients worked, 5 patients were still incapable of working and 6 patients have retired (tab. 2). In accord with those patients in whom torticollis symptoms had improved we observed a reversal of the symptoms in most cases only as late as 6 to 9 months after surgery.

Table 2 Results of BMA for treatment of spasmodic torticollis

	Excellent	Good	Improved	Unchanged	Deteriorated	Died	Side-Effects
Patients Assessment (n = 29)	5 (17%)	7 (24%)	8 (28%)	7 (24%)	1 (3%)		4 (14%)
		20 (69%)		8 (28%)		1 (3%)	
Clinical Assessment (n = 33)	5 (15%)	10 (30%)	12 (36%)	3 (9%)	2 (6%)	1 (3%)	4 (12%)
		27 (82%)		5 (15%)		1 (3%)	

Relating the results to the preoperative torticollis symptoms it can be shown that the purely horizontal torticollis was most susceptible to operation, and 21 out of 22 patients had improved. Also those two patients who had a purely rotatory torticollis did well. The results are bad however, in those 9 patients with combined symptoms. There was no improvement in 5 cases or even in 8 cases in the patient's own evaluation. In 4 of these patients we observed a spread of symptoms in the postoperative course very much like a torsion dystonia (tab. 1).

Discussion

Fitzgerald has shown in rats and mice that the entire motor supply to the sternocleidomastoid as well as to the rostral trapezius was from the SRAN. The sensory supply to the spindles in these muscles however was from the upper cervical spinal nerves. This indicates that the SRAN and the DRCs, DRC 1 and DRC 2 particularly form a closely connected functional system [2].

In humans this is indicated by the existence of intraspinal anastomoses between SRAN and DRC 1/2 [3, 7, 8, 11]. In agreement with other investigators Lang frequently found a small ganglion of DRC 1 next to these anastomoses as well as ganglionic cells within the SRAN [5, 8, 9]. These findings lead to the speculation that those ganglionic cells function as extension receptors of the sternocleidomastoid and trapezius muscle. Therefore the removal of these ganglia may influence torticollis symptoms [9].

It seems therefore justified to assume that a unilateral disturbance of proprioceptive afferents from the upper cervical joints and from the muscle spindles of the AN supplied muscles can cause a centrally controlled compensatory distortion of the head.

When comparing our findings in 50 postmortem evaluations of otherwise normal patients with those in our torticollis patients, we were surprised to find anastomoses between SRAN and DRC 1 intraoperatively twice as often as in the autopsy cases in 87% of the cases [3]. These findings however demonstrate well that this cannot be the only cause for development of ST. One would rather to assume that there is an anatomical disposition towards ST which in adult life will lead to the manifestation of this disease without any obvious cause, affecting men more often than women.

Svien and Cody in 1969 reported exellent results in 6 torticollis patients by means of unilateral iontophoresis of the middle ear. The idea was to suppress afferent impulses from the utriculus to Deiter's nucleus for restoring the balance in the neck-righting reflexes [12]. The fact, that it is possible to influence torticollis symptoms by diminishing afferent impulses from the utriculus shows the complexity of head control. It also indicates the possibility of a peripheral pathogenic factor which may be located in the afferent system of head control.

Based on our operative findings ST can be regarded as a disorder of proprioceptive input, possibly caused by mechanical irritation of the anastomoses between SRAN and DRC 1/2. The histological investigation of some DRC 1 in most cases revealed signs of de- and regeneration probably due to chronic irritation. In addition to a small ganglion next to the anastomosis we sometimes found a small neuroma or significant proliferations of Schwann cells.

Assuming a unilateral irritation or lesion of the afferent system for head control to be a leading cause in the aetiology of ST, our operative aim is to diminish the flow of proprioceptive impulses from the craniocervical region. This has to be done bilaterally to balance the cerebral input from the upper cervical joints as well as from the muscle spindles of the AN supplied muscles.

The delayed reversal of torticollis symptoms is not necessarily contradictory to our hypothesis. It can be explained by the persistance of "wrong" movement patterns which have been established over many years. Therefore we emphasize the importance of a special physical training after surgery for a longer period.

However there is a remarkable clear difference in the operative outcome of those patients with purely horizontal torticollis symptoms indicating involvement of the AN dependent muscles only and those patients with combined torticollis symptoms which suggests also an involvement of muscles supplied by the cervical plexus. It appears justified to separate two different entities which is in agreement also with the postoperative course of four out of nine patients with combined torticollis symptoms. These patients most likely suffer from dystonia of central origin. Only one patient subjectively did well (tab. 1). In those cases a stereotactical treatment has to be considered.

Based on the long-term follow up, we believe, that BMA is justified in those patients with purely horizontal torticollis symptoms. In comparison with other surgical procedures, with the exception of the high cervical DCS, the BMA is relatively less invasive [10]. Moreover it only has a limited risk of adverse side reactions.

In case the operation does not result in a satisfactory improvement, the selective peripheral denervation of single motor branches of the cervical nerves as described by Bertrand might has to be considered, although it is a destructive intervention. Bertrand reported good results in 31 of 35 patients [1]. A repeated exposure of the SRAN should not be performed, because of the increased operative risk. From our own experience the Foerster/Dandy operation, sterotactical procedures or even cervical DCS cannot be recommended because of the bad results or the severe disabling side effects.

Despite a 10% difference in the assessment of postoperative improvement between the involved physicians and the patients in this study, there is a good agreement between external and self evaluation in respect to the benefits from this surgical procedure.

Conclusions

The cause for development of horizontal ST is probably located in the cranio-cervical region. This assumption is supported by the great number of anastomoses between SRAN and DRC 1, which indicates an anatomical disposition. We believe, that an unilateral lesion of proprioceptive afferents in the region of the SRAN can produce torticollis symptoms. BMA consequently should result in a balance of cerebral input and therefore in a suppression of overbearing unilateral motor impulses. The different outcome of patients with horizontal and patients with combined torticollis symptoms indicates a different etiology. In future BMA should be limited to cases with a purely horizontal ST.

References

[1] Bertrand, C., P. Molina Negro, S. N. Martinez: Technical aspects of selective peripheral denervation for spasmodic torticollis. Appl. Neurophysiol. **45** (1982) 326–330.

[2] Fitzgerald, M. J. T., P. T. Comerford, A. R. Tuffery: Sources of innervation of the neuromuscular spindles in sternomastoid and trapezius. J. Anat. **134** (1982) 471–490.

[3] Freckmann, N., R. Hagenah: Relationship between the spinal accessory nerve root and the posterior root of the first cervical nerve in spasmodic-torticollis and common autopsy cases. Zbl. Neurochir. (in press).

[4] Freckmann, N., R. Hagenah, H.-D. Herrmann, et al.: Spasmodic torticollis-follow up and results after microsurgical lysis of the spinal accessory nerve roots. Acta Neurochir. **68** (1983) 154.

[5] Freckmann, N., R. Hagenah, H.-D. Herrmann, et al.: Treatment of neurogenic torticollis by microvascular lysis of the accessory nerve roots-indication, technique, and first results. Acta Neurochir. **59** (1981) 167–175.

[6] Hagenah, R., C. Habich, D. Müller, et al.: Subjektive Beurteilung der Wirkung operativer Therapieverfahren beim Torticollis spasmodicus. Psycho. **9** (1983) 320–321.

[7] Hagenah, R., M. Kosak, N. Freckmann: Anatomic topographical relationship of the intraspinal accessory root to the upper cervical roots and to the vessels of the cranial-cervical region. Acta ant. **115** (1983) 158–167.

[8] Lang, J.: Funktionelle Anatomie der Halswirbelsäule und des benachbarten Nervensystems. In: Halswirbelsäulenerkrankungen mit Beteiligung des Nervensystems (Hohmann, D., B. Kügelgen, K. Liebig, et al., eds.) Springer-Verlag, Berlin – Heidelberg – New York – Tokyo 1983.

[9] Lang, J.: Über Bau, Länge und Gefäßbeziehungen der "zentralen" und "peripheren" Strecken der intrazisternalen Hirnnerven. Zbl. Neurochir. **43** (1982) 217–255.

[10] Motomochi, M., J. Makita, S. Nabeshima, et al.: Spasmodic torticollis – surgical treatments and long-term results. Neurol. Med. Chir. (Tokyo) **23** (1983) 741–746.

[11] Quaknine, G., H. Nathan: Anastomotic connection between the eleventh nerve and the posterior root of the first cervical nerve in humans. J. Neurosurg. **38** (1973) 189–197.

[12] Svien, H. J., D. T. R. Cody: Treatment of spasmodic torticollis by supression of labyrinthine activity. Mayo Clin. Proc. **44** (1969) 825–827.

Irritation of upper cervical nerve roots as a cause of hemicrania

J. Jansen, J. Hildebrandt

Introduction

The causes of many forms of hemicrania (one-sided headache) are unknown; classification is based on varieties of clinical disease progression. A clearer definition is impeded by our lack in understanding the aetiology.

The inclusion of occipital headaches or so-called occipital neuralgias among the cervical radiculopathies is difficult to understand. The reasons for this lie in the shortcomings of the radiological and electrophysiological diagnostic methods available at present. There is no radiological or electrophysiological evidence at all for any compression symptomatics of the C2 roots. Extremely rarely do degenerative changes and disc prolapses occur at the level of the intervertebral spaces between cervical vertebrae 2 and 3, or between 3 and 4 produce a root compression syndrome at levels C3 or C4. These facts only partially explain why irritation of an upper cervical root causing hemicrania is unknown. Frontal and peri-ocular pain do not occur in the area supplied by the upper cervical roots, but rather in the area supplied by the ophthalmic branch of the trigeminal nerve. Nonetheless, the character of fronto-ocular pain, described as unilateral, severe, dull and pessing, but otherwise difficult to differentiate and localise, cannot be mistaken for trigeminal neuralgia.

In 1975 we observed the first indication of a connection between nerve root compression and hemicrania showing mainly fronto-ocular pain. This occured in a patient with a prolapsed disc and a root compression at level C3. The patient complained of intolerable, predominantly fronto-ocular pain; at neurological examination only reduced sensation was found in the cutaneous distribution area of C3. A unilateral pain response was present to pressure at the occipital nerve exit. Disc prolapse was proven by cervical myelography. The patient was free of pain immediately after operation (by the ventral approach) to relieve compression of root C3 by fusion of cervical vertebral bodies 2 and 3.

Findings at operation

In other cases, irritation or compression of nerve roots C3 and C4 were due to: a neurinoma (C3), disc prolapses with arthrotic spondylosis (C3 and C4),

Table 1 Origin of upper cervical nerve root irritation (compression) effecting unilateral hemicrania (operative findings)

Origin of irritation (compression)	Nerve root C_2	C_3	C_4	Total
Vasogenic: network of widened veins	4			4
– with arterial supply	1			1
loop of radicular artery	1			1
Tumor (neurinoma)		1		1
Disc herniation with spondylarthrosis		1	1	2
Spondylarthrosis			1	1
Scar tissue		1		1
Total	6	3	2	11

respectively, and finally, scar tissue surrounding root C 3 in a patient known for many years to have arachnoitis spinalis.

Each example of irritation of root C 2 was due to vasogenic compression. In other cases, irritation of these roots was caused by a plexus of enlarged veins (4 patients); enclosure amongst dilated veins with inflow from an artery (1 patient); and, finally, an arterial sling pressed against the ganglion of C 2 by the close neighbouring arch of vertebra C 1 (tab. 1).

Clinical findings

Which complaints are included under the heading of unilateral hemicrania? (tab. 2).

One-sided headache over the eye or forehead, diffuse and poorly localisable in nature, was foremost in many patients [7]. Less commonly, such headaches were accompanied by occipital pain of equal intensity [2]. Only infrequently did occipital pain outweigh frontal pain [2].

Episodic headaches, beginning slowly, gradually increasing to intolerable levels and lasting for hours, then spontaneously diminishing, were the complains of all patients with a vasogenic compression of root C 2 [6], as also by a patient with the compression by scar tissue. In contrast to this the other 4 patients reported permanent headaches.

Table 2 Symptoms and neurologic deficits in patients suffering from hemicrania

Origin of irritation (compression)	Patients (male = m, female = f)	Unilateral hemicrania fr.	p.-o.	t.-p.	occ.	Ipsilateral: conjunctival injection = ci lacrimation = l blurred vision = by		Neck stiffness = ns reduced motility = rm	Neurological deficits = nd	painful occipital nerve-compression = ponc
Vasogenic: network of widened veins	H. P. 24 f	++	++	++	++	–	hemicrania-attacks = h-a	ns, rm	nd: –	ponc: +
	B. O. 36 m	++	++	+	+	ci, l		ns, rm	nd: –	ponc: +
	D. G. 45 m	+	++	+	+	ci, l, bv		ns, rm	nd: –	ponc: +
	U. W. 45 f	++	++	+	+	ci, l, bv		ns, rm	nd: –	ponc: +
– with arterial supply	R. F. 74 m	++	++	+	+	ci, l		ns, rm	nd: –	ponc: +
loop of radicular artery	I. B. 55 f	++	++	++	++	ci, l		∅	nd: –	ponc: +
Tumor (neurinoma)	G. W. 55 f	+	+	+	++	–	permanent hemicrania	rm	nd: C_3-hypaesthesia	ponc: +
Disc herniation with spondylarthrosis	R. K. 42 m	+	+++	+	+	ci, l, bv		ns, rm	nd: C_3-hypaesthesia	ponc: +
	G. A. 47 m	+	+	++	++	–		ns, rm	nd: –	ponc: +
Spondylarthrosis (multilocalized)	S. N. 62 m	++	++	+	+	–	h-a	ns, rm	nd: –	ponc: +
Scar tissue	G. P. 52 m	++	+++	++	+	–		ns, rm	nd: –	ponc: +

When asked about the character of the pain, the patients unanimously describe the pain in the occipital region as tearing, cutting and sometimes throbbing in synchrony with the pulse. In contrast, pain in the temporal region is described not only as sharp but also as dull. 10 patients described pain in the forehead as dull and pressing; only one patient complained of a tearing pain. In the peri- and retro-ocular region the pain is always dull, pressing, diffuse, and difficult to localize.

The results of neurological examinations provided little information for the diagnosis. All patients had stiffness of the neck and restricted movement of the cervical spine. In all patients the occipital nerve exit points were sensitive to pressure. Sensory disturbances in the form of a hypaesthesia indicated the localization of a root irritation in one patient with a neurinoma of root C3 and in one patient with prolapsed disc at C2/C3. Other neurological features were insignificant.

Diagnostics

X-ray diagnostics with and without contrast media, and including computer tomography, were only of value in those cases where the patient had a tumour. Two patients suffered from prolapsed discs, and in one patient was root compression, caused by arthrotic spondylosis (tab. 3).

Tests to provoke or abolish pain were of benefit in those cases where patients had vasogenic root compression of C2 [6], and for the patient with compression caused by scar tissue around root C3. Ergotamine abolished the pain in 5 patients with vasogenic root compression of C2, and reduced it in one patient.

Oxygen inhalation abolished pain in 4 patients with vasogenic C2 compression, and in one case even reduced provoked as well as spontaneous attacks of pain.

Nitroglycerine (0.8 mg Nitrolingual® sublingually) could trigger unilateral pain attacks together with accompanying symptoms, during pain-free intervals in all patients with vasogenic root compression [6]. In 5 patients with roots enveloped in densely interwoven strongly dilated veins the attack reached full strength; in the patient with a spinal ganglion compressed by an arterial loop, the attack followed an abortive course.

Where irritation of the upper cervical roots was suspected, selective or combined blockade of the roots was carried out, to aid diagnostic differentiation and localization (9 patients). Under radiological control, a local anaesthetic is applied topically to the periganglionic and perineural region of the nerve root. The exact localization of the cannula is checked both by mechanical and electrical stimulation of the root prior to such conduction block. It is possible to provoke

Table 3 Diagnostic findings in patients suffering from hemicrania

Origin of irritation (compression)	Patients (male = m, female = f)	CT or X-ray		Symptoms				
				Loss			Provocation	
		native	contrast	O_2-inhalation	Ergotamine	Root anaesthesia	Nitroglycerine	Root anaesthesia + nitroglycerine
Vasogenic: network of widened veins	H. P. 24 f	–	∅	+	+	+	+	–
	B. O. 36 m	–	∅	+	+	+	+	–
	D. G. 45 m	–	–	(+)	+	+	+	–
	U. W. 45 f	–	∅	+	+	+	+	–
– with arterial supply	R. F. 74 m	–	∅	+	+	+	+	–
loop of radicular artery	I. B. 55 f	–	∅	∅	(+)	+	(+)	–
Tumor (neurinoma)	G. W. 55 f	+	+	∅	∅	∅	∅	∅
Disc herniation with spondyl-arthrosis	R. K. 42 m	+	+	∅	∅	∅	∅	∅
	G. A. 47 m	+	+	∅	∅	+	∅	∅
Spondylarthrosis (multilocalized)	S. N. 62 m	+	+	–	–	+	–	∅
Scar tissue	G. P. 52 m	–	–	∅	∅	+	∅	∅

a pain attack of a kind normally experienced by the patient, during his pain-free intervals. Root blockade was carried out both during such provoked attacks, and also during spontaneous attacks. After 10 – 20 minutes patients were entirely free both of provoked and spontaneous pain. This is accompanied by a numbness in the cutaneous distribution of the nerve root. Freedom from pain and the numbness, both lasted only for as long as the anaesthetic was effective.

During root blockade it was not possible to trigger an attack of pain in any patient by giving nitroglycerine.

Treatment and clinical course

Patients with tumours and those with prolapsed discs were free of pain after surgery. Hemicrania was reduced in the patient with multiple spondylosis (tabl 4).

It was decided to operate patients with vasogenic compression of the nerve root C 2 [6] and scar tissue compression [1] on the basis of the results of pain blockade and provocation; no satisfactory relief had been obtained for these pain-tortured patients during years of conservative treatment.

In the case of the patient with scar tissue compression and a history of arachnoitis spinalis for several years, the root C 3 was freed from the scar tissue. For 12 months after operation the patient was free of this severe pains. Renewed appearance of less intense hemicrania could be reduced by a percutaneous thermorhizotomy; cluster-type headaches remained, which the patient could tolerate without analgesic therapy. In 6 patients a vasogenic nerve root compression of C 2 was discovered at operation: in 4 cases, dilated veins were around the nerve root. In one instance an arterial supply to these veins could be demonstrated. After coagulation of the distended veins the cervical roots were dissected free from the surrounding tissue. In this patient the surrounding veins had deeply indented the root (fig. 1, 1 a). Histological diagnosis was not possible because the tissue removed was totally coagulated. In one patient a U-shaped arterial sling was found, which pressed the ganglion of C 2 against the neighbouring arch of the atlas. Every change in vascular diameter and every pulsation must therefore have been transferred directly to the neighbouring ganglion. This arterial sling was dissected from the ganglion. After partial resection of the arch of the atlas it was cushioned against the ganglion with fibrin foam. In this patient the episodic pulsing hemicrania was absent postoperatively, and she was freed entirely from the remaining permanent hemicrania by thermorhizotomy. It is possible that intraneural fibrotic changes had developed during the period of continual irritation. The patient having a venous root compression with arterial inflow remained free of pain after the operation. Of the 4 patients with venous root compression one patient was freed from pain; one patient experienced

Table 4 Operative treatment and additional thermocoagulation of unilateral hemicrania attacks and permanent hemicrania

Origin of irritation (compression)	Patients (male = m, female = f)	Period of unilateral hemicrania (about)	Post-operative follow-up	Unilateral hemicrania								Preexisting (= p) or remaining (= r) deficits
				Operative treatment				Additional thermo-coagulation (percutan)				
		(years = y, month = m)		Loss	Re-lief	No change	Re-turn	Loss	Re-lief	No change	Re-turn	
Vasogenic: network of widened veins	H. P. 24 f	4 y	8 m	C_2								∅
	B. O. 36 m	4 y	4 y + 5 m		C_2 + C_3					C_3		hemicrania, facial pain region V_{2+3} (p + r)
	D. G. 45 m	2 y	2 y + 1 m	C_2			22 m	will be performed (C_2)				?
	U. W. 45 f	9 y	1 y + 6 m	C_2								tic douloureux V_2, migraine (p + r)
– with arterial supply	R. F. 74 m	25 y	2 y + 6 m	C_2								∅
loop of radicular artery	I. B. 55 f	25 y	9 m		C_2			C_2				∅
Tumor (neurinoma)	G. W. 55 f	2 y	4 m	C_3								∅
Disc herniation with spondylarthrosis	R. K. 42 m	10 y	10 y + 5 m	C_3								∅
	G. A. 47 m	3 y	1/4 m	C_4								∅
Spondylarthrosis (multilocalized)	S. N. 62 m	2 y	1 y + 3 m		C_4							hemicrania (p + r) root compr. syndr. $C_6 + C_7$
Scar tissue	G. P. 52 m	5 y + 8 m	5 y + 6 m	C_3			12 m		C_2			mild temporal cluster headache
Total	11 (4 f + 7 m)			8	3		2	1	2			

reduction of the hemicrania after surgical decompression of C 2 and C 3 and in this case a further improvement was obtained by additional percutaneous thermorhizotomy. But atypical facial pain in the forehead and maxillary region remained. One patient was freed from her episodic severe hemicrania, but not – as could not be expected – from migraine and a tic doloureux which were also present. In the fourth patient with venous root compression pain eventually recurred after 22 months; a percutaneous rhizotomy was performed, after a re-exploration was refused by the patient.

Discussion

11 patients with irritation of an upper cervical nerve root were operated upon. At operation decompression of the root was performed ten times, and in one a tumour was removed. In 3 patients an additional percutaneous thermorhizotomy was necessary. Lasting freedom from pain was achieved in 7 patients, and a further noticeable reduction of pain in two. A recurrence of pain took place in 2 patients, and in both of these percutaneous rhizotomy resulted in improvement. These results indicate that there is a connection between compression or irritation of the upper cervical nerve roots and hemicrania.

The occipital constituent of the pain is easily explained as projected pain caused by an irritation or compression of a root. It is more difficult, however, to understand the fronto-ocular pain. It is distinctly different from to the occipital pain and felt in the distribution of the ophthalmic branch of the trigeminal nerve. However the character of the pain was not comparable to a trigeminal neuralgia.

A number of possible explanations have to be put forward.

1. The subjective impression of a fronto-ocular pain could be projected through afferents, by connections described by Lang [7], between the upper cervical roots (C 2 and C 3) and the vertebral nerves, to the superior cervical ganglion and through the ramus communicans griseus. Alternatively, these afferents could mediate a specific irritation of the fronto-ocular vasculature, which in turn would cause the pain.

2. The following hypothesis seems plausible and is based on investigations by van Valkenburg [8], Escolar [1], Kerr [4, 5] and Kerr and Olafson [6]. Van Valkenburg and Escolar demonstrated functional connections between the afferent neurons of the dorsal horn, the upper cervical nerve roots and the nucleus tracti spinalis of the trigeminal nerve. Kerr could show by means of experimental nerve fibre degeneration that dorsal root neurons terminate in the nucleus tractus spinalis of the trigeminus. Kerr and Olafson showed in the cat that after stimulation of the trigeminal nerve, and after stimulation of the dorsal horn by

microelectrodes, action potentials could be observed in interneurons, suggesting a functional connection.

These investigations explain how an irritation of a nerve root could be transmitted to the lower part of the spinal trigeminal nucleus, which lies at the level of the root entry zone of the upper cervical nerves C 2, C 3, and possibly as low as C 4.

The way in which the facial area is represented in the lower part of the spinal trigeminal nucleus could explain fronto-ocular pain as pain projected to the area of the ophthalmic branch of the trigeminal nerve. The face is represented in an onion-layered fashion in the spinal trigeminal nucleus, the foremost facial region (the fronto-ocular zone) being represented in the lowest part of the nucleus. The representation area of the ophthalmic branch of the trigeminal nerve overlaps with the foremost facial region in the lowest part of the nucleus. This overlap could explain the origin of fronto-ocular pain, since pain transmitted from a nerve root to the lower part of the spinal trigeminal nucleus could therefore be projected to the fronto-ocular region of the face [3].

Summary

The findings at operation show that in addition to the occurance of a tumour, a prolapsed disc, arthrotic spondylosis and/or scar tissue compression, in 6 of 11 patients a vasogenic cause of compression caused nerve root irritation. In five cases the roots were enveloped by dilated and interwoven veins, one vein had an additional arterial feed. In one case a loop of a radicular artery was considered to be the cause of compression. While tumours, a prolapsed disc and arthrotic spondylosis could be largely identified by radiological diagnostics, only root blockade and pharmacological testing were of diagnostic value for vasogenic compression. A connection to the spinal nucleus of the trigeminal nerve probably accounts for the predominantly fronto-ocular pain.

References

[1] Escolar, J.: The efferent sonnections of the 1st, 2nd, and 3rd cervical nerves in the cat. An analysis by Marchi and Radolsky methods. J. Comp. Neurol. **89** (1948) 79–92.

[2] Hildebrandt, J., J. Jansen: Vascular compression of the C 2 and C 3 roots – yet another cause of chronic intermittent hemicrania? Cephalalgia **4** (1984) 167–170.

[3] Jansen, J., O. Spoerri: Atypical frontoorbital pain and headache due to compression of upper cervical roots. In: V. Pfaffenrath, P.-O. Lundberg, O. Sjaastad (eds.): Updating in headache, pp. 14–16. Springer-Verlag, Berlin–Heidelberg 1985.

[4] Kerr, F. W. L.: Atypical facial neuralgias: their mechanism as inferred from anatomic and physiologic data. Proc. Staff. Meetings Mayo Clinic **36** (1961) 254–260.

[5] Kerr, F. W. L.: Structural relation of the trigeminal spinal tract to upper cervical roots and the solitary nucleus in the cat. Exp. Neurol. **4** (1961) 134 – 148.
[6] Kerr, F. W. L., R. A. Olafson: Trigeminal and cervical volleys. Arch. Neurol. **5** (1961) 171 – 178.
[7] Lang, J.: Funktionelle Anatomie der Halswirbelsäule und des benachbarten Nervensystems. In: D. Hohmann, B. Kügelgen, K. Liebig, et al. (eds.): Neuroorthopädie 1, pp. 1 – 118. Springer-Verlag, Berlin – Heidelberg – New York – Tokyo 1983.
[8] Valkenburg, C. T. van: Über die anatomischen und funktionellen Beziehungen der Radix descendens trigemini zum oberen Halsmark. Arch. Neurol. Psychiatr. (Schweiz) **14** (1924) 238 – 254.

V Inflammatory and degenerative lesions

A review of clinical and radiological aspects of rheumatoid arthritis of head joints

F. Schilling

Introduction

The most important inflammations – rheumatic joint diseases of the vertebral column [3] – are chronic polyarthritis (rheumatoid arthritis) with involvement of cervical vertebral and atlanto-axial dislocation and ankylosing spondylitis (Bechterew's disease) resp. the seronegative spondylarthritis. A decisive and important difference between both forms of disease is found in the region of the cervical part of the vertebral column. In case of a spondylarthritis (ASp.) the ankylopoietica type includes the cervical vertebrae but the chronic polyarthritis (RA) is usually limited to the cervical vertebral spine. The incidence in both types (RA and ASp.) of cervical involvement is about 30%.

In order to give a sufficiently complete account of the underlying disease process a description of rheumatoid cervical arthritis will be given first before embarking on destructive and dislocating arthritis of the cranio-cervical function [1] (arthritis of the head and neck joints) (tab. 1).

Table 1 Classification of cervical – medullary syndromes in cervical vertebral arthritis

I. Signs of arterial impairment (vertebral, basilary, spinal and root arteries)	
II. Signs of stenosis the spinal canal at level	
1. Foramen magnum (odentoid process invagination)	upper stenosis
2. Atlas (ventral dislocation)	upper stenosis
3. Subaxial, lower stenosis	
III. Nerve root compression and traction	

Rheumatoid cervical vertebrae arthritis

While the rest of axial skeleton is generally spared from inflammation, the cervical part of the column will be attacked. This is most likely due to the presence of closely associated polysynovial systems of 18 joints, six of those acting in a hinchlike manner in the cervico-occipital region behaving like a '5th extremity' and are the prey of polyarthritic destruction. In view of the static and dynamic speciality of these joints (both vertical load carrying but moveable) and the highly differentiated pattern of movements, the polyarthritic cervical spine loses its function as a stable but mobile component of the vertebral column.

In all chronic cases of polyarthritis 35 – 50% of all patients show clinical vertebral symptoms mainly involving the cervical spine. Signs of an 'inflammatory cervical syndrome' are found in 40% of the patients. These signs involve impairment of (painful) rotation and tilting. In cases of head joints involvement and torticollis in fixed position, clicks when nodding, radiating neural root pains are symptoms of a cervical inflammatory process. Further signs can be an agonising pain in the neck originating from 2nd nerve and extending behind the ears, including radiating pain from corresponding neural segments. These clinical symptoms can be augmented by the pathology of cord compression. The frequency of atlanto-axial dislocation in chronic polyarthritis varies between 10 and 60% depending on the choice of statistical evaluation methods. The dislocation frequency is clearly related to the progress of the disease process. Especially severe clinical cases often endangering life are found when dislocation of the atlas occurs in the 'bipolar type' of adolescent ankylosed spondylitis. It seems likely that the incidence of death following cervical arthritis is higher than usually assumed. Radiological findings are frequently and earlier seen than clinically proven signs. Some of these radiological findings are present in 80% of cases combined with multiple symptoms of definite pictures of cervical vertebrae arthritis and found in 28% of all cases, in more than 50% in later stages and in almost in 100% of patients having reached the final stage [4].

Radiological criteria in assessing primary lesions of rheumatoid cervical arthritis (fig. 1), allowing differentiation from cervical arthrosis are the following points arranged below in order to time their frequent simultaneous development in different combinations and in different segments. However no claim is made concerning the importance of a particular phase or order of severity.

1. Osteoporosis of the vertebral body (atrophy of substantia spongiosa), however this is radiologically problematic and can be combined with a labile loosening of the odontoid joint.
2. Signs of outer vertebral arthritis (arthritis of the joints of vertebral arches): Decreased sharpness of contours, errosion of joint surfaces (a), reduction in the width of joint cavity (atrophy of cartilage in rare instances synostosis occurs) (b) combined with a loosening of segments, instability and dislocation of the joints (fig. 1).
3. Size decrease of intervertebral discs without reactions corresponds to the disease process of discitis or inflammatory slow destruction of intervertebral discs, a process without visible signs of osteophytosis (a). This reaction can develop into so-called spondylodiscitis with endplate erosion and paradiscal sclerosis (b). This condition is either instabile and produces the danger of a

dorsal prolapse of the destroyed material from the disc or it leads to a stabilised state by spontaneous ossification (fig. 1).
4. A rim-erosion of the disc but this is rare (fig. 1).
5. A lysis of the processus spinosus at C7 (fig. 1, 5a–e).
6. Subluxations (fig. 5) in the region of inflammed and instable segments, mainly in central direction, localised atlanto-axial or subaxial.

The stenosis of the spinal canal (fig. 2) is the consequence of ventral dislocation of the atlas, the prolapse of disintegrating material from a disc or/and by dislocation of a vertebral body (fig. 5). The shortening of the spinal canal or

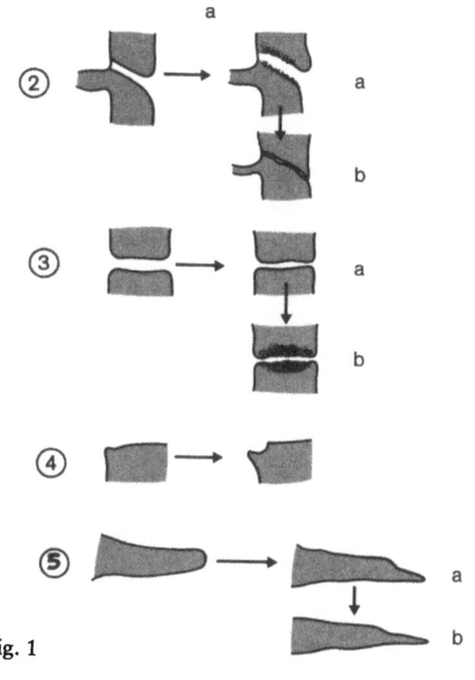

Fig. 1

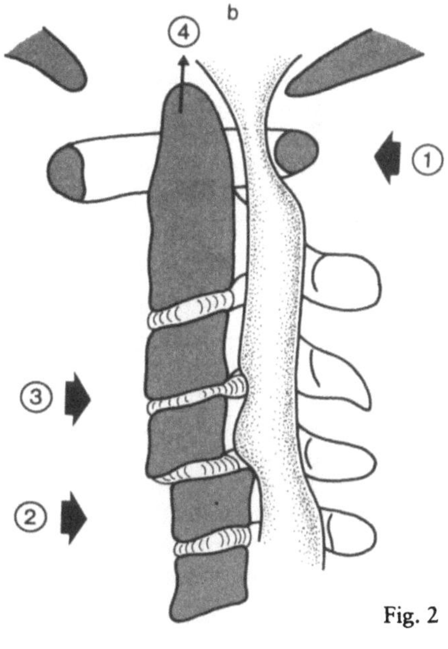

Fig. 2

vertical dislocation by collapse of one or several segments plays an additional patho-mechanical role (tab. 2). We assume that intervertebral arthritis seen as a patho-biomechanical process (tab. 3) is the most likely primary cause. The destruction of the capsule, caused by this primary failure of the instabile segment, leads to a loosening of the segment. This appears to us the pre-condition for the pathology of the disc and its dislocation is highly dangerous for the spinal cord. Within the segment of a subluxated intervertebral arthritis we see either a displacement of the vertebral body and/or a destruction of the disc with segment collapse, fullfilling either the criteria of discitis or (usually rarer) of spondylodiscitis. The segmental detachment caused by destructive cervical arthritis leads in turn to a multi-dimensional shift of vertebrae (tab. 4): the transverse dislocation, is almost exclusively ventrally and asymmetrically combined with a torticollis, a vertical dislocation and a shortening of the spinal canal. We differentiate between the dislocation of the lower head joint and the subaxial dislocation combined with stenosis of the spinal canal or steplike formations. These subluxations occur singly or in various combinations (fig. 5).

Table 2 Pathogenesis (Patho-Biomechanic) of cervical spinal canal stenosis in rheumatoid arthritis

I. Intervertebral arthritis →
  1. Transverse subluxation
    a) ventral – dislocation
    b) dorsal – dislocation (rare) (fig. 6)
  2. Vertical segment collaps →
    Shortening of the spinal canal
II. Segmental ossification →
  damage by overloading adjacent segment
III. Stenosis of the spinal canal

Table 3 Mechanisms responsible for stenosis of the spinal canal

Cervical arthritis → inflammatory subluxating segment detachment
1. Destructive head joint – arthritis
  → atlanto – axial dislocation, transverse or vertical.
2. Intervertebral arthritis
  → subaxial dislocation ←
3. Discitis (Sponylodiscitis) →
  → inflammatory atrophy of intervertebral discs →
4. Vertical shortening of spinal canal. ←

Table 4 Destructive head joint – arthritis

Patho- biomechanical aspects of multidimensional atlanto-axial dislocation
1. Loosening of odontoid joint } mobile,
2. Ventral dislocation of atlas } stable
  asymetrical tilt-gliding → torticollis
3. Head joint collapse – caudal dislocation of atlas occiput
  → pseudo – basilary impression (Dens-invagination) (fig. 8 b)
4. Osteolytic destruction of odontoid process →
  due to arthritis
  a) pseudo – dens aplasia (dens atrophy)
  b) 'os odontoideum' (dens fragment) (fig. 6)
  c) 'pseudo – pseudo-basilary' impression (returning invagination) (fig. 8 c)

The atlanto-axial dislocation

A spontaneous subluxation of the atlas ventrally, usually in conjuction with tilted gliding is the most frequent and often the first dislocation in a series of inflammatory spontaneous shifts of vertebrae. This occurs in children suffering from juvenile chronic arthritis and leads in adolescency to a late-juvenile ankylosing spondylitis of a severe and dangerous nature. This process is frequently encountered in a late stage and in chronic polyarthritis [1, 5] as well as in ankylosing spondylitis [4]. In ankylosing spondylitis, lability is usually present only in the early phase, later on the condition becomes stabilised by ankylosis including an osteolysis of the dens. Due to this ossification in later stages an operation is far less necessary than in chronic polyarthritis. In this disease this symptom can be a relatively early one, but radiologically it can only be verified in an inclined position of the patient.

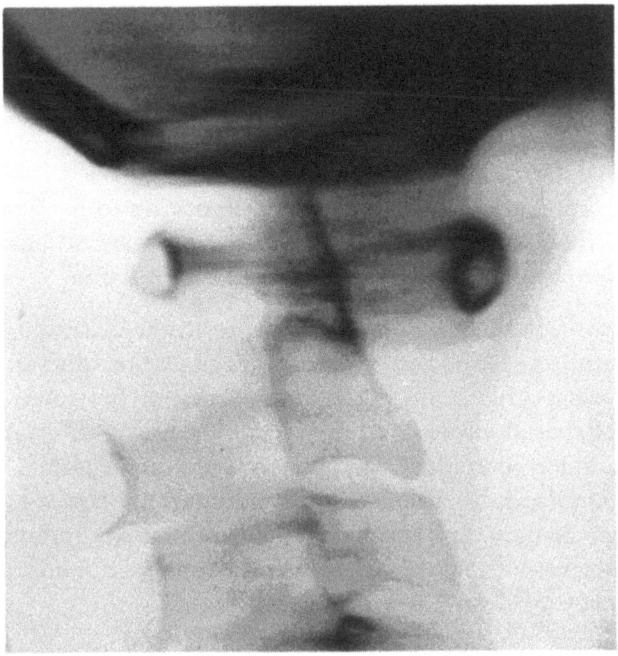

Fig. 3

The multi-dimensional dislocation between atlas and axis develops by successive loosening and eventual destruction of the ligaments of the dens axis in destructive arthritis of the lower head joints composed of six compartments. The first stage of instability in the segment C 1/2, which has no disc, has been termed odontoid slackening. This labile and reversible segment instability shows under dislocation

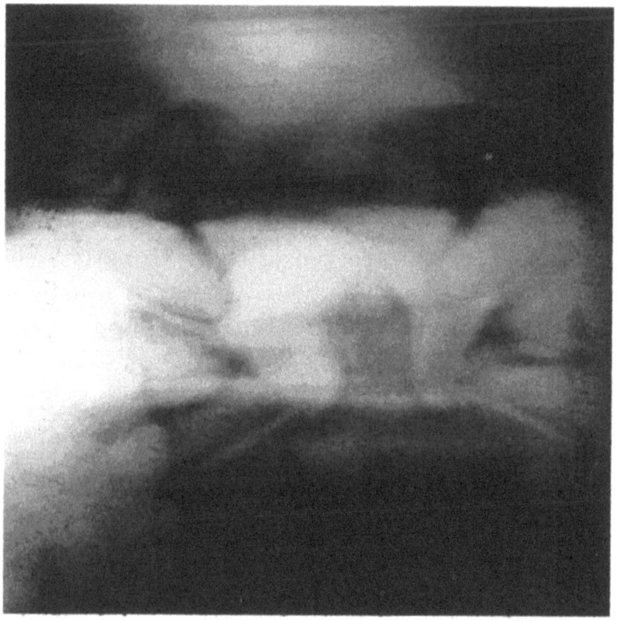

Fig. 4

pressure when inclined, an anterior atlanto-dental distance up to 6–7 mm, but normally only 2 mm in the grown up. It appears that the transverse ligament is still fullfilling its restraining function up to a free distance of 6 mm.

The shift in the atlas position and the eroding changes in the odentoid process are best visible in a lateral projection, ventrally and more marked dorsally at the level of the odontoid process (fig. 3). In the anterior-posterior projection (fig. 4) early erosive changes of the odontoid apex are clearly seen in particular tomographically, the considerablely altered lateral joint surfaces and the lateral dislocation of the lower head joint laterally dislocated. The odontoid process surrounded by synovial membrane changes and probabely undergoing an inflammatory process in the apical bursa will exhibit in a future course a diminishing and reduced size either fracture or totally being resorbed (fig. 5).

The first stage thus includes atlanto-axial instability, slackening in the odontoid joint leading to a complete rupture of the transverse alar and longitudinal ligaments and total instability combined with a mobile luxation of the lower head joint (fig. 6). If a case of a complete deficency of the atlanto-dental ligaments arises combined with tearing off the transverse ligament, the atlas responds with a ventrally directed tilt – gliding up to an anterior – dental distance of 18–20 mm. This instability is enhanced bio-mechanically (tab. 2) by an increase in resisting stability of the upper (atlanto-occipital) head joint. This is especially

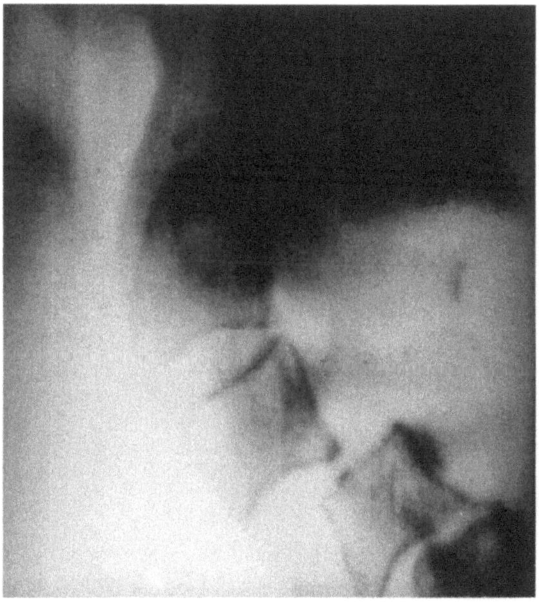

Fig. 5

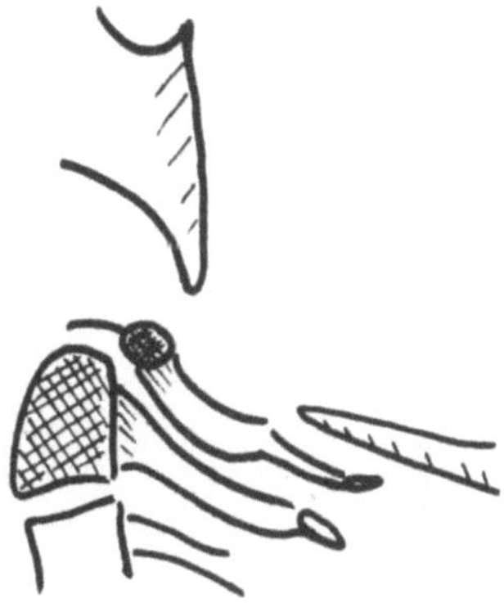

Fig. 6

the case in ankylosed spondylitis both in severe and life endangering cases occuring in adolescence (bipolar type of clinical manifestation) and in presenile cases, when stabilisation has been achieved and is relatively harmless.

The critical distance for a dislocation effect on the spinal cervical cord is about 10 mm and caused by the posterior arch of the atlas. But this depends on the time taken and the degree of compression. Severe degrees of compression and neurologically complicated conditions demand operative intervention and the resection of the posterior arch of the atlas as practised by Schürmann (personal communication) is self evident.

The detachment occuring in the lower head joint has a horizontal but also a vertical component related to the breakdown of segment C 1/2 (tab. 4). The apex of the dens becomes displaced from the palato-occipital line of Chamberlain and from the basilar line of McRae in a cranial direction entering the foramen magnum (fig. 7). This event is refered to as pseudo-basilary impression, a better name would be basal dens invagination. This displacement is a major threat to medullary integrity and function (fig. 2).

This highly threatening situation will be avoided in later stages of the disease, if an absorption of the odontoid process (fig. 6) by osteolytic action is successful and is an incidental 'do it yourself' action in the case of a destructive arthritis: 'pseudo-basal' impression [5] (fig. 8).

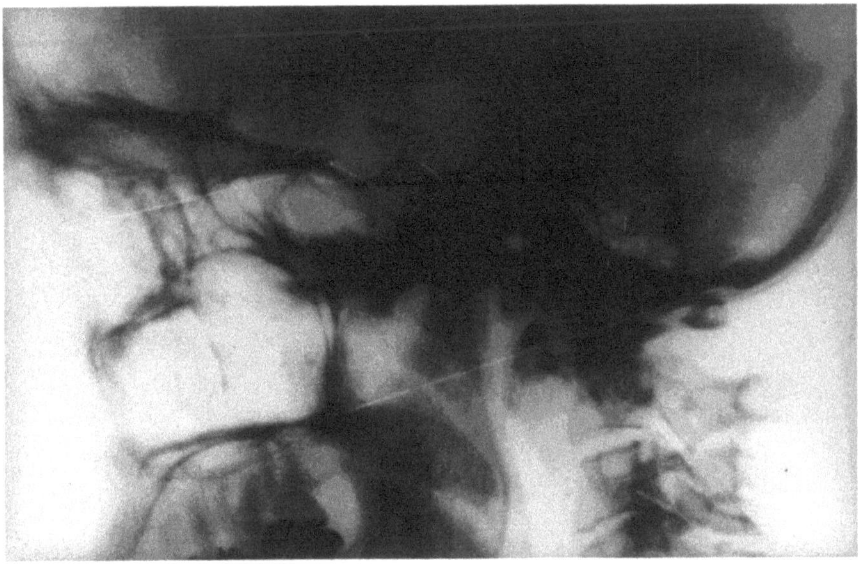

Fig. 7

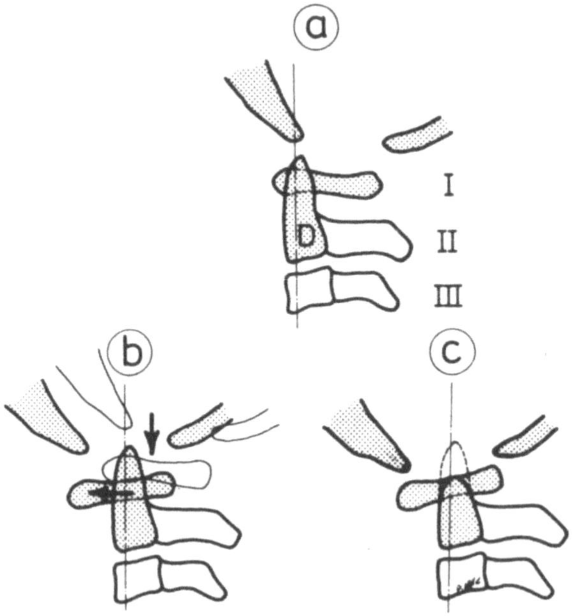

Fig. 8

To be absolutely certain about a odontoid process invagination, it will be necessary to use CT pictures and the data of craniometry (fig. 7) paying attention to the lines of Chamberlain, Mc Rae, Mc Gregor, the basilar line and in particular the measurements of Ranawat if these are below 13 mm a vertical dislocation is present. Helpful are also the bi-mastoid line of Fischgold and the angles of Walker and Boogaart in order not to miss in cases of platybasia the differential diagnostic criteria related to congenital or otherwise acquired cranio-cervical dyplasias [2].

Possible *neurological complications* (tab. 5) can originate from vascular episodes (tab. 6), root irritation (tab. 9), subacute and chronic compression of the spinal cord (tab. 8). The signs of compression can start with conduction failure in long ascending or descending tracts causing paraspastic weakness of lower limbs and bladder signs. The neurological level is not sharply defined but related to the level of the compression. If this occurs at medullary level cranial nerves will be involved (tab. 7).

Table 5 Neurological syndromes in dislocating head joint and cervical vertebrae arthritic

I.	Arterial deficiency in vascular territory of the vertebral and basilar arteries
II.	Cranial nerves and medullary symptoms
III.	Cervical myelopathy caused by compression (spastic syndromes)
IV.	Nerve root irritiation and signs of nerve loss.

Table 6 Neurological syndromes in cervical arthritis I

Intermittent vertebral artery insufficiency
brain stem symptoms in particular:
Rotatory vertigo, nausea, vomiting, nystagmus, episodal loss of consciousness, confusional states

Table 7 Neurological syndromes in head joint arthritis II

Cranial and medullary nerves	
V 1 and V 2:	loss of sensation in face
	diminished corneal reflex
IX	paralysis of soft palate
Sysarthria, bulbar symptoms	
stridor, respiratory dysfunction	
XI	Trapezius paralysis and vagal and hypoglossal symptoms

Table 8 Neurological symptoms in cervical arthritis III

Cervical and medullary compression symptoms
1. Motor weakness can increase to tetraplegia
2. Spastic signs (pyramidal tract) in lower or upper extremities
3. Spinal automatisms, paraesthesia such as tingling sensations in finger tips
4. Anterior horn cells involvement e. g. fasciculation
5. Brown – Séquard syndrome
6. Bladder disturbance

Table 9 Neurological symptoms in cervical arthritis IV

Root signs of neuropathy
1. C II pain → retro-auricular, temporal, frontal
2. Paraesthesia and sensory defects originating from nerve roots

Summary

Collaborative experience since 1966 from the Rheumaklinik Bad Kreuznach (Gamp and Schilling) and the Neurosurgical University Clinic, Mainz (Schürmann, Voth) are the basis for this report. Both these clinics were the first in Germany attempting to alleviate destructive forms of cervical vertebral arthritis by operative intervention. Eventually this collaborative effort developed in a routine treatment programme and so far 50 cases have been treated.

In the course of this collaboration the following operative indications arose:

- Unbearable painful symptoms of nerve root irritation particulary in the area of C 2 in atlanto-axial dislocation.
- Neurological deficits, such as automatism, bladder disturbances or paraspastic symptoms.
- Definite evidence of labile atlanto-axial dislocation, but as yet no signs of neurological symptoms, while the danger of medullary compression is very real.

References

[1] Ball, J., J. Sharp: Rheumatoid arthritis of the cervical spine. In: Modern trends in rheumatology, vol. 2, p. 117. Butterworths, London 1971.

[2] Dirheimer, Y.: The craniovertebral region in chronic inflammatory rheumatic diseases. Springer, Berlin – Heidelberg – New York 1977.

[3] Schilling, F., M. Schacherl, A. Bopp, et al.: Veränderungen der Halswirbelsäule bei der chronischen Polyarthritis und bei der Spondylitis ankylopoetica. Der Radiologe 3 (1963) 483.

[4] Schilling, F., J. P. Haas, M. Schacherl: Die spontane atlantoaxiale Dislokation (Ventralluxation des Atlas) bei chronischer Polyarthritis und Spondylitis ankylopoetica. Fortschr. Röntgenstr. 99 (1963) 518.

[5] Schilling, F.: Röntgendiagnostik der chronischen Polyarthritis. In: Handbuch der Inneren Medizin VI/2 B: Rheumatologie B (1984) 128.

Risk assessment of occipito-cervical involvement in inflammatory rheumatic diseases

H. J. Albrecht, A. Schleich, E. Weller, K. W. Westerburg

In our clinical daily routine we are often confronted with the question of optimal timing for surgical stabilisation of occipito-cervical defects.

Frequency of skull joint involvement in inflammatory rheumatic diseases varies depending on the patients examined. Only some cases are progressive and only a minority are seen to develop spinal cord related neurological symptoms.

The demand for early surgical intervention as such is clearly acceptable. However, what does "early" mean in this case? A too liberal indication may easily result in unnecessary interventions, on the other hand we are often confronted with situations where earlier stabilisation would have been justified.

It is a problem of how to recognize the risk cases. With our patients we have tried to set up a survey of inflammatory changes and conditions, trying to find, which clinical course they may take and in which cases neurological complications may occur or can be expected.

In the absence of a prospective study in this respect (also hoping to receive suggestions for the conception of such a project) we have performed a dominantly retrospective study involving 200 cases with occipito-cervical dislocations of the previous 7 years. These include 174 cases with rheumatoid arthritis and 22 cases with ankylosing spondylitis. The number of 200 should be regarded with reservation however, as a follow up was possible in only 124 cases, the number of computed tomography tests was restricted to 34 more prominent cases (all others were tomographed in the conventional way) and specialized neurological examinations were performed in 53 highly severe cases.

Without listing the various atlanto-dental, atlanto-occipital and atlanto-axial manifestions it should be stated

- that ventral substance loss of the dens will result in a pseudo-widening of the atlanto-dental distance and so this distance is no longer relevant for assessing the width of the bony vertebral canal,
- that this ventral atlanto-dental distance, generally serving as a measure for the dislocation, has turned out not to be representative due to considerable variations of this distance in comparison with the bony sagittal width of the vertebral canal. Therefore we prefer direct measuring of the bony width of the vertebral canal.

In addition we want to point out that a dorsal dens rarefaction creates a space supplement for the spinal cord and that the inflammatory involvement of the occipito-cervical transition usually begins at the atlanto-dental level dorsally. If the skull joints become affected too, this occurs only secondarily, sometimes after several years.

This is the case mainly in rheumatoid arthritis [5, 7, 12], less in ankylosing spondylitis where arthritides of the skull joints can occur without inflammatory changes in the atlanto-dental area. In ankylosing spondylitis [13, 16] as well as in spondylarthropathy psoriatica (the latter with relative rare occipito-cervical involvement) ankylosis may be expected to develop according to the more proliferative tendency of the sero-negative spondyloarthritide – sometimes though in a faulty position.

In rheumatoid arthritis the arthritides of the skull joints may be followed by atrophy of the massae laterales and of the corpus of C 2. This causes vertical dislocation of the atlas which in turn results in raising of the dens epistrophei with pseudo-basilar impression. The latter, however, is reduced in size or non-existent in case of simultaneous inflammatory rarefaction of the dens.

The vertical dislocation of the atlas gradually reduces its mobility and fixes it either in ventral dislocation (whereby in "slip-gliding" the narrowest point of the vertebral canal is to be found between the posterior arch of the atlas and upper corpus edge) or possibly in dorsal dislocation in the rare denslysis or dens rupture but also in normal position in the transversal plane.

Computed tomography allows a direct view of the vertebral canal and simultaneously the intraspinally located dense soft tissue, and gives information on the actual sagittal width of the vertebral canal.

Deformities and displacement of the spinal cord are readily seen with the subarachnoidal space supplement preserved. Differentiation becomes difficult once this extra space has been occupied.

Space-occupying lesions can also be well represented by the dense soft tissue (located dorsal of the dens in the area of the ligamentum transversum) which most probably corresponds to inflammatory proliferation. The longitudinal extent can be assessed in the sagittal reconstruction.

A follow-up of 1 – 12 years (mean 2.92 years) on 124 patients has been performed. 44 patients were observed at least 4 or more years. 45 of these 124 patients presented a vertical dislocation already at start of follow-up, and in 43 cases we observe a fixed atlas in the sagittal plane with increasing pseudo-basilar impression. 74 of the 124 patients presented at start of survey only atlanto-dental dislocation – with atlas mobility according to definition.

In 25 cases this mobility of mean 7 mm (4 – 15 mm) persisted to the same extent for a period of mean 2.5 years (1 – 9 years); in one case a mobility of 8 mm for 9 years. In these cases the small skull joints were mostly uninflamed even though 14 of these cases displayed marked to maximum disease activity.

In 26 of these 74 patients with atlanto-dental dislocation the atlas mobility increased during an observation period of mean 2.6 years (1 – 6 years), once from 4 mm to 11 mm in half a year. Despite marked disease activity the width increase was often just minimal, e.g. in 7 cases during 4 years only 2.1 mm. 4 cases, however, at disease remission still showed an increase of atlas mobility within 2 years of maximal 4 mm to maximal 9 mm. Also in these cases the small skull joints were not involved in the inflammation process.

16 of these 74 patients with atlanto-dental dislocation [17, 19] – with atlas mobility according to definition – developed a vertical dislocation with fixation of the atlas in the transversal plane during an observation period of mean 3.6 years (1 – 7 years). All 16 patients presented a most severe disease courses: atlas fixation occurred 10 × in ventral dislocation, 3 × in dorsal dislocation and 3 × in normal position.

In 2 more of these 74 cases the ventral dislocation occurred without the atlas fixation having become complete within the short observation period of 1 – 2 years.

In 5 cases the initial mobility of 7 – 10 mm, decreased down to 3 mm, partly in disease remission.

5 of the 124 patients whose course we observed developed a vertical dislocation without prior atlanto-dental dislocation. Thus we have courses of greatest diversity without local progression despite marked systemic disease activity on one hand but also local progression rarely without marked systemic inflammatory activity. Inflammatory involvement of the skull joints reduces atlas mobility.

The neurological examination concentrated on all those complaints suggesting a beginning or manifest impairment of the cervical cord and elevated structures. From a pathologico-anatomical standpoint the neurological signs of a neural lesion in the occipito-cervical area were systemized as follows:

1. Impairment of caudal cranial nerves, i.e. with disturbances of the gag reflex, innervation of the uvula, altered speech and pitch of voice, paralysis or atrophy of the musculus trapezius and musculus sternocleidomastoideus, paralysis or atrophy of the muscles of the tongue.
2. Impairment of autonomic centers and pathways.
3. Impairment of central motor pathways (mainly the pyramidal tracts) with flaccid or spastic pareses of the distal extremities.
4. Impairment of sensory tracts.

5. Impairment of upper cervical roots with an 'impulse syndrome' of pains localized behind the ears and tactile disturbances, corresponding to dermatomes C2 and C3.
6. Impairment of the arteria vertebralis with the symptoms of a vertebrobasilar insufficiency like vertigo, tinnitus, nystagmus, transient ocular muscle paralyses and visual field defects.

Bladder function tests were performed only if anamnestic data were present.

Our evaluation covers 53 selected examined marked cases who all had occipital cephalgiae and dysaesthesiae as impulse reactions from the cervical spinal nerves C2 and C3. In 5 of these cases signs of a marked cervical cord affliction were found.

Only once could the neurological symptoms be traced to an exact localisation of the marked spinal cord affliction. It was an impairment of the pyramidal pathway between its crossing over and the pyramid, the cause of which must be seen in the pseudobasilar imprimated dens.

The remaining 4 of the 5 patients with signs of a marked cervical spinal cord affliction had neurological symptoms which can be interpreted as an irritation or impairment of long spinal cord tracts in the dorsal as well as ventral areas. A relation to the type of occipito-cervical pathology could not be established. Common to all 4 cases, however, was a considerable narrowing of the sagittal width of the vertebral canal less than 15 mm even though such constrictions must not necessarily be correlated with neurological symptoms.

Of 19 patients with a sagittal bony residual width of the vertebral canal of less than 15 mm there were 4 with signs of a marked cervical spinal cord affliction, in 3 of whom was the atlas mobile and only in one was the atlas fixed. This point should be stressed.

Conclusions

We have concluded to routinely setting up in the future the CT-examination [2, 3, 8, 11] for direct imaging of the intraspinal situation starting at the latest with 15 mm bony width of the vertebral canal, considering that intraspinal soft tissue is also capable of narrowing the vertebral canal but that on the other hand the spinal cord can evade narrowing by shifting into the lateral space supplements. It should also be mentioned that CT-confirmed changes in form and position of the spinal cord must not necessarily be accompanied by neurological symptoms [9, 14, 15, 20].

It seems that even advanced occipito-cervical defects in general do seldom progress into marked spinal cord afflictions. This view, however, would depend on the length of the observation period and we should not overlook the particular properties of the individual case.

A great local risk is the fast progression of the sole atlas mobility with no involvement of the skull joints, the other risk being the progressive diminishing of the massae laterales with the dens unimpaired. The greatest general risk, however, is the continuous disease process resistent to therapeutic measures [10 18].

The secondary vertical dislocation fixates the mobile atlas, thus reducing the danger element resulting from its mobility in the sense of a defective healing which is apt to persist. On the other hand there is the risk of the pseudo-basilar impression whereby a slow development of the resulting defective positions seems to offer an adaptative location for the spinal cord.

Local progression and systemic disease activity determine the indication for early surgical stabilisation together with the long term results of the operative fusions, especially regarding their effects upon the subaxial segments and with reference to subsequent skull joint arthritides. Of great importance are a careful choice of the various operative methods available and a judicious selection of the suitable surgeon [1, 4, 6].

References

[1] Brattström, H., L. Granholm: Chirurgie der Halswirbelsäule bei Patienten mit rheumatoider Arthritis. Orthopäde **2** (1973) 118 – 120.

[2] Braunstein, E. M., B. N. Weissmann, S. E. Seltzer, et al.: Computed tomography and conventional radiographs of the craniocervical region in rheumatoid arthritis: A comparison. Arthritis Rheum. **27** (1984) 26 – 31.

[3] Castor, W. R., J. D. R. Mller, A. S. Russell, et al.: Computed tomography of the craniocervical junction in rheumatoid arthritis. J. Comput. Assist. Tomogr. **7** (1983) 31 – 36.

[4] Conaty, J. P., E. S. Mongan, C. Downey: Cervical fusion in rheumatoid arthritis. J. Bone Joint Surg. (Am.) **63** (1981) 1216 – 1227.

[5] Dirheimer, Y.: The craniovertebral region in chronic inflammatory rheumatic diseases, pp. 30, 36 – 39, 86, 87. Springer-Verlag, Berlin – Heidelberg – New York 1977.

[6] Gschwend, N., M. Scherer, U. Munzinger: Entzündliche Veränderungen der Wirbelsäule bei der chronischen Polyarthritis. Orthopäde **10** (1981) 155 – 168.

[7] Jäger, M., H. H. Springer: Die entzündlichen Erkrankungen der Wirbelsäule. Orthopäde **10** (1981) 106 – 113.

[8] Kaufmann, R. L., W. v. Glenn jr.: Rheumatoid cervical myelopathy: evaluation by computerized tomography with multiplanar reconstruction. J. Rheumatol. **10** (1983) 42 – 54.

[9] Mathews, J. A.: Atlanto-axial subluxation in rheumatoid arthritis, A 5-year follow-up study. Ann. Rheum. Dis. **33** (1974) 526.

[10] Mikulowski, P., F. A. Wollheim, P. Rotmil, et al.: Sudden death in rheumatoid arthritis with atlanto-axial dislocation. Acta Med. Scand. **198** (1975) 445 – 451.

[11] Raskin, R. J., D. J. Schnapf, C. R. Wolf, et al.: Computerized tomography in evaluation of atlantoaxial subluxation in rheumatoid arthritis. J. Rheumatol. **10** (1983) 33 – 41.

[12] Schilling, F., M. Schacherl: Wirbelsäulenverschiebungen und Blockwirbelbildungen im Bereich der Halswirbelsäule auf rheumatisch-entzündlicher Grundlage: Möglichkeiten und Grenzen in der Röntgendiagnostik der Wirbelsäule. WS Forsch. Praxis **28** (1984) 111.

[13] Schilling, F., M. Schacherl, A. Bopp, et al.: Veränderungen der Halswirbelsäule bei der chronischen rheumatischen Polyarthritis und bei der Spondylitis ankylopoetica. Radiologe **12** (1963) 483.

[14] Schilling, F.: Klinik und radiologische Diagnostik der dislozierenden Cervicalarthritis. 21. Tagung der Deutschen Gesellschaft für Rheumatologie, München 1984.

[15] Schleich, A., H. J. Albrecht, B. Heumann, et al.: Zur Problematik der occipito-cervicalen Manifestation bei chronischer Polyarthritis. 21. Tagung der Deutschen Gesellschaft für Rheumatologie, München 1984.

[16] Schleich, A., H. J. Albrecht, L. Nusselt, et al.: Zur Risikobeurteilung occipito-cervicaler Dislokationen bei entzündlich-rheumatischen Krankheiten. Z. Rheumatol. **44** (1985) 120–132.

[17] Thabe, H.: Atlantodentale Dislokation bei chronischer Polyarthritis. Korrelation klinischer, röntgenologischer, neurologischer und elektromyographischer Befunde. Z. Rheumatol. **40** (1981) 6–11.

[18] Vandenbroucke, J. P., H. M. Hazevoet, A. Cats: Survival and cause of death in rheumatic arthritis: A 25-year prospective followup. J. Rheumatol. **11** (1984) 158–161.

[19] Weissmann, B. N. W., P. Aliabadi, M. S. Weinfeld, et al.: Prognostic features of atlanto-axial subluxation in rheumatoid arthritis patients. Radiology **144** (1982) 745–751.

[20] Winfield, J., D. Cooke, A. S. Brook, et al.: A prospective study of the radiological changes in the cervical spine in early rheumatoid disease. Ann. Rheum. Dis. **40** (1981) 109–114.

Surgical treatment for instability in cranio-cervical bones and their joints in rheumatoid arthritis

U. Steiger, N. Gschwend

Introduction

Inflammatory destructive alterations of the spine in rheumatoid arthritis, particularly of the cervical spine, occur more frequently than is assumed. Since the cranial segments of the cervical spine are mostly involved, rheumatoid arthritis is different from other inflammatory rheumatoid disorders, mainly from Morbus Bechterew, where the pathologic alterations become more significant distally. The main initial site of the disease process concentrates on the synovia and the lesions of the small vertebral joints producing all the consequences regarding stability and the mutual relationship of vertebral positions.

Reviewing the relevant publications [2, 6, 8, 13, 14, 17, 20, 22], the spine is involved in 50 to 93% of patients with rheumatoid diseases. The atlanto-axial subluxation [15, 16, 21] is a definite characteristic of a cervical spine in rheumatoid arthritis. A subluxation is suggested, when the distance between the dens and the arch of the atlas is greater than 4 mm. No definite correlation exists between the extension of a subluxation and the occurrence of neurological dysfunctions. Smith [22] reports neural symptoms in 30 of 150 patients with atlanto-axial subluxation. The pseudo-basilar impression, which in radiography extends beyond the McGregor line by 4.5 mm, corresponding to the apex of the dens, is the cause of sudden death owing the pathologic displacement in the cranio-cervical part or upper part of the cervical spine. In autopsies it could be ascertained that 10% of deaths in rheumatoid arthritis patients in a hospital for chronic diseases were caused by medullary compression [18]. The literature between 1980 and 1984 summarily reports on 129 surgical fusions in patients with rheumatoid arthritis [1, 5, 7, 11, 12, 19, 23]. Preoperatively, neurologic deficiency was found in 1/4 of the cases. The postoperative fixation with a cast after different surgical techniques lasted usually 3 months. Using conservative management, such as a cervical collar, complaints can be reduced but a further increase of the subluxation by a progressive destruction of the joints, particularly of the ligamentous structures, cannot be prevented.

What made orthopaedic surgeons rather hesitating giving indications for surgical intervention, and what has kept them waiting for irreversible neurological impairment? The main reasons are:

1. The ignorance about the frequency and prognostic significance of pathological alterations of the cervical spine in rheumatoid arthritis.
2. The great number of additional problems related to rheumatoid arthritis.
3. The apprehension of the difficulties and hazards of complication caused by surgical intervention.
4. The high rate of failure in a bony fusion and in permanent reposition.

Material and approach

The patient, provided by a halo-brace, is fixed in a device for support constructed by us (fig. 1) and various additional mechanical and corrective adjustments are provided. Preparation of the aid is facilitated by a longitudinal pull and flexion of the head; this refers also to the reposition by extension of the head. Patients who have to be operated for their cervical spine disorders, have mostly suffered from rheumatoid arthritis for many years. Consequently, we have to deal with people whose general condition is severly reduced and often maxillary joints are involved too. Anaesthesia by intubation is then indispensable, since surgery has to be performed in a ventral position. Where the mouth can be opened only a little, a nasal intubation with flexible fibre-glass optics may be necessary. The longitudinal pull can be appropriately exerted thanks to the aforementioned device of support. Thereby soft movements are required.

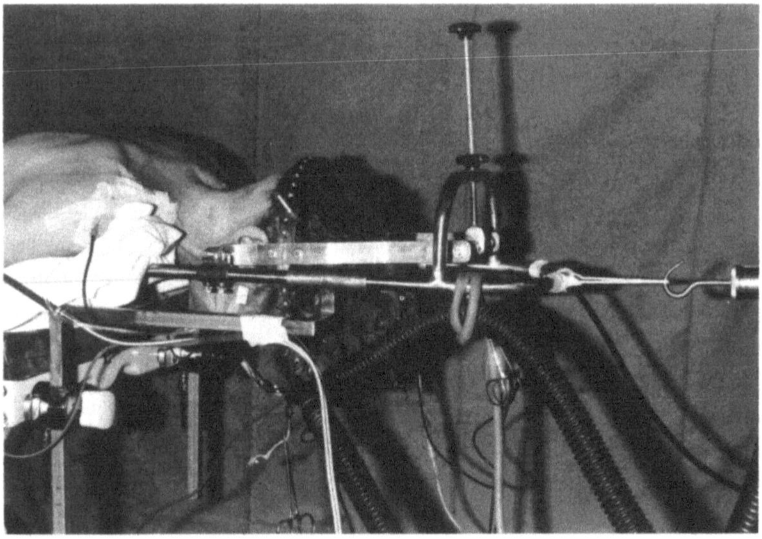

Fig. 1 Special device for the patient's positioning, providing several facilities for adjustment and longitudinal pull.

Surgery aims at the optimal removal of any subluxation position and elimination and prevention of symptoms of compression of the spinal cord and the nerve roots. Furthermore a permanent stabilization of the spinal segments concerned is desirable which will enable the patient to be mobilized as soon as possible. Specially applied wire loops proved appropriate for the reposition and stabilization, and the same refers to autologous graft material for a permanent fixation as well as to the simultaneous use of bone cement to facilitate mobilization as early as possible [8, 9]. In cases of basilar impression, stabilization does not concern C 1/C 2 only, but the occiput has as well. Only in cases with an isolated severe subluxation of C 1/C 2 (more than 4 mm) does the wire loop include the arch of the atlas and the spinous process or the arch of C 2. In the presence of subluxation and instability with pain distal to C 2, we include those segments into the fusion, because experience has proved that a stabilization of the segments near the head may result in additional overloading of the distal ones, occasionally with neurologic complications due to subluxation of the vertebrae beneath the spondylosed portion.

In the fusion of C 1/C 2, the vertebral arches of the atlas as well as the spinous processes and the arches of the 2nd vertebra are exposed. Cerclage wires are passed around the vertebral arches and a cancellous graft is inserted (fig. 2). This procedure is performed with a slight flexion of the head and a longitudinal pull of 10 to 12 kg. The reposition takes place with the head increasingly extended; the wires are tightened. An additional cortico-cancellous graft is notched in H-form and put on spinous process II. This graft is fixed by 2 additional crossing wires around the vertebral arches.

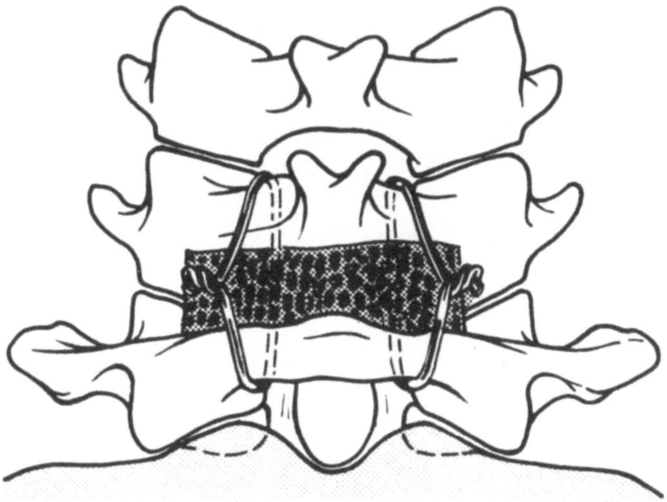

Fig. 2 Our method for the fusion of C 1/C 2 with wire loops and autologous cancellous graft.

We have constructed a self-cutting screw to fix the cerclage wires in the fusion between the occiput and C 2 (fig. 3). The screws are twisted 1 cm laterally to the midline. The cortico-cancellous graft is inserted from the spinous process to the occiput and stably fixed by crossing cerclage wires carried around the screws (fig. 4). Additional stability is obtained by using Palacos cement on the left side in the region of the wire-whirl.

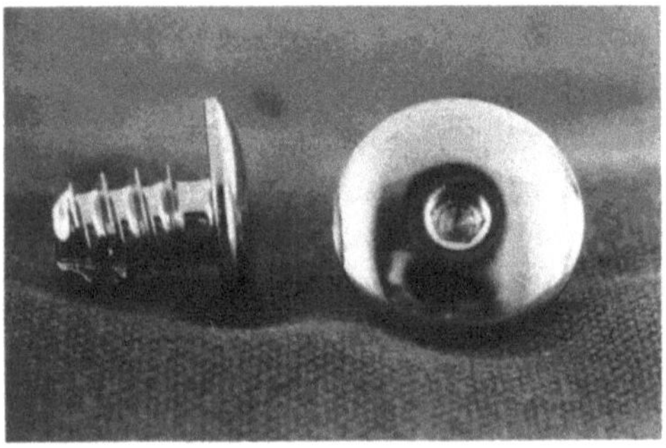

Fig. 3 Self-cutting screw with a broad top for anchoring the wire slings at the occiput.

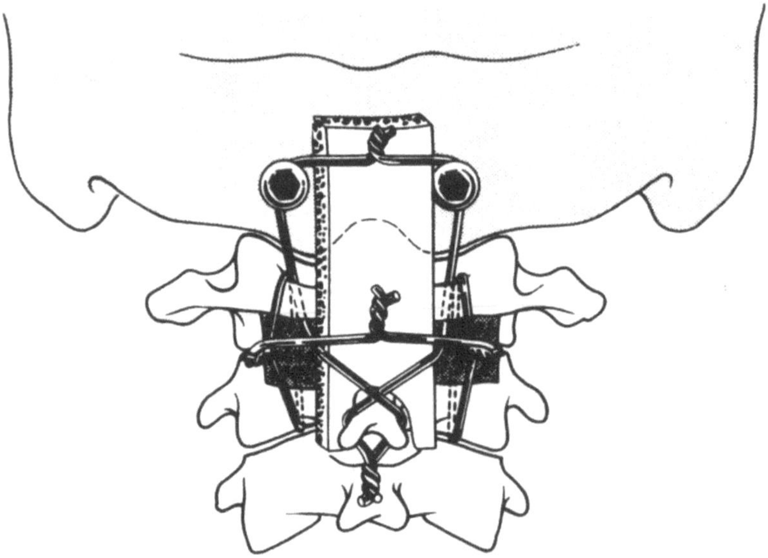

Fig. 4 Fusion technique between occiput and C 2 with autologous bone grafts, special screws and 4 wire loops.

At the end of the operation a light cervical collar is provided; mobilization usually follows at first postoperative day. A removable cervical collar provides for additional support during the first 6 weeks.

Between 1967 and 1984 we performed fusion of the upper part of cervical spine, i.e. between C0/C1 or C1/C2, in 39 patients with rheumatoid arthritis. 32 patients were female. The average age at the time of surgery was 55 years. The postoperative follow-up was on the average 3,7 years.

The majority of the patients were in a severe and progressive phase of disease (Larson's phase III and IV was found in 32 cases). The sedimentation rate was distinctly increased even under Cortisone, i.e. more than 30 mm in 28 cases. A total of 160 other surgical measures had been undertaken in the patients prior to the spinal fusion.

Preoperatively, 37 patients complained of pain. In 7 cases a vertebral insufficiency was present, and in 5 cases a central myelopathy with impaired sense of vibrations, paresis of the upper extremities, weakness and sensory loss as well as hyperreflexia. In 19 cases a subluxation of C1/C2 of 6–20 mm was found. In 10 cases there was precence of a pseudobasilar impression and in 7 cases destruction of the dens. In 17 cases the spinal fusion was undertaken between occiput/C2, and in 19 cases between C1/C2.

Results

A reduction of pain in all cases operated on and followed up was noticeable. A bony consolidation was obtained in 33 cases and no neurological complications occured in this group of 39 patients operated on. Postoperative reposition by our method proved to be satisfactory. The atlanto-axial dislocation was:

<3 mm	26 patients
4–5 mm	5 patients
>6 mm	5 patients

Two patients died in the postoperative period. The first one due to a poor general condition with ensuing gram-positive sepsis two weeks after the operation, without local involvement of the fusion. The second patient died 4 weeks postoperatively because of a gram-negative urosepsis. Three other patients died within 3 years; in none of them the cause of death was related to an instability of the upper part of spine.

Pseudoarthrosis was found in 4 patients, in 3 with fusion of C1/C2 and in one of C0/C2. Other complications were wound infection in one case which healed spontaneously, and in another case reoperation was performed due to instability of the inferior segment.

Discussion

Pathological dislocations in the superior cervical region in rheumatoid arthritis patients are of major, and sometimes even of vital significance. As a rule, a ventral subluxation of C 1/C 2 is present. Dorsal subluxation occurs associated with a destruction of the dens epistrophei but is less common. The vertical displacement of C 0/C 1, known as pseudobasilar impression, is of no less importance. Reviewing international literature, we notice a considerable discrepancy between the frequency of those pathological alterations and the rather infrequent but effective surgical management. The reason for real consideration is, than on one hand, in the few publications, there is only a small number of patients. On the other hand, namely in Scandinavian centres for rheumatism, where the number of patients with RA is markedly higher, numerous neurologic complications existed already preoperatively [2, 3, 10, 24].

Conservative measures [4], such as supporting collars, are only of a limited efficacy in view of preventing a progressive displacement.

Our clinical experience forced us to broaden the indications and to choose an earlier period for operation. We find that the indication for reposition and fusion of one or several segments of the cervical spine is given:

1. In cases with persistant pain which do not respond to conservative treatment.
2. In cases with neurological symptoms of irritation and dysfunction caused by compression.
3. In cases with progressive (sub)luxation of C 0/C 1 and C 1/C 2.

Unfortunately, many patients are sent rather late by rheumatologists for surgical treatment. Despite the negative selection, a relatively low rate of complications exists. Our surgical technique achieves a rather high fusion rate without additional external fixation and allows immediate mobilization. The special support which we have devised helps to reduce the risks and facilitates surgery, particularly in view of a complete reposition (fig. 5).

Conclusion

The presence of pathological displacements in the upper part of cervical spine in patients with rheumatoid arthritis should be carefully considered. Progressive and painful subluxations should be surgically treated before the occurrence of neurological symptoms or vertebral pathology.

Modern surgical techniques, even without external fixation, allow satisfactory high fusion rates with a relatively low rate of complications.

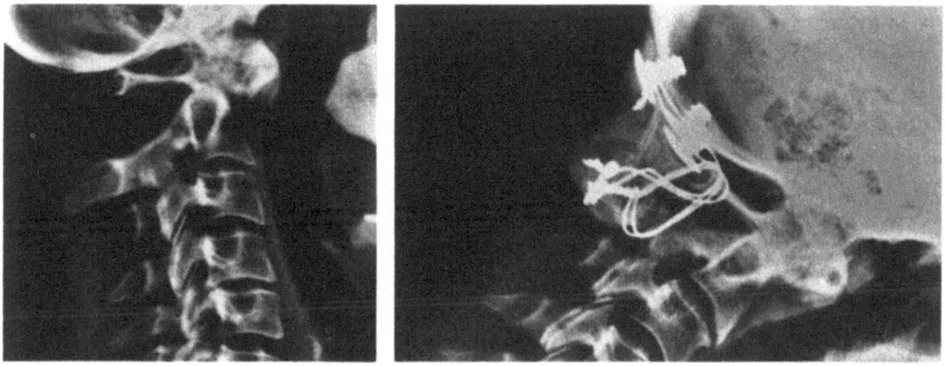

Fig. 5 Considerable subaxial displacement in a 48 year-old patient with rheumatoid arthritis and pseudobasilar impression. The postoperative picture shows a fusion between the occiput and C2 with good reposition.

References

[1] Awerbuch, M. S., D. R. Henderson, S. C. Milazzo, et al.: Longterm follow-up of posterior cervical fusion for atlanto-axial subluxation in rheumatoid arthritis. J. Rheumatol. **8** (1981) 423 – 432.

[2] Brattstroem, H., L. Granholm: Atlanto-axial fusion in rheumatoid arthritis. A new method of fixation with wire and bone cement. Acta Orthop. Scand. **47** (1976) 619 – 628.

[3] Brattstroem, H., L. Granholm: Chirurgie der Halswirbelsäule bei Patienten mit rheumatoider Arthritis. Orthopäde **2** (1973) 118.

[4] Brattstroem, M.: Gelenkschutz bei progredient chronischer Polyarthritis. Studentenliteratur, Lund 1972.

[5] Cregan, J. C. F.: Internal fixation of the unstable rheumatoid cervical spine. Ann. Rheum. Dis. **25** (1966) 242.

[6] Garrod, A. E.: A treatise on rheumatism and rheumatoid arthritis. Griffin, London 1980.

[7] Glynn, M. K., J. M. Sheehan: Fusion of the cervical spine for instability. Clin. Orthop. **179** (1983) 97 – 101.

[8] Gschwend, N.: Surgical treatment of rheumatoid arthritis. Thieme, Stuttgart – New York 1980.

[9] Gschwend, N.: Die operative Behandlung von Wirbelsäulenveränderungen bei Polyarthritis. Akt. Rheumatol. **5** (1980) 281 – 291.

[10] Hopkins, J. S.: Lower cervical rheumatoid subluxation with tetraplegia. J. Bone Joint Surg. **49-B** (1967) 46.

[11] Koop, S. E., R. B. Winter, J. E. Lonstein: The surgical treatment of instability of the upper part of the cervical spine in children and adolescents. J. Bone Joint Surg. (Am) **66** (1984) 403 – 411.

[12] Lesoin, F., B. Duquesnoy, A. Destee, et al.: Complications neurologiques cervicales de la polyarthrite rhumatoide. Indications du traitement chirurgical. Sem. Hop. (Paris) 59 (1983) 1806 – 1809.

[13] Lispon, S. J.: Rheumatoid arthritis of the cervical spine. Clin. Orthop. (1984) 143 – 149.

[14] Martel, W., J. Page: Cervical vertebral erosions and subluxation in rheumatoid arthritis and ancylosing spondylitis. Arthr. Rheum. **3** (1960) 546.

[15] Martel, W., M. R. Abell: Fatal atlanto-axial luxation in rheumatoid arthritis. Arthr. Rheum. **6** (1963) 224.

[16] Mathews, J. A.: Atlanto-axial subluxation in rheumatoid arthritis and ankylosing spondylitis. Arth. Rheum. **3** (1960) 546.
[17] Meikle, J. A., M. Wilkinson: Rheumatoid involvement of the cervical spine. Radiological assessment. Ann. Rheum. Dis. **30** (1971) 154.
[18] Mikulowski, P.: Sudden death in rheumatoid arthritis with atlanto-axial dislocation. Acta Med. Scand. **198** (1975) 445–451.
[19] Ranawat, C. S., P. O-Leary, P. Pellicci, et al.: Cervical spine fusion in rheumatoid arthritis. J. Bone Joint Surg. (Am) **61** (1979) 1003–1010.
[20] Sharp, J., D. W. Purser, J. S. Lawrance: Rheumatoid arthritis of the cervical spine in the adult. Ann. Rheum. Dis. **17** (1958) 303.
[21] Sharp, J., D. W. Purser: Spontaneus atlanto-axial dislocation in ancylosing spondylitis and rheumatoid arthritis. Ann. Rheum. Dis. **20** (1961) 47.
[22] Smith, P. H., R. L. Benn, J. Sharp: Natural history of rheumatoid cervical luxations. Ann. Rheum. Dis. **31** (1972) 431.
[23] Teinturier, P., J. P. Levai, J. P. Collin, et al.: La luxation atloido-axoidienne au cours du rheumatisme inflammatoire chronique. Résultats de 16 arthrodèses occipito-axoidiennes. Rev. Chir. Orthop. **68** (1982) 529–538.
[24] Whaley, K., W. C. Dick: Fatal subluxatial dislocation of cervical spine in rheumatoid arthritis. Br. Med. J. **II** (1968) 31.

Operative stabilization of atlanto-axial dislocation combined with cervical cord compression (myelopathy) in rheumatoid arthritis

K. Schürmann

Introduction

Since 1967, a period of almost 20 years, the neurosurgical department of the Johannes Gutenberg University of Mainz has carried out fusion operations on the cervical spine in more than 500 patients. In about 50 of these cases, bone grafts after partial or total removal of the vertebral body were performed.

Since 1969, we have observed 43 cases atlanto-axial dislocation with cervical cord compression and myelopathy, most of which in progressive chronic polyarthritis (PCP). In order to decompress the cervical cord and to stabilize the unstable cranio-cervical junction, the indication for a dorsal suboccipito-cervical decompression operation was unavoidable. This operation was carried out together with a stabilization of the cranio-cervical junction by fusion.

The techniques [12] elaborated for this operation were tried by us for the first time in 1969 and its early results in 16 cases were published in 1979 [13]. The complications and results in our recent series of 43 patients have been reviewed in this issue of the Mainz proceedings. Following the request of the editors the special surgical technique and its indication in PCP in the atlanto-axial articulation are fully communicated below.

Etiology and differential diagnosis

In nosology [1, 2] we distinguish between Juvenile Bechterew Disease (JBD) and Progressive Chronic Polyarthritis (PCP), following the classification of Schilling [10].

Differential diagnosis between JBD and PCP is not difficult as the average age of patients with JBD is between 18 and 30 years, whereas the PCP patients have an average age of 50 to 70 years. Moreover, it must be emphasized that the atlanto-axial dislocation in JBD patients is an *early* symptom of the so-called bipolar manifestation of the disease, namely caudal pelvic lesion (iliosacral ankylosis) concomitant with the cranial spinal lesion (destruction of atlas-axis ligaments).

On the other hand, in the elderly PCP patients there is more or less a long history of generalized PCP affecting all joint capsules with arthro-deformities, tendinous luxations, peripheral neuropathy with resulting muscular atrophy. That means, in PCP patients, the atlanto-axial dislocation [5, 6, 8, 11] is a *late* symptom in the long progress of this chronic disease. In general, the chronic proliferative inflammation of all synovial tissue leads to severe lesions of discs, bone, joint capsules, and ligaments. These lesions are more frequently found at the atlas-axis level (20 – 34% in the literature) than is commonly known.

The destructive inflammatory process of the atlanto-axial articulation (fig. 1) affects mainly the transverse and the cruciform ligaments of the atlas, the alar ligaments of the axis *(ligamentum apicis dentis),* the anterior and posterior atlanto-occipital membranes, and especially the odontoid process of the axis itself (tab. 1, fig. 2). As a result of this destruction, there is severe instability of the atlas-axis articulation and a ventral dislocation of the atlas in certain cases (figs. 2, 3).

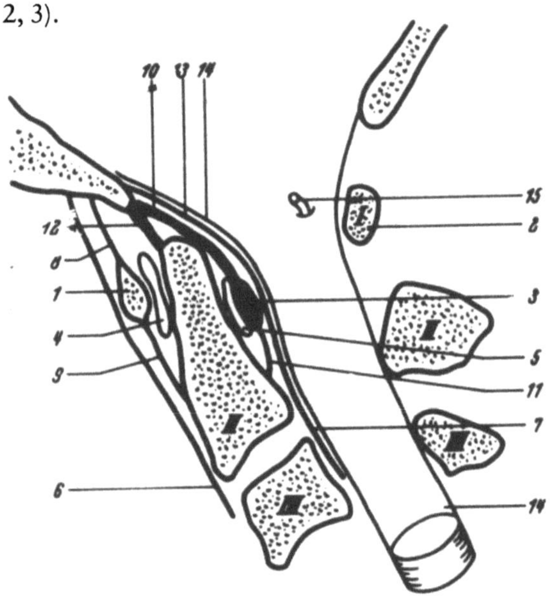

Fig. 1 Normal anatomy of the suboccipitocervical region (modified after Spalteholz, Lehrbuch für Anatomie), with distinguishings marks of the most important ligaments of the atlas-axis and axis-clivus: 3 = Transverse ligament of the atlas; 10 = Cruciform ligament of the atlas; 12 = Apical ligament of the odontoid process of the axis *(Ligamentum apicis dentis).*

Clinical signs

The clinical signs are characterized in the early stage by dorsal neck pain, combined with rigidity of the neck and followed by a rigid torticollis caused by blocked rotatory movements. These very early signs are already alarming

Table 1 Short summary of the clinical differential diagnosis between JBD and PCP

Nosology

Juvenile Bechterew-disease JBD Age: from 18 – 30 years	*Progressive chronic polyarthritis* PCP Age: from 50 – 70 years
Atlantoaxial dislocation = *early* (first) symptom	Atlantoaxial dislocation = *late* symptom
Bipolar manifestation *caudal* pelvic lesion = ileosacral ankylosis *cranial* spine lesion = Atlas-axis	Together with generalized PCP of all joint capsules, tendinous luxations, peripheral neuropathy and other signs

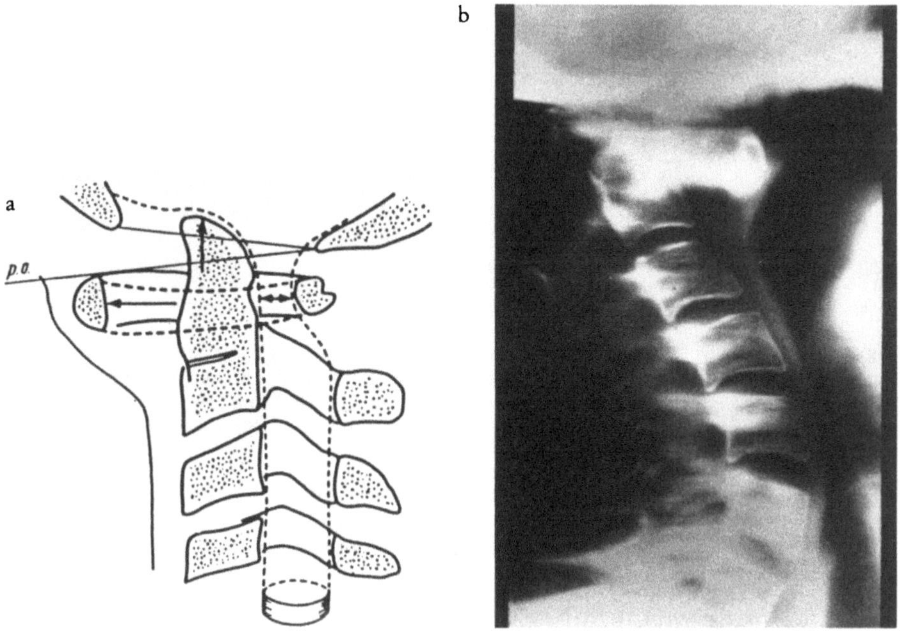

Fig. 2 a Shows the severe instability of the atlas-axis articulation and a ventral dislocation of the atlas in JBD. If the dislocation amounts to more than 12 mm (up to 20 mm), then a more or less severe myelopathy is seen.

Fig. 2 b X-ray to figure 2 a: 18 years old boy with JBD and myelopathy (Quadrispasticity). Good remission after surgery.

symptoms and the medical profession must promptly warn the patient seeking help from "chiropraxis" or manipulation therapy. The subsequent symptoms are caused by incipient cord compression. Patients complain of dysesthesia in hands and fingers, sandpaperlike sensations, and/or sudden shooting pains into the legs caused by compression of the posterior columns of the cord by the anteriorly dislocated dorsal arch of the atlas. These alarming symptoms require urgent diagnostic measures [7]. In a high percentage of cases, the diagnosis is not made before further myelopathic symptoms appear, generally in the following sequence: disturbed bladder function, urinary incontinence or urinary retention, then weakness in arms and legs with diminishing motor power in the four limbs, and finally quadri-spasticity. We did not observe total quadriplegia.

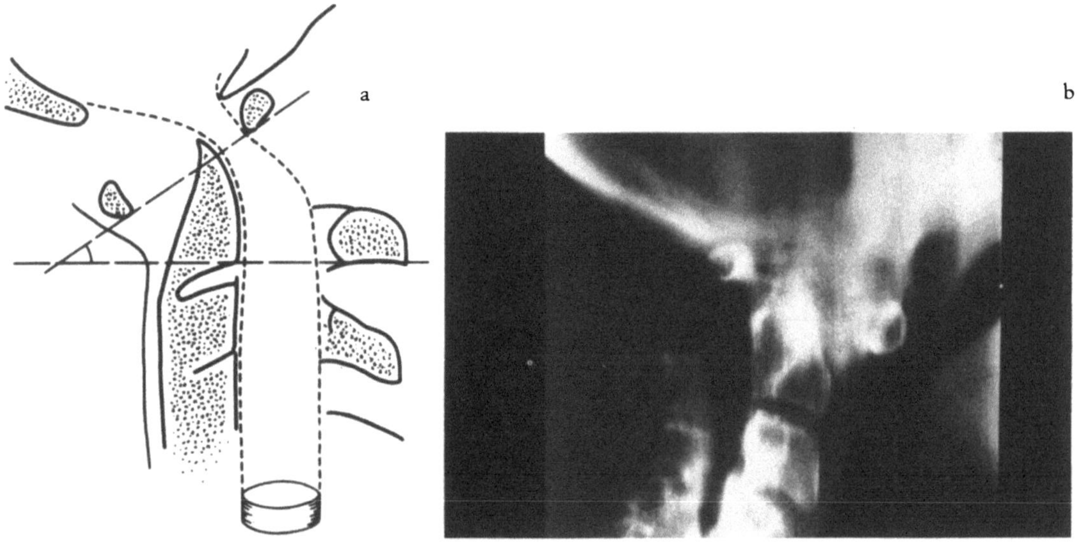

Fig. 3 a Shows the often very severe instability of the atlas-axis articulation, combined with a not seldom extreme tilt gliding of the atlas in PCP patients. The narrowing of the high cervical channel is in our series to be found between 13 and 5 mm (the normal width is 22 mm). In the majority of PCP patients we saw also a remarkable rarefaction of the dens of the axis.

Fig. 3 b X-ray to figure 3 a: 62 years old lady with severe PCP, peripheral arthropathies and -deformities, peripheral neuropathy and muscle atrophy as well as a high grade myelopathy with tetraspasticity. Significant amelioration of quadrispasticity after surgery and postoperative conservative treatment in a rehabilitation centre for rheumatic diseases.

Radiologic signs

In most cases a rarefaction of the odontoid process of the axis can be seen. The ventral dislocation of the atlas varies from 4 to 20 mm. If the dislocation did not amount to more than 9 mm, then we did not find any neurological deficits. On the other hand, if the dislocation amounts to more than 12 mm (up to 20 mm), then a more or less severe myelopathy is seen. In our series we found a narrowing of the high cervical canal to between 13 and 5 mm (the normal width is 22 mm). A tilt gliding of the atlas by more than 10° is not infrequent (fig. 3). "Pseudobasilar invagination" (penetration of the dens into the foramen magnum) is occasionally observed.

Indication for surgery

- Instability with local signs, severe suboccipital pain and headache and slow progression of the dislocation in a certain time interval during observation. Indication should be made before the beginning of cord compression symptoms.
- Instability and slight signs of myelopathy.
- Instability with severe signs of myelopathy.

Surgical treatment

The aims of the treatment are:
- decompression of the cervico-bulbar transition
- permanent stabilization of the unstable atlas-axis particulation (figs. 4, 5).

Surgical technique

Patient is positioned on the operating table in the prone position. Crutchfield traction is applied in order to achieve retroflexion of the cervical spine to avoid a sliding movement of the atlanto-axial articulation during surgery. A bone block is taken from the posterior iliac crest (figs. 6, 7). A midline skin incision is made into the dorsal neck, the arch of the atlas removed, and the foramen magnum enlarged.

Then follows resection of the narrow atlanto-occipital cicatricial tissue ring. This is absolutely necessary, since without its removal, decompression of the dura is inadequate. The spinous processes of C2 and C3 are removed. The posterior cortical wall of the arches of C2 and C3 are resected up to free spongious bone. Burr holes are applied bilaterally and suboccipitally. Steel wires are to be inserted through these as well as epidurally through the arches of C2 and C3. The two bone blocks are placed on the arches of C2 and C3 with the upper ends

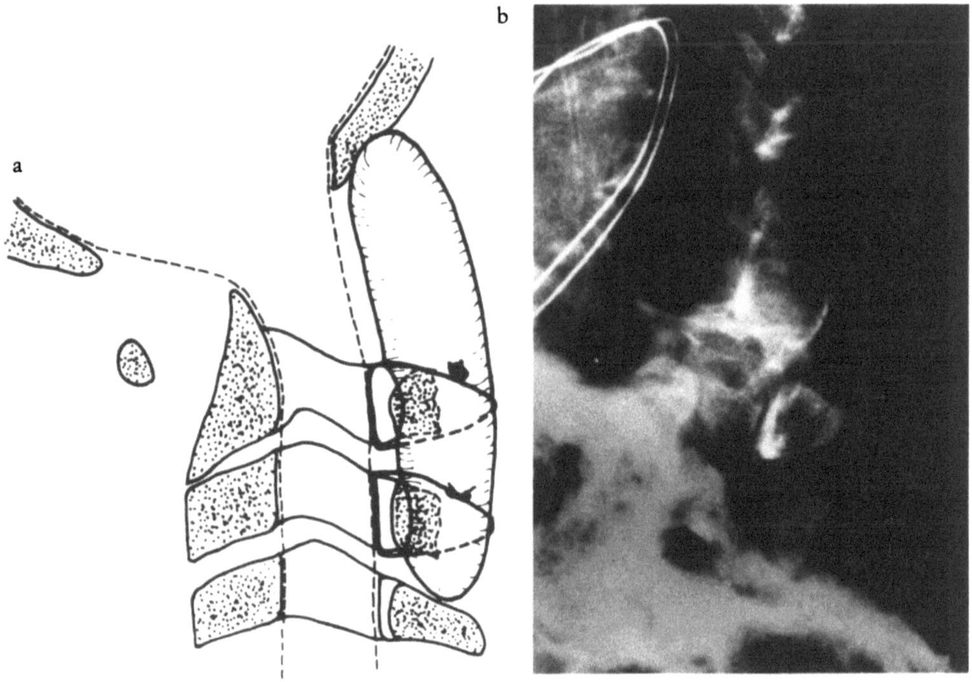

Fig. 4a Shows the result of surgical treatment: (1) the decompression of the cervicobulbar cord and (2) the permanent stabilization of the unstable atlas-axis articulation by the inserted bone-blocks for the dorsal suboccipitocervical fusion (surgical technique see text).

Fig. 4b Postoperative x-ray to figure 4a.

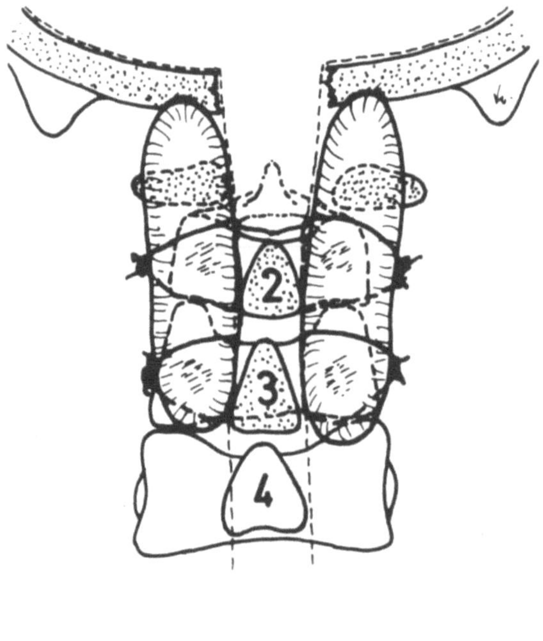

Fig. 5 The sketch shows the situation of figure 4 in a posterior view.

projecting into the burr holes on each side. They are then fixed by the previously inserted steel wires. The wound is now closed and a 'Baycast'-jacket is applied for 6 to 8 months. When this jacket has become hard (2 – 3 days), the Crutchfield tong is removed. The patient can then leave the bed and walk, provided that the neurological status allows movements (figs. 8, 9).

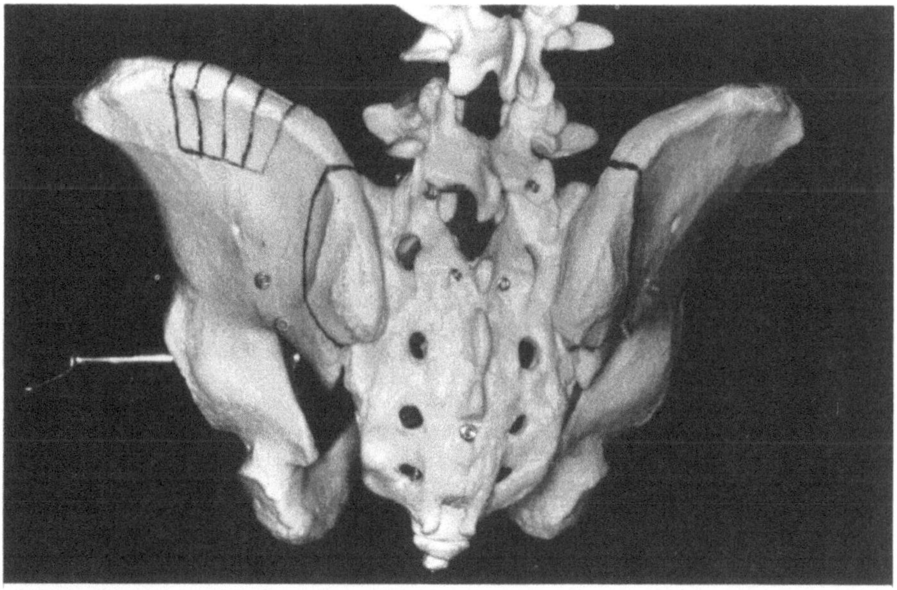

Fig. 6 The pelvis model shows the posterior iliac spine, from which the strong bone blocks are taken.

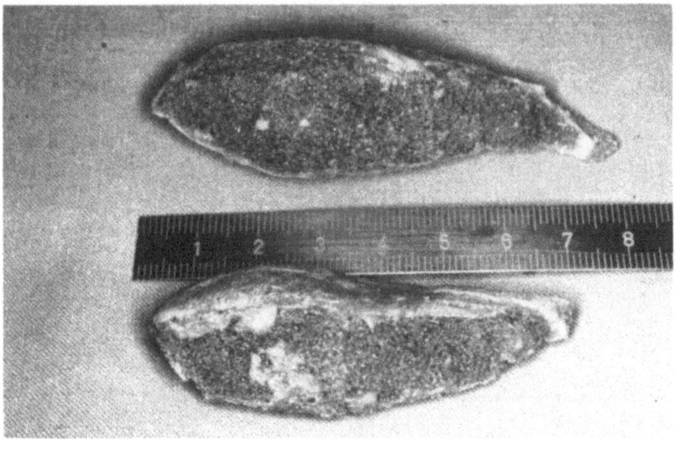

Fig. 7 The original bone blocks from the posterior iliac spine used for the dorsal fusion. The length amounts to 70 – 80 mm.

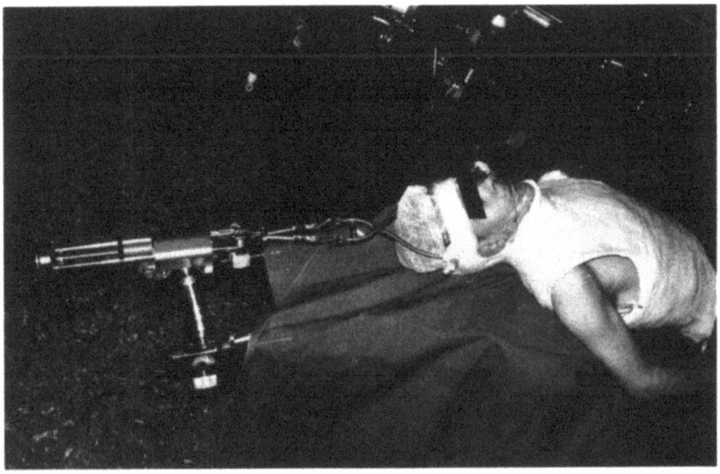

Fig. 8 Patient on the operating table after surgery, turned on his back for finishing the plaster of Paris diadem jacket resp. "Baycast"-jacket. The Crutchfield-tong is connected with a mechanical winch (constructed by Maquet AG, Kehler Straße 31, D-7550 Rastatt, FRG), which can increase the traction up to 30 kg and more. The winch is attached to the operating table with revolving arms, so that the traction can easily be changed in ante- or retroflexion position and the traction force can be changed as needed.

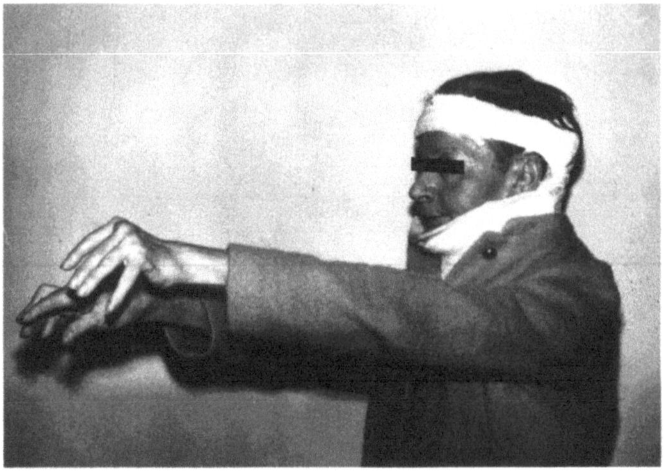

Fig. 9 A 62 year-old-lady with a severe PCP, ventral atlanto-axial dislocation and gliding, myelopathy (quadrispasticity), generalized arthrodeformities, tendinous luxations, peripheral polyneuropathy with consequent muscular atrophy, 6 days after surgery (see figs. 3, 4 and 5).

Discussion

Our experience has shown that in the majority of cases reposition of the atlanto-axial dislocation in rheumatoid-arthritis is not possible due to the chronic inflammatory fibrosis in the affected articulation. In our opinion it is necessary to decompress the cervico-bulbar transition by enlarging the foramen magnum and by removal of the dorsal arch of the ventrally dislocated arch of the atlas (figs. 10a–c). This is absolutely necessary, as well as the resection of the narrowed atlanto-occipital cicatritial tissue ring between the dorsal circumference of the atlas. Without these measures, decompression of the cord is inadequate, and when this is done, the dorsal decompression of the cord disappears and a good dural pulsation is seen.

The techniques by Brattström [4], Gschwend and Roosen [3, 9] do not decompress the cord and are only practicable in cases without severe cord compression. These techniques are restricted to stabilisation of the unstable cranio-cervical joint.

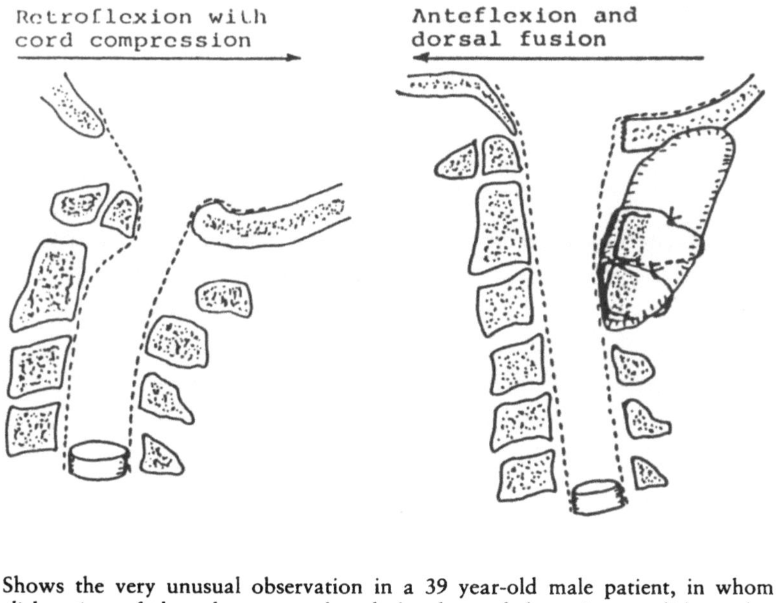

Fig. 10a Shows the very unusual observation in a 39 year-old male patient, in whom a *dorsal dislocation of the atlas* occurred and the dens of the axis was dislocated posteriorly and lies within the high cervical canal producing a cord compression and myelopathy (quadrispasticity). After reposition by traction and anteflexion, the dorsal fusion operation with our technique was performed. After surgery quadrispasticity improved in about 3 to 4 days so that the patient could walk with the plaster of Paris diadem jacket. Patient was operated upon on the 28th of September 1978 and left the hospital on the 5th October 1978, i.e., 7 days postoperatively, to celebrate the 80th birthday of his father.

b c

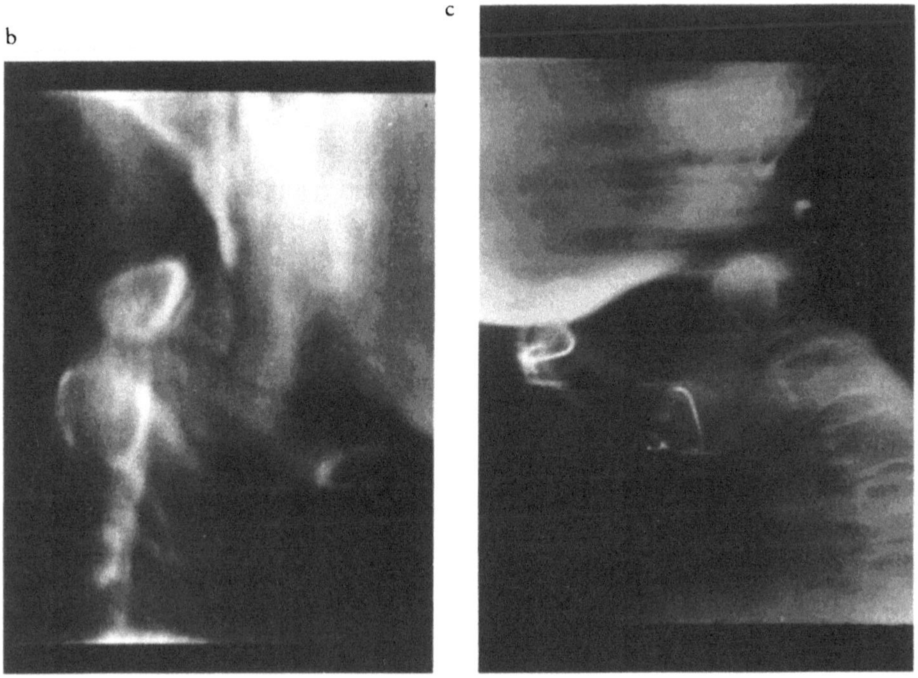

Fig. 10 b, c X-ray to figure 10 a: Pre-operative and post-operative situation (c).

Summary

A special and preferable technique has been elaborated for alleviating the symptoms of atlanto-axial dislocation in rheumatoid arthritis with cervical cord compression, which is suitable for two reasons, as it achieves

- decompression of the cervico-bulbar cord and
- permanent stabilization of the unstable atlas-axis articulation.

The results in our operational series of 43 patients have been reviewed by my coworkers in this issue of our proceedings. The two first groups considered for surgical intervention show that the obtained results were more favourable than in the last, the third group, suffering from severe myelopathy.

References

[1] Ball, J.: Pathology of the rheumatoid cervical spine. Ann. Rheum. Dis. **17** (1958) 121.

[2] Ball, J., J. Sharp: Rheumatoid arthritis of the cervical spine. In: Modern trends in rheumatology. Hill, A. G. S. (ed.) **117**. London: Butterworths 1971.

[3] Brattström, H., L. Granholm: Atlanto-axial fusion in rheumatoid arthritis. Acta orthop. Scand. **47** (1976) 619–628.

[4] Brattström, H.: Surgery in atlanto-axial dislocation in rheumatoid arthritis. Reconstr. Surg. Traumat. **18** (1981) 16–29.

[5] Dunbar, H. A., B. S. Ray: Chronic atlanto-axial dislocation with late neurological manifestations. Surg. Gynecol. Obstet. **113** (1961) 757–762.

[6] Meyers, K. A. E., G. Th. van Beusekom, W. Luyendijk, F. Duytjes: Dislocation of the cervical spine, with cord compression in rheumatoid arthritis. J. Bone Joint Surg. **56** (1974) 608–680.

[7] Newman, Ph., R. Sweetnam: Occipito-cervical fusion. J. Bone Joint Surg. **51-B** (1969) 423–428.

[8] Patterson, F. P.: Instability of the upper cervical spine. J. Bone Joint Surg. **55-B** (1973) 456–457.

[9] Roosen, K., A. Trauschel, W. Grote: Posterior Atlanto-Axial Fusion: A new compression clamp for laminar osteosynthesis. Arch. Orthop. Traumat. Surg. **100** (1982) 27–31.

[10] Schilling, F., J. P. Haas, M. Schacherl: Die spontane atlanto-axiale Dislokation (Ventralluxation des Atlas) bei chronischer Polyarthritis und Spondylitis ankylopoetica. Fortschr. Geb. Röntgenstr. Nuclearmed. **99** (1963) 518–538.

[11] Sharp, J., D. W. Purser: Spontaneous atlanto-axial dislocation in ankylosing spondylitis and rheumatoid arthritis. Ann. Rheum. Dis. **20** (1961) 47–77.

[12] Schürmann, K.: Rekonstruktive Chirurgie bei Wirbelkörperdestruktionen mit begleitenden Stabilisierungsmaßnahmen. Zbl. Neurochir. **37** (1976) 216.

[13] Schürmann, K.: Atlanto-axial dislocation in rheumatoid arthritis with cervical cord compression (myelopathy). Adv. Neurosurg. 7 (1979) 151–159.

Atlanto-axial dislocation in rheumatoid arthritis – signs and symptoms, radiographic pathology, operative techniques and results

H. Brattström, L. Brandt, B. Ljunggren

Introduction

In his monograph "A Treatise on Rheumatism and Rheumatoid Arthritis" of 1890 Garrod presented the first report ever on rheumatoid arthritis of the cervical spine as a clinical entity [9]. He stated that out of 500 patients with rheumatoid arthritis, 178 (36%) showed evidence of cervical spine involvement. This frequent involvement of rheumatoid dislocations of the upper cervical vertebrae has subsequently been verified by many more recent investigators [1, 2, 7, 8, 10, 14]. Such findings represent a continuum from slight degrees of subluxation at the CI – CII level and/or odontoid upward migration without symptoms to severe subluxation and/or pronounced cranial settling with secondary myelopathy or brain stem compression causing total physical incapacitation of the patient [11, 15]. Furthermore it has been recognized that spinal cord damage secondary to a previously proven occipito-atlanto-axial dislocation is not an infrequent cause of sudden death in afflicted patients [12].

This report is focused on long-term results after posterior occipito-cervical fusion performed with a follow-up of at least 4 years and describes our operative techniques and complications.

Patient Material

This report includes a consecutive series of 47 patients, who presented rheumatoid subluxation at the CI – CII level, and who were operated upon with a posterior fusion in the years 1971 – 1976. Thirty-six were female, and 11 male; age ranged from 27 to 74 (mean: 61), and 40 patients were rheuma-seropositive (85%). Thirty-four patients (72%) had received treatment with steroids for one year or more prior to surgery.

Signs and symptoms

Occipito-atlanto-axial dislocations may cause a wide spectrum of signs and symptoms including brain stem and cranial nerve root dysfunction, cervical myelopathy and cervical nerve root involvement with poorly localized motor abnormalities ranging from fatigability to paraparesis or quadriparesis and sensory dysfunction usually manifested as severe suboccipital headaches in the sensory C II root distribution. Vascular disturbance may also be encountered with symptoms including syncopé, vertigo, transient hemiparesis and episodic loss of visual fields.

There is also a group of patients who show no or very slight symptoms which may be eliminated by a simple neck collar. In the present series the patients could be divided in 4 symptom-groups:
1. Symptoms ascribed to cervical root compression, mostly involving the sensory C II root with intense sub-occipital headaches,
2. Unpleasant experience of instability in the neck manifested as audible crepitation when the patients rotates or moves his/her head forwards/backwards,
3. Symptoms caused by compression of the cervical cord, which includes limb paraesthesias, variable weakness in the upper and lower extremities ranging from slight weakness to an obvious quadriparesis. In this context it should be stressed that neurological symptoms may be quite difficult to evaluate in patients who are already severely crippled by a generalized rheumatoid arthritis with severe and widespread chronic joint pathology and muscle atrophies. In severe cases spasticity and sphincter disturbances were encountered,
4. Symptoms due to vertebral arterial insufficiency, such as vertigo, syncopé, and transitory loss of visual fields.

Radiographic findings

The radiological examination should include lateral radiographs of the whole cervical spine, in both flexion and extension. A distance from the lower posterior border of the anterior arch of the atlas to the nearest part of the dens epistropheus exceeding 3 mm is regarded as pathological indicating an anterior or horizontal atlanto-axial dislocation. On reviewing previous radiographic examinations it was noted that a horizontal atlanto-axial dislocation almost without exception precedes any vertical (occipito-) atlanto-axial dislocation [13] or "cranial settling". In cases with advanced dislocations and with erosions and destruction of the odontoid process it may be difficult to estimate any vertical dislocation of the C I and C II vertebra. We used a method recently described in a thesis from the University of Lund [13]: The distance between the palato-occipital line

(McGregor's line) and the lower end plate of the C II vertebra is measured. This measurement can easily be performed with high accuracy. The measurement points are easily defined as the arthritic destruction of the lower end plate of the C II vertebral is extremely rare. A measured value below 34 mm in males and below 29 mm in females is regarded as indicating the presence of a vertical dislocation and the progress of such dislocation can, thus, be recognized by comparing consecutive radiographs. Symptoms are usually aggravated when vertical dislocation is superimposed upon an already existent horizontal atlanto-axial instability and the patient no longer experiences a relief from his/her symptoms by conservative treatment with a neck collar.

Computerized tomography (CT) offers good information concerning the bony cervical spine and joints as well as impediment of the cervical spinal canal and should be the method of choice in examinations of patients with advanced rheumatoid arthritic changes involving the upper cervical spine.

Indications for surgery

One or more of the following criteria should be fulfilled:

1. Severe suboccipital pain/headache despite external fixation by neck collar treatment.
2. Neurological symptoms (cord compression and/or symptoms attribute to vertebral artery compression).
3. Great difficulties in wearing a cervical neck collar or a patient who simply is so crippled that he/she can not apply a collar him/herself.
4. Instability.

Operative procedure

Patients were considered eligible for surgery when an atlanto-axial luxation with or without a vertical dislocation had been verified according to the radiographic criteria given above and when one or more of the above clinical criteria were fulfilled. Antibiotic prophylactic treatment is now routinely used (not in the first 15 patients). In cases with vertical dislocation, skull traction with a Gardner-Wells tong is applied some days prior to surgery with the patient in a Stryker turning frame so as to obtain the best possible realignment. In cases with only horizontal dislocation, skull traction is applied the day before surgery or immediately prior to operation. General anaesthesia is used and administered via an endotracheal tube, introduced with the patient in the supine position on the Stryker frame. Traction prevents hazardous movements of the cervical spine when the patient is positioned on the operating table in the prone position. The head is placed on a cerebellar headrest, which ensures that no inadvertent pressure is placed around the eyes. A midline incision is made from the inion to the spinous process of C IV and the paracervical musculature is then dissected off the spinous processes and laminae. The suboccipital musculature is dissected from the occipital bone in a subperiosteal plane with cutting current and sharp-blunt dissection. An occipito-cervical fusion is then performed (fig. 1) [3, 4, 5].

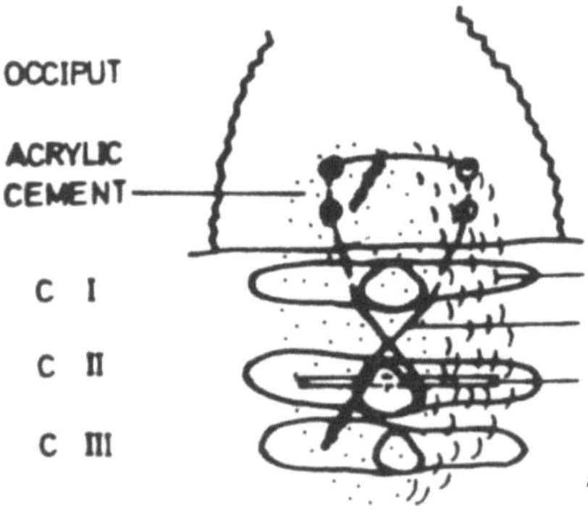

a

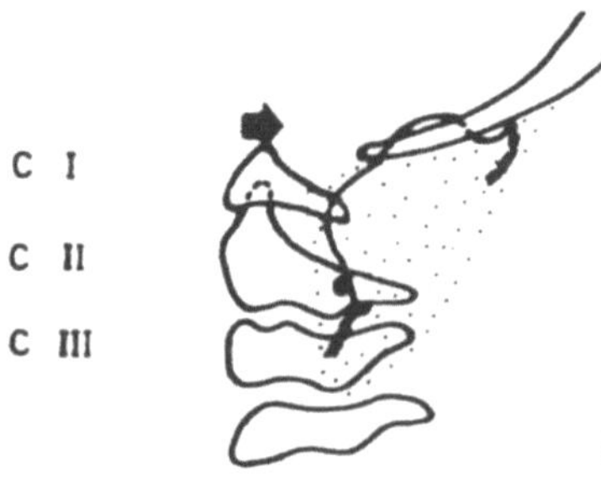

b

Fig. 1 a Schematical drawing of the operative procedure with twisted wire ends on one side embedded in acrylic cement and bone chips on the opposite side to result in bony fusion.

Fig. 1 b Schematical drawing of operative procedure; side view.

c

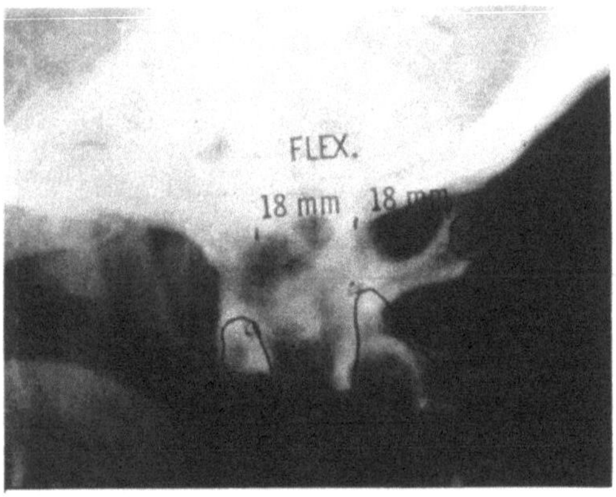

d

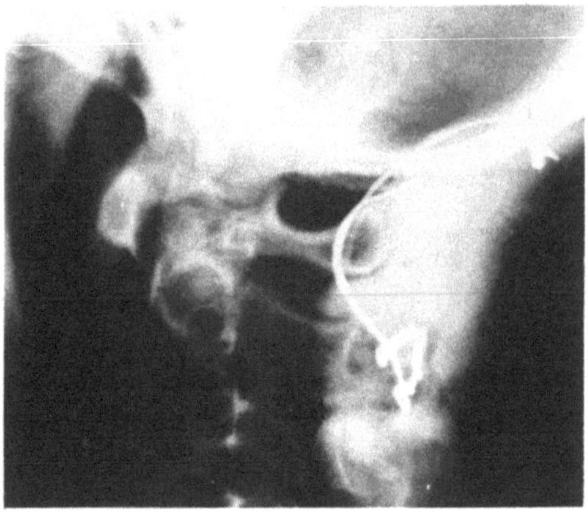

Fig. 1 c Roentgenological side view prior to surgery demonstrating a severe posterior dislocation of dens epistropheus; actual distance between posterior atlas arch and dens: 18 mm.

Fig. 1 d Roentgenological side view after reposition and posterior fusion.

Four burr holes are made in the occipital bone with a trephine, two on each side of the midline, the lower two holes approximately 7 – 8 mm above the edge of the foramen magnum. The posterior arch of the atlas is dissected free and a nylon thread is passed extradurally and ventral to the posterior arch. By means of this nylon thread a stainless loop of steel wire is pulled under the arch. The loop is then cut and the two free wires are crossed, whereupon one cranial wire end is bent and passed in and out through the burr holes on one side and the other wire is similarly passed through the burr holes on the other occipital side. The upper wire ends are then twisted in the midline below the occipital protuberance. A pin, originally designed to fix a fractured medial malleous, is then passed through the spinous process of C II, its way through the process having been prepared by introducing both ends of a heavy towel clamp. One end of the pin is bent so as to improve later incasement in bone cement and to prevent the wire from slipping. One caudal steel wire end is now passed dorsal to the pin and twisted with the other wire end passed identically on the other side. When the atlas arch is very thin or retracted in the foramen magnum, a laminectomy is preferred and the steel wires instead passed ventrally to the pin in the C II spinous process (fig. 2).

On one side the two occipital burr holes, the proximal and distal wire twistings, the C II spinous process and the bent end of the pin in the process were encased in acrylic bone cement. Heat production during polymerisation was counteracted by heavy rinsing with physiologic saline solution. The uncovered occipital bone on the other side and laminae on that side were partly decorticated with a chisel and covered with bone chips obtained from the iliac crest and bone meal from the burr holes so as to result in a future bony fusion. After closure of the wound in several layers (without drainage), skull traction tongs and the endotracheal

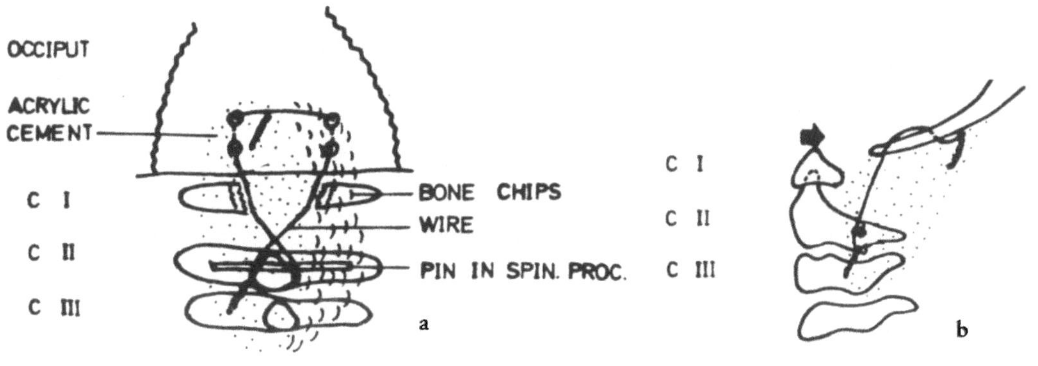

Fig. 2a Schematical drawing of the operative procedure when laminectomy has been performed.

Fig. 2b Schematical drawing when laminectomy of C I was performed. Note that the wire is pulled ventral to the pin in the C II spinous process in such cases.

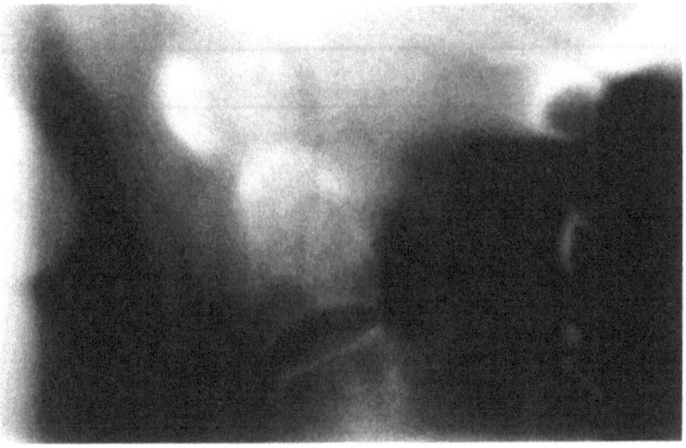

Fig. 2c Roentgenological side view prior to surgery. Note that the posterior atlas arch is immediately anterior to the posterior rim of the foramen magnum necessitating laminectomy.

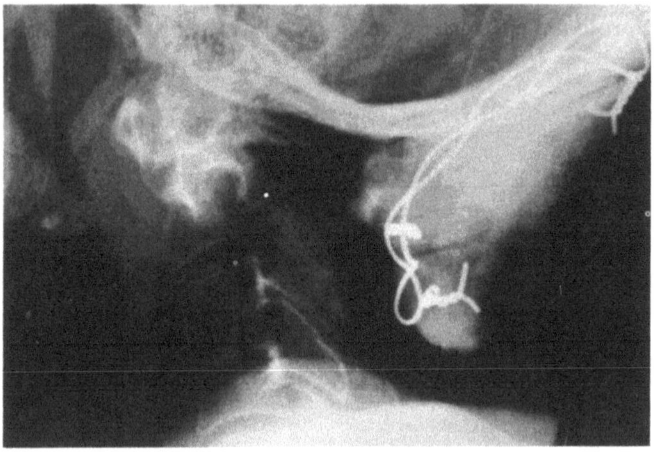

Fig. 2d Roentgenological side view after posterior fusion with wire pulled ventral to the pin in the C II spinous process.

tube are removed and the patient returned to the neurosurgical intensive care unit. After a postoperative radiographic check-up the patient is mobilized on the following day in a soft neck collar.

Operative results

Fracture of the spinous process of C II occurred within the first two months in two patients, who had a second exploration with extended fusion to lower spinous processes with favourable end results. Fracture of the steel wire visualized on radiographic check ups occurred in three patients, in whom however the fusion appeared radiographically stable. Five patients had late infectious complications, in four cases necessitating reoperation with exstirpation of the acrylic cement whereupon the infection cleared off and the bony fusion appeared stable. Reluxation occurred in one patient, who was not subjected to further surgery.

Pain relief and amelioration of preoperative symptoms was experienced postoperatively in 45 patients. One patient with an acute tetraplegia markedly improved and could manage her wheelchair, eat by herself and showed restored bladder function.

Discussion

Mikulowski and coworkers from the University of Lund in 1975 presented a study based on systematic post mortem examinations of rheumatoid arthritis individuals with sudden death [12]. This study revealed an unexpectedly high and not previously reported incidence (11%) of fatal cord compression in rheumatoid arthritis patients with atlanto-axial dislocation. This study points to the necessity of early recognition of this complication in RA patients and to evaluation and selection of patients amenable to surgical correction and stabilization [6]. Since extended periods of time in bed are particularly harmful for RA patients, an operative procedure allowing immediate mobilization is highly desirable. Ideally the fusion should furthermore permit the patient not to be dependent on the use of any external fixation. In our mind the described method has these advantages. The favorable experiences of the described operative procedure in combination with the low complication rate and the fact that the horizontal instability, if not controlled, usually proceeds to the more harmful vertical dislocation, are all indices in favour of an active surgical approach.

References

[1] Ball, J., J. Sharp: Rheumatoid arthritis of the cervical spine. In: Modern trends in rheumatology, vol. 2 (A. G. S. Hill ed.). Butterworth, London 1971.

[2] Bland, J. H.: Rheumatoid arthritis of the cervical spine. J. Rheumatol. 1 (1974) 319 – 342.

[3] Brattström, H., L. Granholm: Chirurgie der Halswirbelsäule bei Patienten mit Rheumatoider Arthritis. Orthopäde 2 (1973) 118 – 120.

[4] Brattström, H., L. Granholm: Atlanto-axial fusion in rheumatoid arthritis. Acta orthop. Scand. 47 (1976) 619 – 628.

[5] Brattström, H.: Surgery in Atlanto-axial dislocation in rheumatoid arthritis. Reconstr. Surg. Traumat., vol. 18, pp. 16 – 29. Karger, Basel 1981.

[6] Conaty, J. P., E. S. Mongan: Cervical fusion in rheumatoid arthritis. J. Bone Joint Surg. (Am) 63 (1981) 1218 – 1227.

[7] Conlon, P. W., I. C. Isdale, B. S. Rose: Rheumatoid arthritis of the cervical spine. Ann. Rheum. Dis. **25** (1966) 120–126.
[8] Dirheimer, Y.: The craniovertebral region in chronic inflammatory rheumatic diseases, pp. 173. Springer Verlag, Berlin–Heidelberg–New York 1977.
[9] Garrod, A. E.: A Treatise on rheumatism and rheumatoid Arthritis, pp. 1–342. C. Griffin, London 1890.
[10] Martel, W., J. W. Page: Cervical vertebral erosions and subluxations in rheumatoid arthritis and ankylosing spondylitis. Arthritis Rheum. **3** (1960) 546–556.
[11] Menezes, A. H., J. C. van Gilder, C. J. Graf, et al.: Craniocervical abnormalities. A comprehensive surgical approach. J. Neurosurg. **53** (1980) 444–455.
[12] Mikulowski, P., F. A. Wollheim, P. Rotmil, et al.: Sudden death in rheumatoid arthritis with atlanto-axial dislocation. Acta Med. Scand. **198** (1975) 445–451.
[13] Redlund-Johnell, I.: Dislocations of the cervical spine in rheumatoid arthritis. Academical Thesis from the Department of diagnostic radiology, Allmänna sjukhuset, pp. 1–140. University of Lund, Malmö 1984.
[14] Smith, P. H., R. T. Benn, J. Sharp: Natural history of rheumatoid cervical luxations. Ann. Rheum. Dis. **31** (1972) 431–439.
[15] Gilder, J. C. van, A. H. Menezes: Craniovertebral abnormalities and their treatment. In: H. H. Schmidek, W. H. Sweet (eds.): Operative neurosurgical techniques; indications, methods, and results, vol. I, pp. 1221–1235. Grune & Stratton, Orlando, FL-London 1982.

The role of the compression clamp for dynamic posterior fusion in rheumatoid atlanto-axial dislocation

K. Roosen, W. Grote, A. Trauschel, R. Kalff, W. Castro

Introduction

Hardly any of the surgeons operating in this vital area can be free from anxiety, when wires or autogenous tendons have to be guided around the vertebral arches passing through the spinal canal. Cracks occuring in those cerclage wires and even vertebral arch fractures have been reported by tightening the wires [8, 14, 21]. These complications gave rise to the idea for clamping the vertebral arches at the posterior aspect. The method is simple, safe, biomechanically reliable and variable, dependent on the individual anatomical conditions. This approach can be added to the already large number of treatments [1, 4, 5, 9–16] and is especially useful for correcting the instability caused of rheumatoid arthritis [18–22, 24–27].

The new device [21–23]

The first model, based on the Harrington conceptions, proved to be on theoretical grounds inadequate. Only the introduction of a spring into a hookbarrel allowed a constant contact pressure in the system (fig. 1). Reparative alteration procedures

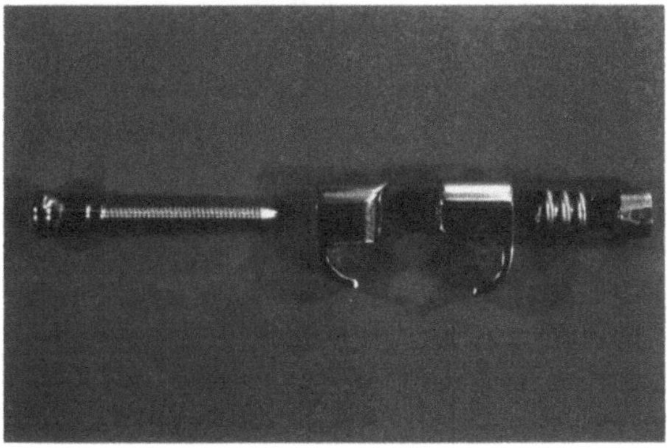

Fig. 1 The single parts of the device (explosion figure).

at the bony structures usually cause a loss of contact pressure necessary for the exact and solid osteosynthesis. This reduction is effectively compensated for by the permanent force of the internal spring.

The spring is held firmly in the hookbarrel by a nut that is moveable in a longitudinal axis but is safe from twisting and cannot be detached from the barrel (fig. 2). Three pieces have to be tightened together by the surgeon: two hooks and the screw.

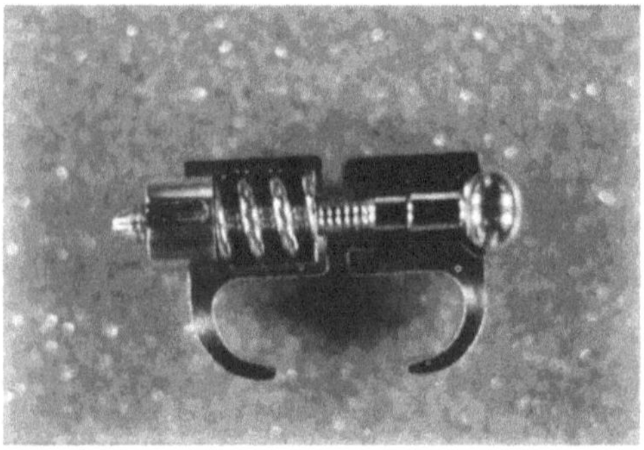

Fig. 2 Median section of the device.

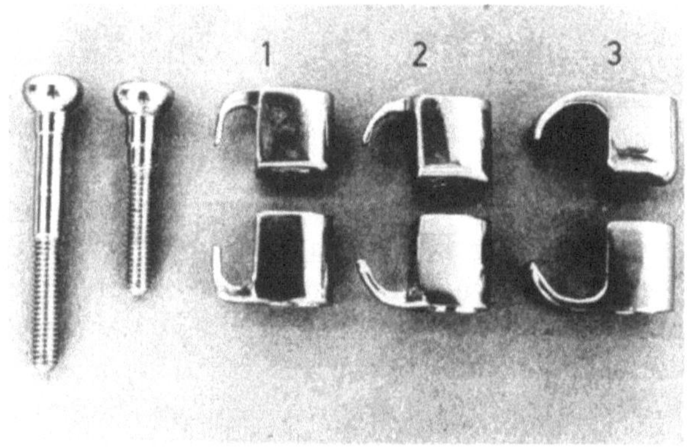

Fig. 3 Varying sizes of the screw and the hook.

All pieces are variable (fig. 3), the length of the screw, the size of the barrel of the clamps, the width and the depth of the hooks, allowing the implant to be adapted to the bone structures of children as well as of adults (fig. 4 a, b). In case of thin bone structures, common in patients with rheumatoid arthritis, wide hooks are recommended to ensure a more even distribution of pressure.

a

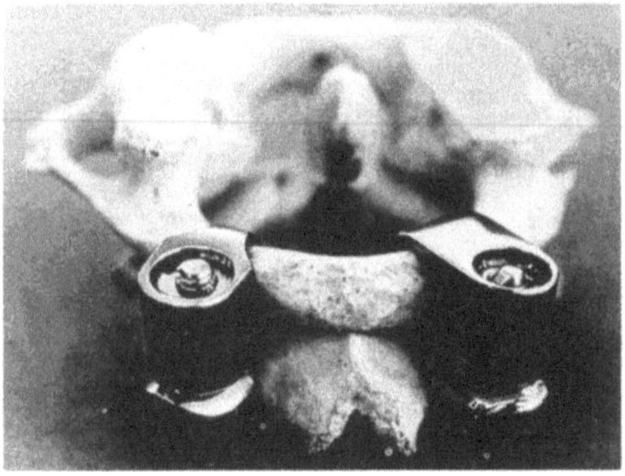

b

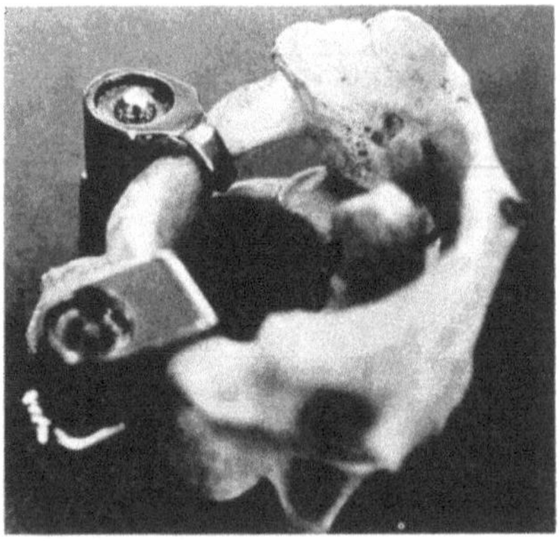

Fig. 4 a, b The clamp applied to an anatomical model at the C 1/C 2 segment.

Even if in the case of a maximum spring tension of 250 N, only one third of the possible metal-bone-contact area is used, which is conceivable in a rough vertebral arch relief, and only pressure peaks of 6 and 9 N per mm² respectively based on the size of the model, are recorded (fig. 5).

To ensure a better contact with the bone, the inner side of the hooks is roughened. The embedding of the head of the screw in a concave cavity and the different diameter of the screw barrel and the inner hook drilling permits an oblique position of the screw (fig. 2); Due to this an optimum adjustment to the vertebral arches is assured preventing deviation from the horizontal plane and a load on the screw causing it to become bend is impossible.

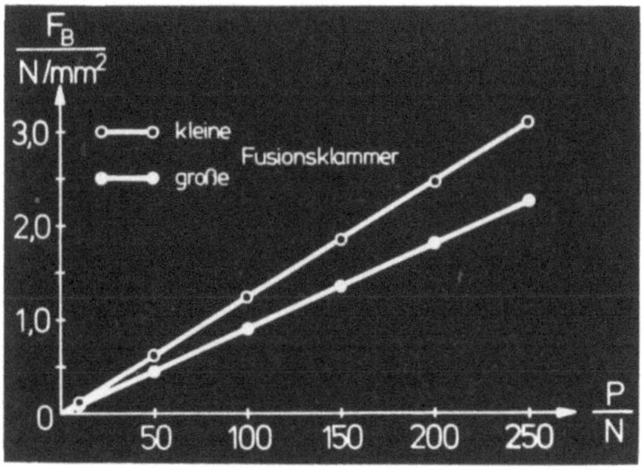

Fig. 5 Pressure/surface relationship.

Surgical technique (fig. 6)

The segment is brought into focus under radiological control. After planing of the contact areas of the bone, a solid cortico-cancellous bone-graft is implanted in the interlaminar space. As an autogenous bone-graft only the iliac crest or portion of the tibia should be used. Presected spinous processes are indeed big enough but not sufficiently stable to carry the stress and by shrinking caused by the spring load and are the reason for unavoidable future instability. Micro-movements are frequently found to be the cause of loosening of the clamp.

In the diseases listed in table 1, we have implanted the device 32 times; among these were 11 patients with rheumatoid arthritis and a five-year-old boy with Grisel's syndrome and imminent instability C 1/2.

Figures 7 a – c demonstrate the clinical example of a 49-year-old female patient with rheumatoid arthritis, who for 3 yrs. had complained of occipital headache and who had developed a progressive cervical myelopathy for 12 months. The extremely thin arches are pathognomonic for rheumatoid arthritis patients. After

Table 1 Indications

Atlanto-axial instability caused by
– Malformation (f. e. os odontoid)
– Trauma
– Primary chronic polyarthritis
– Tumor

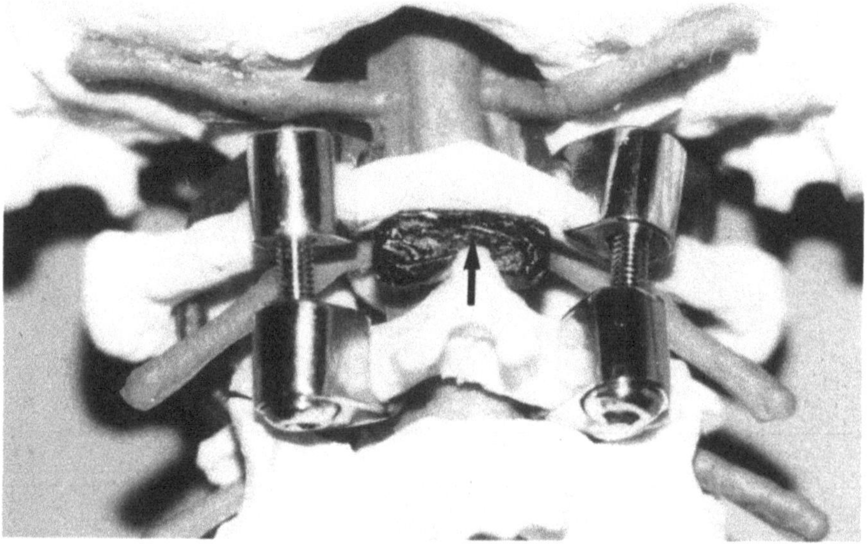

Fig. 6 Model of a C1/C2 interlaminar spondylodesis by interlaminar bone-graft and bilateral dynamic clamps (Roosen – Trauschel). → = graft (cortico-cancellous hip-bone).

the operation (figs. 7 b, c) the pain subsided; the chronic myelopathy improved to such an extent that the patient who had been bedridden before became again a wheelchair patient. Whether the occipito-axial fusion had now been better can only be proven by the long-term result. The oblique view (fig. 7 c) however shows how precisely the clamp hook can be adapted to the individual arch width.

In figure 8 we demonstrate the possibility to extend the spondylodesis caudally by choosing longer screws. The solid cortico-cancellous bone-graft that cushions the pressure on the system and preserves the interlaminar space heals within 6 months.

If the dislocation cannot be eliminated functionally, an extension therapy of variable length should precede the compression spondylodesis.

Complications listed in table 2 occurred in a total of 32 patients. Sensibility disorder and the torticollis however did not decrease but were not harmful to

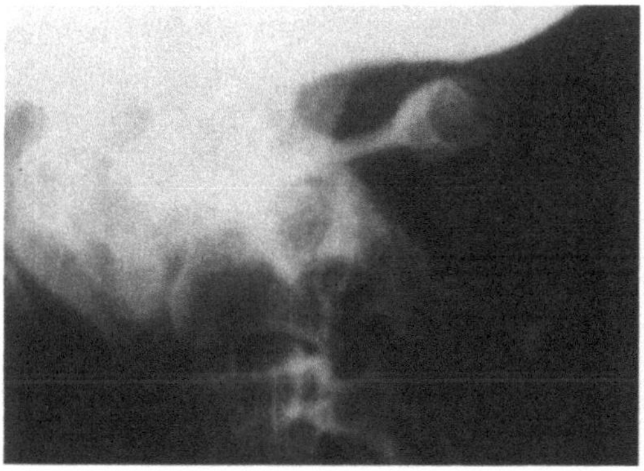

a

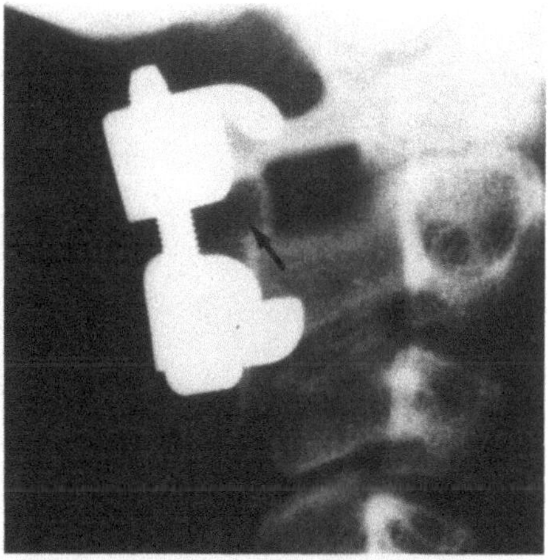

b

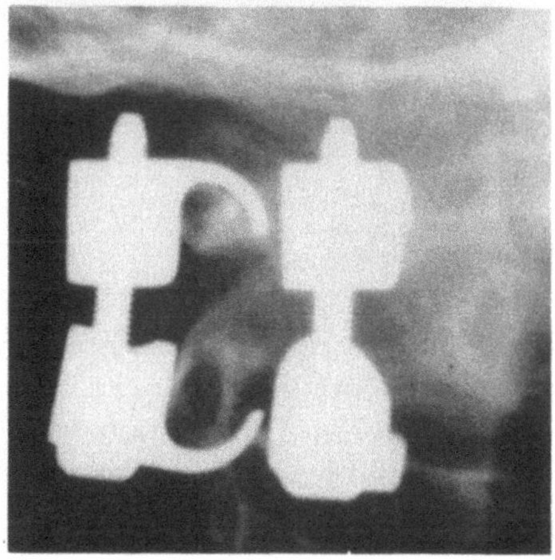

c

Fig. 7a–c a) Rheumatic atlanto-axial dislocation; b) Postoperative situation (→ = graft); c) Oblique view.

Table 2 Complications (n = 32 patients)

Early	Infection – superficial	1
	Hypaesthesia C2	1
	Torticollis	1
Late	loosening – clamp (tumor)	1
	– screws (1 reop.)	3

the patients. In another patient loosening of a screw was observed seven weeks after implantation. Clinically, the preoperative symptoms of cervical neck pain had again increased. She was operated upon again and the system was secured with an additional locking nut between the hooks. Since this incidence an improved design of the clamps will prevent this complication.

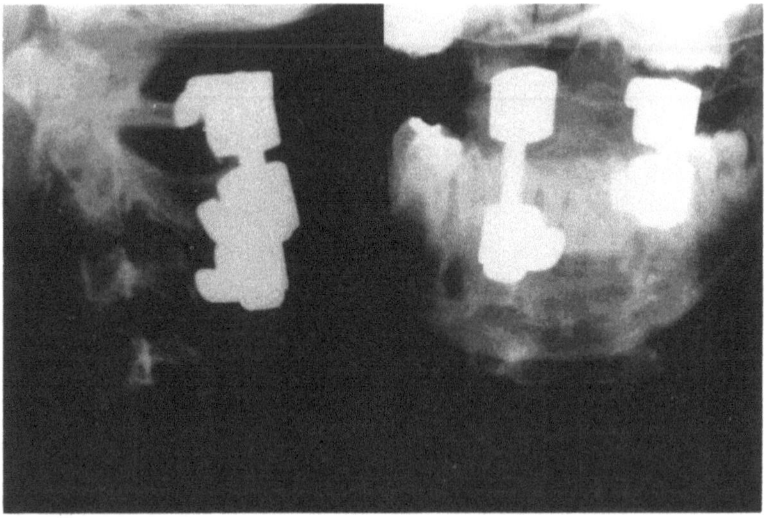

Fig. 8 Spondylodesis caudally extended to C 3 on the right side.

Results

The long-term results are satisfactory. With 9 out of 12 patients the operation dates back more than one year. In all cases, a solid laminar osteosynthesis was achieved (fig. 9). The rotation was limited to 1/3. The impediment could be compensated for by the patients in an acceptable way by moving the body.

Only in three patients, who were operated upon because of other diseases, were the clamps explanted at their own personal wish. There were no load damages of the material according to the metal investigations. In our view the implant can be left in situ without any risk.

During the operation as well as radiologically, the solid bony interlaminar bridge could be assured (fig. 9).

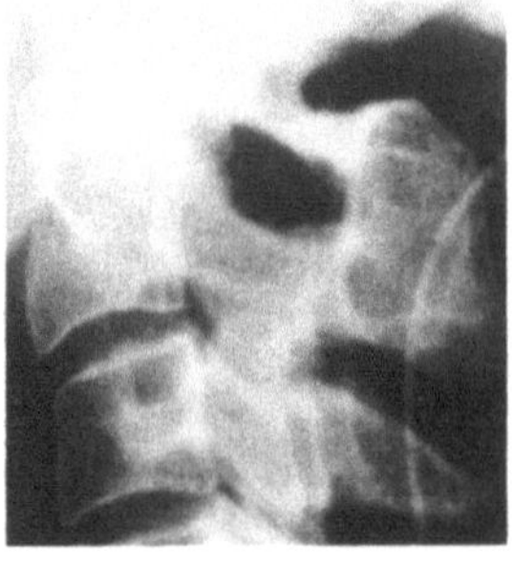

Fig. 9 Solid interlaminar osteosynthesis. 1 year after implantation; immediately after explantation.

Conclusions

As a disadvantage of this procedure as well as of all other posterior fixation methods is the loss of rotation of more or less 2/3 of the rotation capability (which harms the patients differently) should be mentioned as a matter of course. In certain cases of fractures of the odontoid process the anterior screwing technique published by Böhler [3] should definitely be preferred since it preserves rotation function of the C 1/C 2 segment.

The compression clamp method depends on the integrity of the laminar osseous structures, a necessity that can be avoided with the technically problematical transpeduncular screwing. Simple median fractures of the arch of the atlas and congenital anterior or posterior arch defects do not naturally mean a contraindication against the clamp-spondylodesis. After implementation of solid bone-grafts bridging the congenital clefts of the arch the clamp can safely be applied on both sides next to the graft inactivating pathological motion within the defect.

The first stage of a 5-year-old clinical experience with the device has shown that the implant, but especially the auxiliary instruments, needed to be improved. The newest models of the compression clamp have taken care of the negative experiences.

The disadvantages are opposed to those qualities that are rated as positive. Application is safe and, with a little patience, simple to perform. For all sizes of the arches, there are suitable models. For the first time the principle of a dynamic spondylodesis by integration a spring into the design has been realised.

The shape of the hooks guarantee wide pressure distribution, for the thin bone structures of patients suffering from rheumatoid arthritis have little carrying capacity. It must be emphasized that not a single vertebral arch was fractured when fixing the device. Additional external fixation usually is superfluous; the patients can be mobilised after the first post-operative day provided there are no neurological deficits. As a rule, a useful stable interlaminar fusion is achieved after 3 – 4 months.

Based on these results, the appeal to the rheumatologists is justified, to send their patients with atlanto-axial dislocation at an early stage for further treatment. This allows a corrective procedure at a stage when the dislocated segment is still mobile. Once luxation of the C 1/C 2 segment is solidly fixed, laminectomy of C 1 and occipito-cervical fusion [6, 17, 20, 25] will be indicated.

The dynamic compression spondylodesis after Roosen and Trauschel is an alternative and practical method in the treatment of rheumatoid arthritis patients.

References

[1] Alexander, jr. E., H. F. Forsyth, C. H. Davis, et al.: Dislocation of the atlas on the axis: the value of early fusion of C1, C2 and C3. J. Neurosurg. **15** (1958) 353–371.

[2] Bachs, A., L. Barraquer-Bordas, L. Barraquer-Ferre, et al.: Delayed myelopathy following atlanto-axial dislocation by separated odontoid process. Brain **78** (1955) 533–537.

[3] Böhler, J.: Schraubenosteosynthese von Frakturen des Dens axis. Unfallheilkunde **84** (1981) 221–223.

[4] Brattstroem, H., L. Granholm: Atlanto-axial fusion in rheumatoid arthritis. A new method of fixation with wire and bone cement. Acta Orthop. Scand. **47** (1976) 619–628.

[5] Brooks, A. L., E. B. Jenkins: Atlanto-Axial arthrodesis by the wedge compression method. J. Bone Joint Surg. **60-A** (1978) 279–284.

[6] Brussatis, F., M. E. Müller: Okzipito-zervikale Arthrodese durch Verriegelungsspan. Z. Orthop. **84** (1954) 369–373.

[7] Dunbar, H. S., B. S. Ray: Chronic atlanto-axial dislocation with late neurological manifestations. J. Surg. Gynecol. Obstet. **113** (1961) 757–762.

[8] Fried, L. C.: Atlanto-axial fracture dislocations. Failure of posterior C1 to C2 fusion. J. Bone Joint Surg. **55-B** (1973) 490–496.

[9] Gallie, W. E.: Fractures and dislocations of the cervical spine. Am. J. Surg. **46** (1939) 495–499.

[10] Griswold, D. M., J. A. Albright, E. Schiffman: Atlanto-axial fusion for instability. J. Bone Joint Surg. **60-A** (1978) 285–292.

[11] Guillaume du Toit, M. B.: Lateral atlanto-axial arthrodesis – a screw fixation technique. South African J. Surg. **14** (1976) 9–12.

[12] Hentzer, L., M. Schalimtzek: Fractures and subluxations of the atlas and axis. Acta Orthop. Scand. **42** (1971) 251–258.

[13] Holness, R. O., W. J. Huestis, W. J. Howes, et al.: Posterior stabilization with an interlaminar clamp in cervical injuries: Technical note and review of the long-term experience with the method. Neurosurgery **14** (1984) 318–322.

[14] Hupfauer, W., K. F. Schlegel: Unsere Technik der atlanto-axialen Fusion. Chirurg **43** (1972) 476–479.

[15] Karimi, A.: Indikation, Technik und Ergebnisse der operativen Behandlung von Halswirbelsäulen- (HWS) Verletzungen. Fortschr. Neurol. Psychiat. **48** (1980) 183–206.

[16] Kelly, D. L., jr. E. Alexander, H. D. Courtland, et al.: Acrylic fixation of atlanto-axial dislocations. Technical note. J. Neurosurg. **36** (1972) 366–371.

[17] Lipscomb, P. R.: Cervico-occipital fusion for congenital and post-traumatic anomalies of the atlas and axis. J. Bone Joint Surg. **39-A** (1957) 1289–1301.

[18] McGraw, R. W., R. M. Rusch: Atlanto-axial arthrodesis. J. Bone Joint Surg. **55-B** (1973) 482–489.

[19] McLaurin, R. L., R. Vernal, J. H. Salomon: Treatment of fractures of the atlas and axis by wiring without fusion. J. Neurosurg. **36** (1972) 773–780.

[20] Rathke, F. W., K. F. Schlegel: Surgery of the spine. Atlas of Orthopaedic Operations. Vol. I (M. Hackenbroich, A. N. Witt eds.) G. Thieme, Stuttgart 1979.

[21] Roosen, K., A. Trauschel, W. Grote: Posterior atlanto-axial fusion: a new compression clamp for laminar osteo-synthesis. Arch. Orthop. Traumat. Surg. **100** (1982) 27–31.

[22] Roosen, K., W. Grote, A. Trauschel: Modern treatment of the symptomatic os odontoideum. Neurosurg. Rev. **6** (1983) 229–232.

[23] Roosen, K., W. Grote, A. Trauschel: Dorsale Verklammerungsspondylodese der oberen Halswirbelsäule – ein neues technisches Konzept. Med.-orthop. Techn. **103** (1983) 18–21.

[24] Schlesinger, E. B., J. M. Taveras: Lesions of the odontoid and their management. Am. J. Surg. **95** (1958) 641–650.

[25] Schürmann, K.: Atlanto-axial dislocation in rheumatoid arthritis with cervical cord compression (myelopathy). Adv. Neurosurg. 7 (1979) 151 – 158.
[26] Sherk, H. H., B. Snyder: Posterior fusions of the upper cervical spine: Indications, technique, and prognosis. Orthop. Clin. NA **9** (1978) 1091 – 1099.
[27] Stöwsand, D., U. Muhtaroglu: Dorsale Stabilisierung bei Luxationsfrakturen des 1. und 2. Halswirbels mit Palacos und Drahtumschlingung. Neurochirurgia **18** (1975) 120 – 126.
[28] Stratford, J.: Myelopathy caused by atlanto-axial dislocation. J. Neurosurg. **14** (1957) 97 – 104.

Late results in cases of atlanto-axial dislocations after dorsal fusion

N. Brito, P. Klawki, M. Schwarz, D. Voth

Introduction

Cervical myelopathy is caused by a cranio-cervical instability, especially in the segment of atlas-axis, the so-called atlanto-axial dislocation. The myelopathy produces critical symptoms, making surgical intervention necessary [1, 4, 5, 7, 8].

The atlanto-axial dislocation is mainly found in combination with a disease of rheumatic nature, leading to the destruction of joints, as well of the syndesmoses of the osseous activators [2]. It may also originate from a trauma, an instability as result of the operation or from a congenital malformation [11, 13, 16, 19].

Method of treatment

Among the various operative procedures we prefer the dorsal fusion with autologous bone material [17]. We present the late surgical results of 43 dorsal fusions focusing attention on those cases where rheumatoid arthritis was the initial disease (fig. 1).

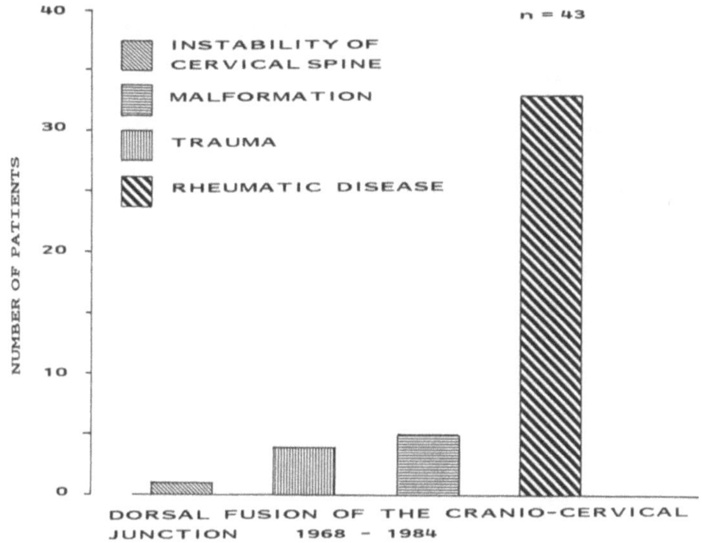

Fig. 1 Patients after dorsal fusion in the region of cranio-cervical junction.

For evaluation of the case material we used

1. pre-operative and postoperative objective neurological findings including continuous postoperative neurological control examination,
2. subjective report of clinical symptoms of the patient,
3. results of radiological pre-operative and postoperative diagnostics and control examinations.

Case material

Figure 1 shows the distribution of etiology referred to in our case material, performing from 1976 to 1984 a total of 43 dorsal fusions. In one patient with a severe instability of the upper head joint after laminectomy of C 1 – C 4, which had been carried out to alleviate an arachnitis, a clinic-neurologically state of tetraplegia existed. But after surgery the patient died of a severe pneumonia.

In 4 patients with malformations in the area of cranio-cervical junction were stabilized by dorsal fusion. These patients suffered from 2 congenital atlanto-axial dislocations, one patient with os odontoideum and a boy (11 years) with chondrodystrophic nanism.

In 5 cases with traumatic dens fracture and the development of a pseudoarthrosis, the postoperative course was without complications.

The patients with chronic rheumatoid diseases – PCP and Morbus Bechterew – and the resulting atlanto-axial dislocation represent the most important group.

Findings and results

In the following we concentrate especially on patients with a chronic rheumatoid disease. The incidence of the atlanto-axial dislocation in the disease increases with advancing years and is most frequently observed at the age between 50 and 70.

Table 1 shows the tabulated presentation not only of the local symptoms but also the symptoms of a cervical myelopathy. The neurological picture can be explained by the different patho-physiological mechanisms. The ventral gliding of the atlas caused a stenosis and compression of the cord. The fact that most cases of atlanto-axial dislocations, even those of more than 12 mm, remain clinically silent, indicates a lateral evading shift of the medulla.

The relative width of the spinal canal in this area of 22 to 24 mm makes this possible. This is also helped by the presence of an epidural venous plexus and the epidural adipose tissue.

Table 1 Clinical symptoms of atlanto-axial dislocation and the resulting myelopathy

	Local symptoms
	1. Pain in the neck
	2. Restricted movement
Cervical myelopathy	*Neurological symptoms*
	1. Dysesthesia
	2. Tingling paresthesia
	3. Motoric lesion { Monoparesis Paraparesis Tetraparesis }
	4. Pathological reflexes
	5. Spinal ataxia
	6. Autonomic dysfunction (Disturbance of micturation and motion)
	7. Signs of vertebro-basilar insufficiency

The structural atlanto-axial weakening can lead to a disturbed blood supply of the vertebro-basilar system due to additional stenosis and compression. The deficits caused by the intermittently reduced blood supply manifests itself in transitory giddy attacks, dysopias and disturbances of consciousness. A further pathogenic factor, increasing the signs of a severe, high cervical myelopathy, is the pseudobasilar impression which can be observed in many cases. This is a penetration of the dens into the foramen magnum causing an increased compression of the medulla and by the slipping of the atlas.

We have divided our case material of atlanto-axial dislocations caused by a chronic-rheumatoid arthritis into 3 groups:

The *1st group* includes patients with local symptoms like rigidity of the neck and painfully restricted movements in the cervical spine without neurological deficits.

The *2nd group* refers to patients with the clinical signs of a cervical myelopathy, which we differentiate, according to the degree of severity of the neurological condition, between a slight, i. e. a beginning cervical myelopathy.

The *3rd group* refers to patient with a severe myelopathy and aggravating neurological deficits.

The *1st group* – only local symptoms – includes 10 patients (fig. 2). The time interval between making the diagnosis of a rheumatoid disease and developing of local symptoms was on the average 15 years at an individual time span of 5 to 25 years. The period from the definite diagnosis of an atlanto-axial dislocation to operation was on the average 1.9 years. The distance of the atlanto-axial dislocation was preoperatively at 9.5 mm. In 4 cases a pseudobasilar impression could radiologically be proved.

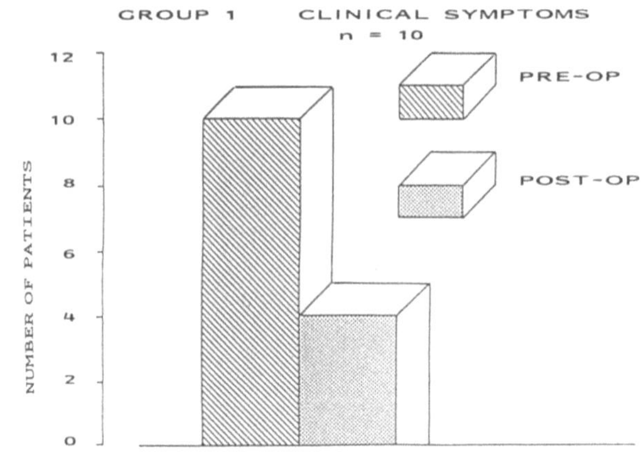

Fig. 2 Pre- and post-operative local symptoms in patients of the 1st group.

In 10 patients only local symptoms were reported in our clinical examination. Postoperatively only 4 patients complained of local pain, 6 patients were without pain. One patient died 16 days postoperatively as a result of bilateral pneumonia. One patient showed 2 weeks after operation a distinct deterioration of consciousness. The computerized tomography showed an intracranial inclusion of air in the base of the skull to the left and medially. The 4th ventricle could not be outlined anymore, but a hydrocephalus occlusus of the 1st – 3rd ventricle had developed. After application of a CSF-drainage system the symptoms receded quickly and the ventricular sizes became normal. During the postoperative X-ray controls the atlanto-axial distance was on the average 7.3 mm compared to 9.5 mm preoperatively. A sufficiently strong osseous structure was seen after 6 – 7 months and the plaster of Paris diadem jacket could be removed.

The *2nd group* – suffering from a slight, i. e. incipient cervical myelopathy – consisted of 7 patients (fig. 3). The duration of chronic polyarthritis until the appearance of cervical vertebral column symptoms was on an average 13.4 years and the time between identified atlanto-axial dislocation and operation 2.1 years. The extent of the dislocation was preoperatively 9 mm, postoperatively 6.4 mm. One patient showed additionally a pseudobasilar impression. A 49-years old patient of this group suffered from neurosurgical complications and showed a delayed healing of an epidural empyema and a tetraparesis forcing the removal of the inserted bone blocks for stabilization. After recovery an external stabilization was achieved using a plaster of Paris diadem jacket. The neurological symptoms did not show further deterioration, although 5 1/2 years later the atlanto-axial dislocation had increased from 5 to 9 mm. After about 4 1/2 months a radiologically demonstrable bony junction was present.

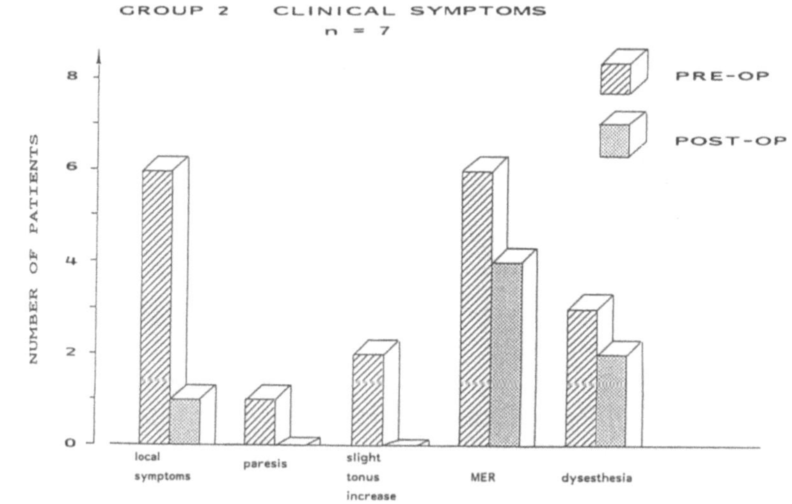

Fig. 3 Clinical symptoms in patients of the 2nd group.

The *3rd group* of 16 patients included mainly older patients with severe cervical myelopathy (tab. 2). The period from the definite diagnosis of PCP to the onset of complaints in the cervical vertebral column region was 21 years on the average and from a diagnosed atlanto-axial dislocation to operation 1.8 years. The extension of dislocation preoperatively had a mean value of 9.9 mm. In 11 patients an additional pseudobasilar impression could be proved.

Table 2 Pre- and postoperative clinical symptoms of 16 patients with severe myelopathy

Group 3 Clinical Symptoms	Pre-op.	Unchanged	Postop. Complete remission	Partial remission
Local	16	1	13	2
Neurological symptoms				
Caudal cranial nerves	2	–	2	–
Medulla oblongata	2	–	2	–
Tetraspasticity	16	6	1	5
Paresis	5	–	2	3
Pathological reflexes	9	5	4	–
Spinal ataxia	7	2	5	–
Dysesthesia	8	3	3	2
Hypesthesia	9	5	3	1
Autonomic	5	–	5	–

n = 16 (from these 4 patients died)

The following complications were seen in this group. A delayed healing process developed in one patient in the region of the donor area of the bone, the dorsal iliac pelvic crest. Retarded healing in the area of cervical spine was observed in 2 patients. For this reason the inserted bone chips had to be removed from the cranio-cervical area in one case and the patient died of a sepsis. Another patient also died of pneumonia and in a further patient the cause of death could not be determined, even after autopsy.

A 70 years old patient died 2 months after the intervention of a severe broncho-pneumonia and additionally signs of a chronic medullar compression were found at autopsy.

The four deceased patients had an average age of 60 3/4 years. The average wearing of the plaster of Paris diadem jacket until a radiological examination showed a bony junction was 5 months. The radiological pictures showed post-operatively an average reduction of atlanto-axial dislocation of 9 mm; pre-operatively 9.9 mm. On the average 4 postoperative control examinations were made during a period of about 2 years (tab. 3).

Table 3 Results of the dorsal fusion (n = 33)

	Group 1 No Neurology	Group 2 Slight cervical Myelopathy	Group 3 Severe cervical Myelopathy
Complete Remission	5	3	1
Partial Remission	1	2	5
Unchanged	3*	2	6**
Aggravated	–	–	–
Deceased	1	–	4**
Total	10	7	16

* From these, 2 patients with pseudobasilar impression
** 3 patients with pseudobasilar impression
*** Pseudobasilar impression in all patients

Discussion

We have examined the results, in particular the late results, of 33 patients who underwent a dorsal vertebral fusion for an atlanto-axial dislocation caused by rheumatoid arthritis [17]. It was clear that those cases with a severe and manifest myelopathy combined with a pseudobasilar impression improve [3, 6, 10, 12, 18].

Even in cases where a pseudobasilar impression is not present, the postoperative course showed unsatisfactory neurological results. Whether a possible second intervention – transoral dens resection – can improve the results is debatable.

On the other hand we found much better operational results in the groups 1 and 2 and we believe that the results can only be improved if
1 – radiologically a progressive atlanto-axial dislocation is proved and
2 – only local symptoms are present without neurological deficits [9, 14, 15].

Summary

We surveyed 43 cases of dorsal fusion in relation to late operational results. The majority of 33 cases refers to an acquired atlanto-axial dislocation caused by rheumatoid arthritis. We have divided these cases related to their clinical neurological symptoms into 3 groups:
a) only local symptoms,
b) local symptoms with beginning cervical myelopathy and
c) local symptoms with distinct myelopathy.

In view of the unsatisfactory late operational results in group "c" to improve an already manifest cervical myelopathy by dorsal fusion, an early operation should be carried out to avoid the development of a cervical myelopathy (operation if only local symptoms are present). In cases of already present or the beginning of even slight neurological signs of a cervical myelopathy an operation is necessary.

References

[1] Ahlgren, P., J. Fog: Atlanto-epistrophical subluxation in rheumatoid arthritis. Acta Rheum. Scand. **14** (1968) 210–221.

[2] Ball, J., J. Sharp: Rheumatoid arthritis of the cervical spine. In: Modern trends in rheumatology, Vol. 2, p. 117. Butterworths, London 1971.

[3] Cregan, J. C. F.: Internal fixation of the unstable rheumatoid cervical spine. Ann. Rheum. Dis. **25** (1966) 242–252.

[4] Crellin, R. Q., J. J. Maccabe, E. B. D. Hamilton: Severe subluxation of the cervical spine in rheumatoid arthritis. J. Bone Joint Surg. **52** (1970) 244–251.

[5] Davis, F. W., H. E. Markley: Rheumatoid arthritis with death from medullary compression. Ann. Met. Med. **35** (1967) 451–458.

[6] Schürmann, K.: Atlanto-axial dislocation in rheumatoid arthritis with cervical cord compression (myelopathy). Adv. Neurosurg. 7 (1970) 151–159.

[7] Hopkins, J. S.: Lower cervical rheumatoid subluxation with tetraplegia. J. Bone Joint Surg. **49-B** (1967) 46.

[8] Martel, W., M. Abell: Fatal atlanto-axial luxation in rheumatoid arthritis. Arth. Rheum. **6** (1963) 224–231.

[9] Meienberg, O., A. Bischoff, F. Regli, et al.: Polyneuropathie bei progressiv chronischer Polyarthritis. Dtsch. Med. Wochenschr. **42** (1972) 1595–1598.

[10] Moore, H. D.: Death from vertebral artery thrombosis in rheumatoid arthritis. Medical Memoranda 2 (1968) 537–538.
[11] Polyzoides, A. J., J. R. Pearson: Tetraplegia in rheumatoid arthritis with complete recovery after surgery. Br. J. Surg. **60** (1973) 327–329.
[12] Robinson, H. S., M. D. Vancouver: Rheumatoid arthritis – atlanto-axial subluxation and its clinical presentation. Can. Med. Ass. J. **94** (1966) 470–477.
[13] Schilling, F., J. P. Haas, M. Schacherl: Die spontane atlanto-axiale Dislokation (Ventralluxation des Atlas) bei chronischer Polyarthritis und Spondylitis ankylopoetica. Fortschr. Röntgenstr. **99** (1963) 518–523.
[14] Schilling, F., M. Schacherl, A. Bopp, et al.: Veränderungen der Halswirbelsäule (Spondylitis cervicalis) bei der chronischen rheumatischen Polyarthritis und bei der Spondylitis ankylopoetica. Radiologe **12** (1963) 483.
[15] Schilling, F.: Die schwergradigen Formen der Spondylitis ankylopoetica, pp. 4511–4522. Verlag G. Braun, Karlsruhe 1980.
[16] Schilling, F.: Die Affektion der oberen Halswirbelsäule bei der Spondylitis ankylopoetica. Z. Rheumaforsch. **22** (1963) 342–348.
[17] Schürmann, K.: Ventrale und dorsale Fusionsoperationen an der Halswirbelsäule bis zum Wirbelkörperersatz. Indikation, Operationstechnik und Ergebnisse, Band 81. Ber. Physikal.-Med. Ges. Würzburg 1973.
[18] Störig, G., F. Schilling: Die Fraktur der Halswirbelsäule bei Spondylitis ankylopoetica. Z. Orth. Grenzgeb. 97 (1963) 492–502.
[19] Vogelsang, H., H. Zeidler, A. Wittenborg, et al.: Rheumatoid cervical luxations with fatal neurological complications. Neuroradiology **6** (1973) 87–92.

Clinical features of Lyme disease: Immunological and neurological aspects

K. M. Goebel, A. Krause, H. H. Goebel

Introduction

Recent clinico-epidemiological studies and microbiologic-immunological research provided conclusive evidence that varying reactive oligoarthritides may be triggered by various bacteria and viruses which, based on genetic predisposition, may frequently follow the pathogenic pattern of an immune complex arthritis. Among the seronegative oligoarthritides a recently (1976) rediscovered and described infection may be placed that was termed "Lyme" disease due to the small community of Lyme (Connecticut/USA) where a cluster of such patients had been observed by Yale University scientists [3, 5, 9 – 14].

The clinical symptomatology comprises erythema chronicum migrans [7, 9, 13, 16], occasionally life-threatening cardiac [8] and neurological [1, 15] complications and a rheumatoid symptomatology [4, 5].

Finally, thorough investigations revealed that "Lyme" disease is a bacterial infection caused by tick bite and by numerous immunolocally related transmitted spirochetes [2, 3, 9, 11]. This report deals with the broad clinical spectrum of "Lyme" disease and the correlation between different rheumatologico-immunological and neurological complications of this disease.

Patients

This study comprises 24 patients, 22 to 54 years old (mean age 48.5 years), 14 men and 10 women whose clinical symptoms started between 3 and 6 months after the tick bite. According to clinical activity at the time of the first examination, patients were placed in stages I or II of "Lyme" disease. 10 patients already had advanced to stage III associated with the clinical spectrum of complicated visceral involvement.

Based on differential diagnostic examination the diagnosis could finally be ascertained by demonstrating antibodies against Ixodes ricinus spirochetes in serum or cerebrospinal fluid.

Methods

Blood samples were mixed with either ACD solution or with EDTA and then submitted to various tests. Several rheumatic factors, inflammatory proteins and immune complexes were determined immuno-nephelometrically using a Laser as the light source. Data were plotted on a reference curve which was produced by employing standardized dilutions. Analysis of biochemical parameters was routinely performed according to standard techniques. Quantitative determination of antibodies against borrelia of Ixodes ricinus spirochetes was based on an enzyme-linked immunoassay (ELISA). The applied biological procedure is predicated on the test system of a solid ELISA that utilizes the sandwich technique. The antibodies present in the blood sample adhere to substances which are fixed on the spheres. The conjugate then reacts with the antigen antibody complex adherent to the sphere. The non-adherent components are then removed by washing the spheres. During the subsequent reaction a colour develops the intensity of which (proportional to the antibody level in the blood sample) is measured spectrophotometrically. All our data were controlled in outside reference laboratories.

Results

All 24 patients came from an epidemic district surrounding the Marburg-Biedenkopf area in Northern Hessen where, particularly during the summers of 1983 to 1985, numerous tick-bite infections were registered.

All 24 patients regularly developed, at the site of the tick-bite, a very painful erythema of partly annular expansion and central pallor which sometimes enlarged to palm size, and retrospectively could be considered an erythema chronicum migrans. While 14 patients developed additional symptoms when under observation at the outpatient rheumatology clinic of Marburg University, 10 patients already presented with the complete pattern of an extensive visceral involvement, stage III of Lyme disease. Clinical details and subclassification of individual patients' Lyme disease according to stages I and II (early) and stage III (late) are listed in table 1. As regards neurological complications, 8 patients demonstrated transient cranial nerve palsies. Simple non-invasive diagnostic procedures sufficed in these 10 patients to document cardiac complications (tab. 1). Numerous patients of the entire group developed such cardiac symptoms only after a symptom-free interval and showed rheumatological complications which partly started as mild polyarthralgia and finally resulted in partly erosive-destructive oligoarthritides. The typical distribution pattern of inflammatory joint involvement in all patients is illustrated in figure 1. During long-term observation, 4 patients showed radiculoneuritis and also central neural pathway deficits.

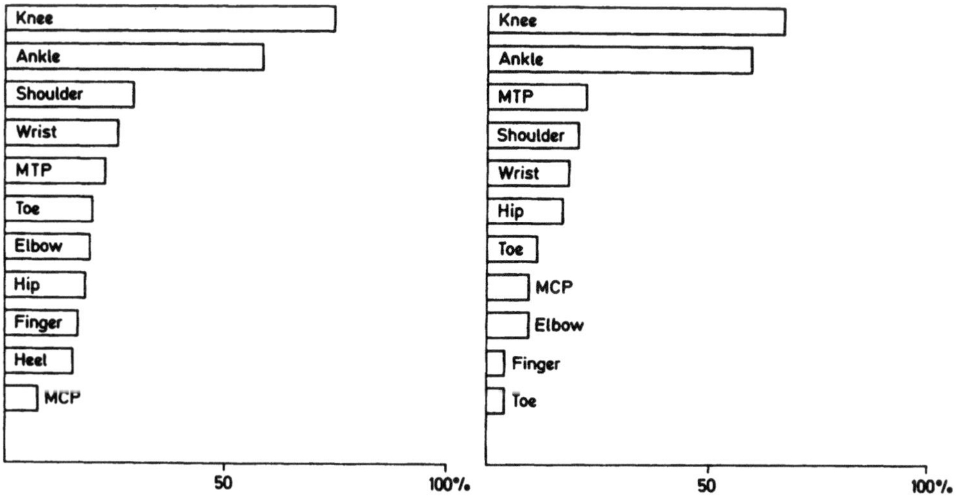

Fig. 1 Distribution of joint symptoms in pauci-articular oligoarthritis in Lyme disease. The joint symptoms may be acute, short-lived and transient. 52 patients in the literature, including 24 patients observed at the University Hospital of Marburg, are considered. 39 had an acute onset (left side), and in 13 patients the onset was insidious (right side). Weight bearing joints, particularly the knees and ankles, are most frequently involved.

In addition, electromyography showed secondary muscular involvement. While simultaneously antibodies against cross striated muscle were demonstrated in these patients' sera, histopathology of a muscle biopsy gave evidence of type II muscle fibre atrophy (fig. 2). Each patient had general clinical symptoms of varying intensity (tab. 1). They had sometimes considerably elevated erythrocyte sedimentation rates. In their sera, nephelometry revealed abnormally high immune complexes (IK 32.4 ± 11.2 g/l). Antibodies against yersinia, salmonella, chlamydia, brucella, staphylococci, and streptococci were absent. The diagnosis of Lyme disease was based on the serological evidence of high IgG antibody titres against Ixodes ricinus spirochetes (Ixodes ricinus borrelia-ELISA-IgG 545 ± 112 IU) indicating a tick-transmitted infection.

Discussion

On principle, differential diagnostic aspects of seronegative oligoarthritis ought to include Lyme disease. Diagnosis of atypical cases of Lyme disease is particularly difficult when typical clinical findings which may allow exact classification frequently only develop during long periods of observation. Non-characteristic dermatological, rheumatological and neurological symptoms encountered by

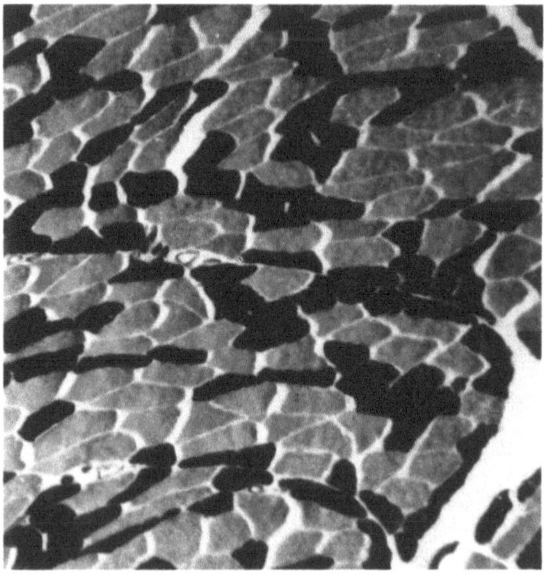

Fig. 2 Type II fiber (dark) muscle atrophy which sometimes may be observed particularly in those patients with Lyme disease who suffer from serious neurological complications.

Table 1 Lyme-Disease-Scale. Evaluation derived from 24 patients with different clinical stages of Lyme-Disease

Early Manifestation Stage I and Stage II	
Organic Involvement	*Symptoms and Signs*
General Aspects	Fatigue, Headache, Fever, Stiffness, Myalgia, Malaise, Vomiting, Lymphadenopathy
Skin	Erythema Chronicum Migrans
Joints	Migratory Polyarthralgia, Attacks of pauci-articular Oligoarthritis
Nervous System	Paraesthesia, Hyperaesthesia, Sensory Disturbances
Late Manifestations Stage III	
Heart	Myocarditis, Pericardial Inflammation, Atrioventricular Block, T-Wave-Inversions, Complete Syncopes
Joints	Chronic Oligoarthritis with Erosions of Cartilage and Bone
Nervous System	Chronic Meningitis, Progressive Encephalomyelitis, Cranial-Nerve-Paralysis (f. i. facial, optic, oculomotor, abducens, auditory nerves)

paediatricians, internists, orthopaedists, neurologists and general practitioners ought to be considered in the differential diagnosis.

Non-specific lesions of skin, mucus membranes, eyes and peripheral nerves may point in the correct diagnostic direction when signs of joint involvement developed which altogether are part of the broad clinical spectrum of Lyme disease [1, 4, 5, 7, 8, 10, 12]. Joint involvement differential diagnostically alerts us to the extra-articular symptoms of sero-negative spondylarthritis, Reiter's syndrome, spondylarthritides associated with intestinal diseases, the varying entero-arthropathies such as colitis ulcerosa, Crohn's disease, Whipple's disease, reactive arthritis caused by Yersinia enterocolitica, and sarcoidosis (fig. 3).

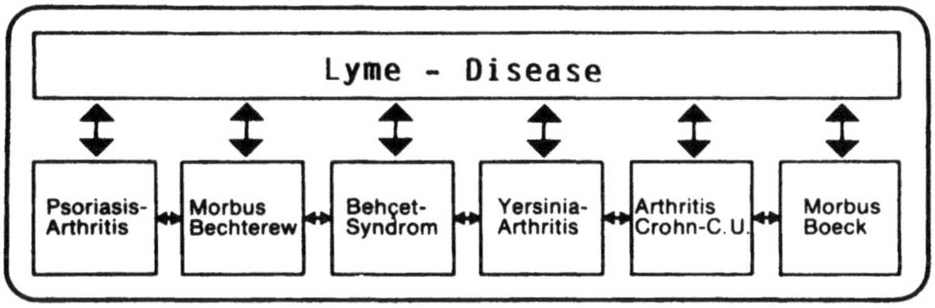

Fig. 3 Differentialdiagnostic features of Lyme disease.

Typical Lyme disease is frequently marked by non-specific symptoms such as malaise, fatigue, headache, neck stiffness, lymphadenopathy, myalgia, arthralgia and fever [5, 6, 15]. The observation that both erythema chronicum migrans and Lyme disease are caused by tick-bite inflicted infection of various spirochetes and borrelia species explains why such infections occur especially frequent during summer months in tick-infested regions [7, 12, 15] as documented in several instances of this study. The variegated picture of Lyme disease particularly concerns the often protean spectrum of neurologic complications as recently documented in 39 Swedish patients with chronic meningitis owing to Lyme disease [15]. The occasionally life-threatening heterogenous clinical symptomatology of progressive borrelia encephalomyelitis has also recently been convincingly documented in 8 cases [1].

Our study emphasizes the necessity to include the search for Lyme disease in the extensive diagnostic program concerning syndromes marked by dermatological, rheumatological, and neurological complications, because a correct diagnosis of Lyme disease requires specific therapy.

Summary

Lyme disease has recently been recognized as a separate entity due to its close geographic clustering of affected patients within specific areas in Europe, UK and USA.

This article reviews the causal, clinical and laboratory features of this inflammatory disorder with its wide spectrum of clinical manifestations. 24 patients are recorded in detail with their clinical features of an erythema chronicum migrans, meningoradiculitis and carditis associated with oligoarthritis which definitely were triggered by Ixodes ricinus spirochetes.

Since Lyme disease may closely be linked with transient autoimmune phenomena occurring in serum specimens of the patients it is pointed out that Lyme disease spirochetes might also be able to produce a strong polyclonal stimulation of B-cell activity thus signalling a non-specific autoimmune process.

References

[1] Ackermann, R., E. Gollmer, B. Rhese: Progressive Borrelien-Enzephalomyelitis. DMW 110 (1985) 1039 – 1042.

[2] Benach, J. L., E. M. Bosler, J. P. Hanrahan, et al.: Spirochetes isolated from the blood of two patients with Lyme disease. N. Engl. J. Med. **308** (1983) 740 – 742.

[3] Burgdorfer, W., A. G. Barbour, St. F. Hayes, et al.: Lyme disease – a tick-borne spirochetosis? Science **216** (1982) 1317 – 1319.

[4] Goebel, K. M., A. Krause, H. H. Goebel: Acquired autoimmunity in Lyme disease. Inn. Med. **12** (in press, 1985).

[5] Myerhoff, J.: Lyme-disease. Amer. J. Med. **75** (1983) 663 – 670.

[6] Moffat, C. M., L. H. Sigal, A. C. Steere, et al.: Cellular immune findings in Lyme disease. Amer. J. Med. **77** (1984) 625 – 632.

[7] Muhlemann, M. F.: Thirteen British cases of erythema chronicum migrans, a spirochaetal disease. Br. J. Dermat. **111** (1984) 335 – 339.

[8] Steere, A. C., S. E. Malawista, D. R. Snydman, et al.: Lyme arthritis: an epidemic of oligoarticular arthritis in children and adults in three Connecticut communities. Arthr. Rheum. **20** (1977) 7 – 17.

[9] Steere, A. C., S. E. Malawista, J. A. Harin, et al.: Erythema chronicum migrans and Lyme arthritis: the enlarging clinical spectrum. Ann. Intern. Med. **86** (1977) 685 – 696.

[10] Steere, A. C., T. F. Broderick, S. E. Malawista: Erythema chronicum migrans and Lyme arthritis: epidemiological evidence for a tick vector. Amer. J. Epidem. **108** (1978) 312 – 321.

[11] Steere, A. C., A. Gibofsky, M. E. Patarrago, et al.: Chronic Lyme arthritis. Clinical and immunological differentiation from rheumatoid arthritis. Ann. Intern. Med. **90** (1979) 896 – 901.

[12] Steere, A. C., S. E. Malawista: Cases of Lyme disease in the United States: locations correlated with distribution of Ixodes dammini. Ann. Intern. Med. **91** (1979) 730 – 733.

[13] Steere, A. C., W. P. Batsford, M. Weinberg, et al.: Lyme carditis: cardiac abnormalities of Lyme disease. Ann. Intern. Med. **93** (1980) 8 – 16.

[14] Steere, A. C., R. L. Grodzicki, A. N. Kornblatt, et al.: The spirochetal etiology of Lyme disease. N. Engl. J. Med. **308** (1983) 733 – 742.

[15] Stiernstedt, G. T., B. R. Sköldenberg, B. Vandvic: Chronic meningitis and Lyme disease in Sweden. Yale J. Biol. Med. **57** (1984) 491 – 497.

[16] Weber, K., A. Puznik, Th. Becker: Erythema migrans Krankheit. DMW **108** (1983) 1182 – 1190.

Laminoplasty as a method for enlargement of the spinal canal in spondylotic cervical myelopathy

O. Hey, Th. Wallenfang

The osseous stenoses developing in the course of a spondylarthrosis, are quite frequently found in the area of the cervical canal. These osseous serrae cause a number of pathophysiological changes, when situated ventrally in the spinal canal. In time there may finally even occur a cervical spondylotic myelopathy.

Calcifications of the posterior longitudinal ligament may also cause a cervical myelopathy. This form of myelopathy was reported by Key as early as 1838 in Guy's Hospital Report and similar papers have appeared in the literature concerning spinal column pathology [5, 11]. Ossification of the posterior longitudinal ligament of the spine however was recognized as a homogenous syndrome in 1960 by Tsukimoto. The etiology of ossification of the posterior longitudinal ligament remains obscure. The incidence of ossification of the posterior longitudinal ligament is higher in the Mongolian subjects than in white subjects.

In monosegmental causes of the spinal canal stenosis of the cervical region, surgical treatment can be performed by an anterior approach: anterior direct decompression with removal of the ossified foci followed by interbody fusion. This is performed to stabilize the spine. However, in our opinion an anterior approach is limited to three vertebral bodies. In multisegmental stenosis of the cervical canal (three levels or more) we advocated in earlier days a decompression of the spinal cord by posterior approach. This method did not have any such limitation. However, a multisegmental laminectomy revealed the instability of the spine caused by the removal of posterior structures. The long-term follow-up evaluation after laminectomy were in general not satisfactory.

The third surgical treatment is a dorsally performed spinal canalwidening operation, the so-called laminoplasty. We recently performed this method in patients with cervical spondylotic myelopathy.

Technique of laminoplasty

Various surgical procedures to enlarge the spinal canal are being developed by Japanese surgeons [13]. In our clinic we evolved a modified method of laminoplasty. In these procedures the neural laminae are not removed but are rather opened with double hinges, with bone grafting, as shown in figure 1. Patient is operated on in prone position, undertaking a light flexion of cervical spine. Skin incision is performed in the midline between protuberantia occipitalis externa and the spinous process of C7, followed by exposure of the dorsal cervical spine together with the laminae of the dorsal facet joints. Important is the complete removal of the fibromuscular tissue of the laminae. After resection of the spinous processes on the baseline a 3 mm wide bone channel is fraised on the left side with high-speed air drill, paramedian of the facet joints into the laminae. The inner plates of the laminae are maintained, followed by complete fraising of the

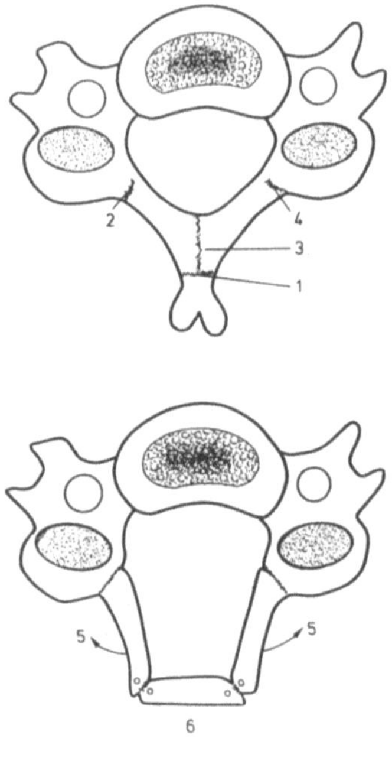

Fig. 1 Technique of laminoplasty.
1 = Resection of the spinous process; 2 and 4 = bone channel in the laminae; 3 = complete fraising of the laminae in the midline; 5 = tipped up semi-laminae; 6 = fusion of semi-laminae.

laminae in the midline of the area in which the spinous process was removed before. Finally fraising of a groove into the laminae right paramedian is performed. So, two semi-laminae are formed being folded to lateral and dorsal. In this course the inner plates of the laminae are breaking. However, the continuity of bone structures remains. The adjusted spinous processes are positioned between the semi-laminae and fixed with thread so that the widened spinal canal remains open, and the semi-laminae right and left are fixed to the interarticular ligaments and to the musculature. This procedure provides the conditions for a stabile osteosynthesis.

Materials and results

Laminoplasties were applied to seven patients, three females and four males. The youngest patient was 47 years old and the oldest 75 years old. Length of history from the beginning of initial symptoms to the operation was between 14 and 1 year (fig. 2). All patients were treated conservatively during this time and showed progression of neurological deficits. Neurological findings on admission listed in table 1. Patients were divided into categories according to the predominant cord syndrome. The pathological findings were categorized into symptoms with evidence of corticospinal tracts involvement (paresis, spasticity, hyperreflexia and

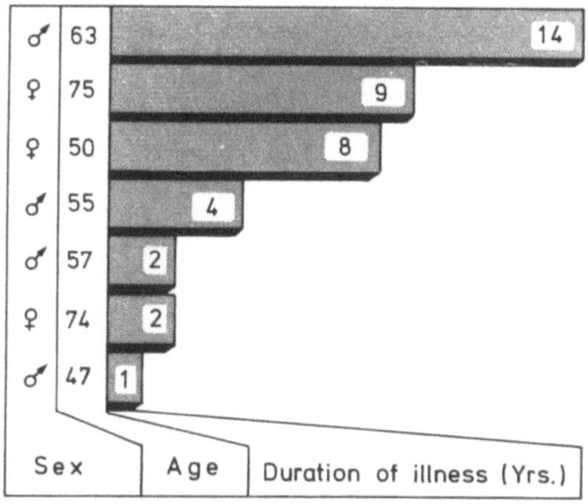

Fig. 2. Preoperative duration of illness in operated patients.

Table 1 Neurological findings in patients operated on cervical canal stenosis

Neurological findings	Patients 1.	2.	3.	4.	5.	6.	7.
Paresis	Para	Tetra	–	–	–	–	–
Spasticity	Tetra	Tetra	Tetra	Tetra	Para	Para	Para
Hyperreflexia	+	+	+	+	+	+	+
Babinski	+	+	–	–	–	–	–
Ataxia	–	–	+	+	+	+	+
Sensory deficits	legs	legs	legs	legs	–	legs	–
SEP	+	+	+	+	+	+	+
Sphincter Disturbances	+	+	–	+	–	–	–

+ = proved; – = not proved; SEP = sensory evoked potentials

Babinski-phenomenon), posterior column or spinothalamic tract involvement (spinal ataxia, sensory deficit, pathologic (sensory evocated potentials) SEP) and neurogenic sphincter disturbances. Results of neurological examination on admission revealed a variety of signs. All patients showed signs and symptoms of a cervical myelopathy. Most prevalent were spasticity and weakness in the lower extremities. However, spasticity and weakness in the proximal and distal parts of the upper extremities were also observed. Preoperative ability to walk was diminished in two patients (Patients No. 1 and 2). SEP showed in all patients typical findings for a lesion of the cervical part of the medulla.

Table 2 Antero-posterior diameter of cervical canal in operated cases

Patient No.	Diameter of spinal canal	Operated Segments
1	10 mm	(C2 – C6) = 5
2	6 mm	(C3 – C6) = 4
3	11 mm	(C3 – C5) = 3
4	9 mm	(C3 – C6) = 4
5	8 mm	(C3 – C6) = 4
6	10 mm	(C4 – C7) = 4
7	10 mm	(C3 – C6) = 4

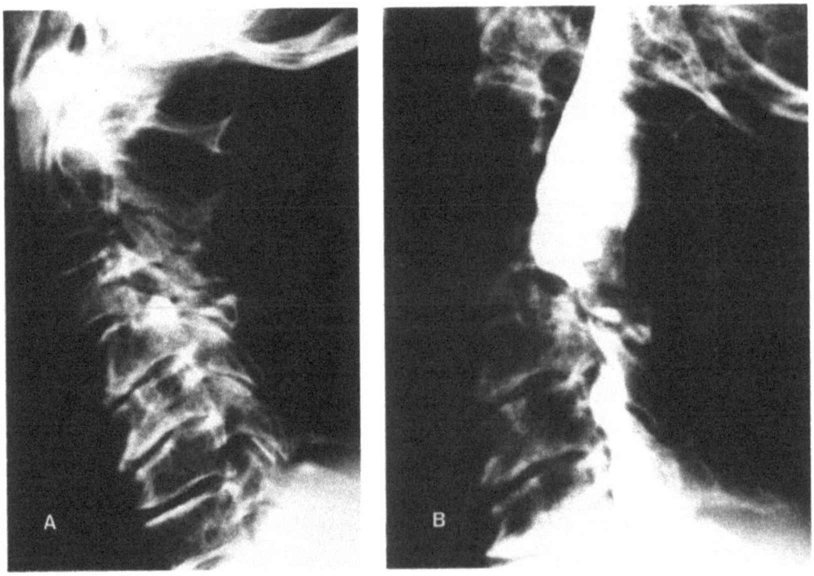

Fig. 3 (A) Subluxation between C3 and C4 vertebrae; (B) Stenosis of spinal canal in myelography.

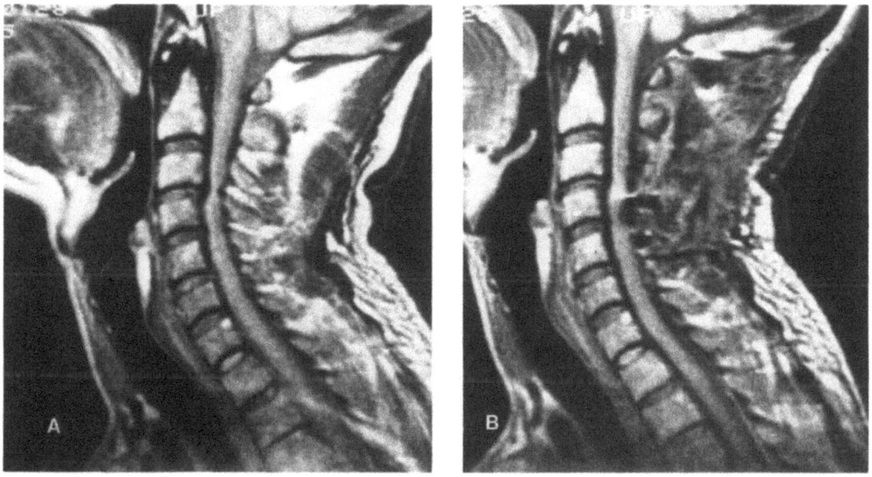

Fig. 4 (A) Spondylotic compression of spinal cord preoperative; (B) Condition after laminoplasty of C2–C5.

Measured values for the diameter of the cervical canal of operated patients are compiled in table 2. The antero-posterior diameter of the spinal canal was measured for each vertebra by the method of Nurick [9]. The least of these measurements in each case was termed the Minimum Antero-posterior Diameter (Min. APD). The values of the minimum APD were measured between six and eleven mm. Narrowing of spinal canal was expanded over three segments and more in the operated cases. Laminoplasty was performed in five cases over four segments and in one case each over three respective five segments.

Surgical results are based on control examinations performed 12 months after the operation. No aggravating complications were present, except in one patient. This patient showed preoperatively a severe paraparesis and was unable to walk for 2 years. After laminoplasty from C2–C6 a tetraparesis could be proved. Cause was a spinal cord lesion, probably arising from a reactive edema of spinal cord after surgical decompression. In the further postoperative course the neurological deficits decreased and at present this patient is able to walk again.

In the other patients an impressive postoperative improvement of functional capacity and a subjective reduction of symptoms was observed. Patients stated an improvement in walking and reduction of sensory paralgesia. The postoperative neurological control examinations showed that the spastic signs and symptoms were reduced in six of seven patients and ataxia in five patients. All patients with a preoperative neurogenic sphincter disturbance (three patients) had postoperatively normal findings. Figures 3 to 5 demonstrate the radiological findings of three cases being operated on cervical myelopathy.

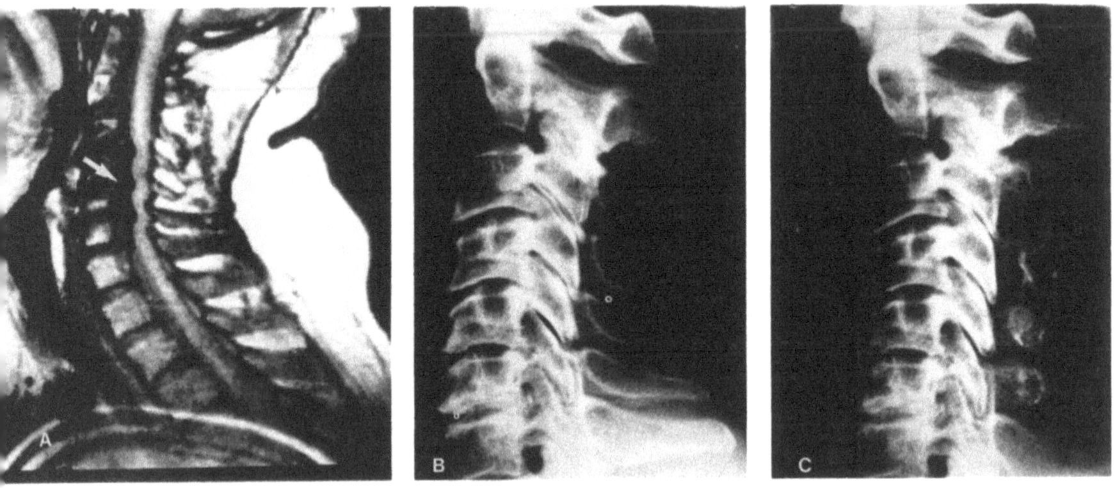

Fig. 5 (A) Spondylotic compression of spinal cord preoperative; (B) Preoperative radiographic study; (C) Radiographic study after laminoplasty of C3 – C6.

Discussion

The spondylotic stenosis of spinal canal over several segments can lead to severe disturbances of the dynamic interactions between the wall of spinal canal, dura, and spinal cord. Experiments on normal human spinal cords have shown that by effects of flexion and extension various changes can appear on these structures [8]. The flexion movements of the cervical spine causes an elongation of the cervical spine canal by 28 mm. In addition an elongation of the dural sac appears through which its transverse diameter and the antero-posterior diameter narrows. Furthermore it can be seen that an axial spinal cord reposition in the caudal as well as in the cranial direction occurs. The caudal shifting is largest in the region of C1 and the cranial displacement in Segment C7. The relation of the position between spinal canal, meninges and spinal cord, however, remain unchanged in segment C6. In contrast, a forced extension of cervical spine causes a shortening of the cervical spinal canal by 15 mm, a transverse folding of the dura and pia as well as an enlargement of the transverse and AP-diameter of the dural sac. This results in an increase of the transverse diameter of the spinal cord.

In conclusion we can state: the cervical spine transfers its changes in length and curvatures to the meninges and the spinal cord causing traction- and gliding movements. It is understandable that the deformity of the spinal cord in spondylotic cervical canal stenosis leads to severe disturbances by compressing the structures of spinal canal. The pain appearing after cervical spine movements and the neurological lesions can be explained by the pathological process due to a narrowing of the canal. Surgical treatment for cervical spondylotic myelopathy with spinal canal stenosis has yielded a wide range of results. Analysis of these data has indicated that several preoperative factors may play a part in the outcome [1, 2, 3, 6, 7, 9, 10].

The most common indication for operation was progressive decline in spinal cord function. With chronic cervical intervertebral degeneration at multiple levels (three or more), narrow sagittal diameter of the spinal canal (< 13 mm), lordosis, and telescoping of the laminae, or "shingling", the operation of cervical laminectomy was generally carried out. When radiographic studies indicated chronic cervical degenerative disease with impingement on the spinal cord at one to two interspaces, the operation of anterior cervical disc excision and interbody fusion by the Cloward technique was generally performed. In addition, if the radiographic studies demonstrated fixed cervical kyphosis, despite the multiple-level involvement, the anterior approach was selected to relieve the anterior cord pressure. The comparison of these surgical procedures and the results of long-term follow-up evaluation showed that many years after operation instabilities with severe deformities on the cervical spine may occur.

Kawai [4] and other surgeons from the Japanese Society for Spine Surgery [12] have reported on several types of laminoplasty with or without posterior fusion for the enlargement of the cervical spinal canal. These surgeons advocated the use of spinal canal-widening procedures to avoid destructive laminectomy for cervical myelopathy. We developed in our clinic a modified form of laminoplasty and applied it to suitable patients.

The investigations of Louis [8] reveal that the stability of cervical spine is mainly founded on three vertical columns. These columns are additionally anchoraged together with horizontal bars. The vertical columns are constructed by the cervical bodies situated ventrally from the spinal canal, and dorsally herefrom are the second and third columns, consisting of the right and left articular processes. These columns are horizontally braced with two diagonal bars through the pediculi and the laminae. The spinal processes and transverse processes do not count much for stability.

After extensive laminectomy with resection of facet joints, laminae and ligaments the horizontal stability system is seriously disturbed. For this reason after laminectomy a kyphosis or a luxation in the cervical spine region may occur. An additional factor is that a firm post-laminectomy membrane develops around the epidural space which again changes the flexibility and deformability of spinal cord. On the other hand, after laminoplasty the total stability of cervical spine only changes minimally at the beginning. In the further course, after about six to eight weeks, a stable osteosynthesis in the laminae region develops. Only during this time do patients need to wear a neck support which should avoid extreme movements of cervical spine.

In summary, indication for laminoplasty exists in our opinion only in cases when a spondylotic cervical canal stenosis of multiple levels (three or more) has been proved with signs and symptoms for spinal cord compression. Laminoplasty leads to a decompression of spinal cord by enlarging the spinal canal, but changes the stability of the spinal cord only minimally and represents an alternative operation to the laminectomy.

References

[1] Dalle, ore, G., G. Vivenza: Cervical spondylotic myelopathies: Long term results of surgical treatment. Adv. Neurosurg. **8** (1980) 78 – 82.

[2] Gregorius, F. K., T. Estrin, P. H. Crandall: Cervical spondylotic radiculopathy and myelopathy. A long-term follow-up study. Arch. Neurol. **33** (1976) 618 – 625.

[3] Hohmann, D., B. Kügelgen, K. Liebig: Chronische spondylogene zervikale Myelopathie. Pathogenese, Prognose, Therapie. Orthopäde **14** (1985) 101 – 111.

[4] Kawai, N., S. Hattori, Y. Shigetomi: Enlargement of the cervical canal – Indication and the technique. Orthop. Trauma. Surg. **23** (1980) 23.

[5] Key, C. A.: On paraplegia depending on disease of the ligaments of the spine. Guy's Hosp. Rep. **3** (1838) 17 – 23.

[6] Kuhlendahl, H.: Cervical myelopathy. In: Surgery of cervical myelopathy (W. Grote, M. Brock, H. Clar, M. Klinger, H. Nau, eds.), pp. 34 – 39. Springer, Berlin – Heidelberg – New York 1980.

[7] Liebig, K., B. Kügelgen: Results of treatment of patients affected by chronic cervical myelopathy by surgical decompression and ventral fusion according to Cloward. Adv. Neurosurg. **8** (1980) 100 – 103.

[8] Louis, R.: Surgery of the spine. Springer, Berlin – Heidelberg – New York 1985.

[9] Nurick, S.: The pathogenesis of the spinal cord discorder associated with cervical spondylosis. Brain **95** (1972) 87 – 100.

[10] Nurick, S.: The pathogenesis of cervical spondylotic myelopathy. Acta Neurol. Belg. **76** (1976) 274 – 275.

[11] Oppenheimer, A.: Calcification and ossification of vertebral ligaments (spondylitis ossificans ligamentosa). Roentgen study of pathogenesis and clinical significance. Radiology **38** (1942) 140 – 146.

[12] Tsukimoto, H.: On an autopsied case of compression myelopathy with a callus formation in the cervical spinal canal. Nihon-gekahokam **29** (1960) 1003.

[13] Tsuyama, N.: Ossification of the posterior longitudinal ligament of the spine. Clin. Orthop. **184** (1984) 71 – 84.

VI Tumors of the cranio-cervical junction

Neuropathology of tumors in the craniospinal region

H. H. Goebel, J. Bohl, S. Al-Hami

Introduction

Assessing pathological processes in the craniospinal region one may assign such processes to the following categories: malformations, trauma, vascular disorders, infection and inflammation, degenerative processes, and lastly tumors. This presentation concerns the very latter group which may be numerically extremely infrequent when compared with the entire spectrum of neuropathologic tumors but may nothwithstanding encompass a variegated gamut of different neoplasms.

Topography

The clinical importance of the craniospinal region is largely evinced by the peculiar topography of the only significant pressure outlet of the entire cranial cavity, the foramen occipitale magnum (FOM), the pressure through which is directed one way, rostrocaudally. Although being the largest of all cranial foramina lack of complimentary space in the cranium is the chief reason why minor space occupying lesions not only of neoplastic but also of traumatic or inflammatory origin may quickly result in fatal disaster.

The FOM is a rigid osseous ring of the occipital bone bordered rostrally by the bony, meningeal and brain stem structures of the infratentorial cavity and caudally by the upper cervical spine and its inherent functionally complex tissue of interacting vertebral joints, inwardly vested by the meninges which surround the slender cervical cord.

Thus, only a small complimentary topographic space may be compromised by tumefaction of mesenchymal and neuroectodermal neoplasms. Contrary to the adverse aspects of limited availability of spatial reserve, the individual patient may benefit from the general experience that tumors of the craniospinal region are generally benign and slow growing, more often resulting in non-invasive compression than in destructive infiltration and thus giving the skillful and attentive clinician an opportunity to exercise his diagnostic ability to his patient's early benefit.

Furthermore, as more spacious cavities vicinal to the FOM, the infratentorial and cervical cavities, are richly endowed with smaller outlets passing through rigid bone, the cranial nerve and cervico-spinal root foramina, some parts of an expanding life threatening tumor within the cranio-cervical region may be diverted from the medullo-spinal junction to the peripheral nerve outlets.

Individual tumors of the craniospinal region

When looking at tumors of this region from a topographic point of view those originating in or around the FOM proper may be separated from those extending from neighboring areas into the FOM.

Adding a histological aspect to this topographic approach neuro-ectodermal tumors of the medullospinal transition zone may be distinguished from tumors of or within the meninges and from extradural neoplasms, respectively.

By far, the most frequent tumors of the FOM occur in the subarachnoid space [3, 4].

Fig. 1

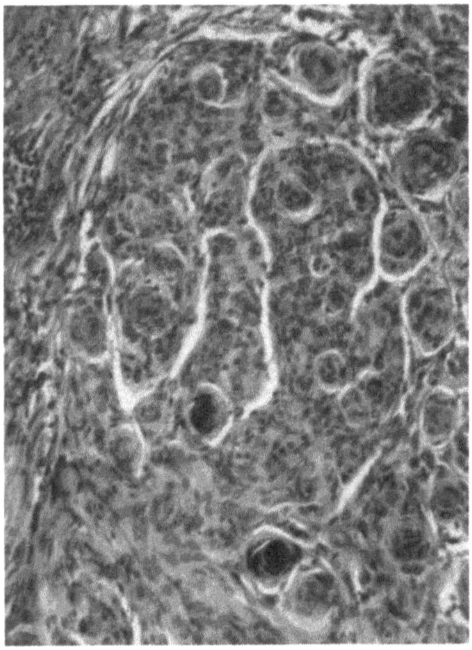

Fig. 2

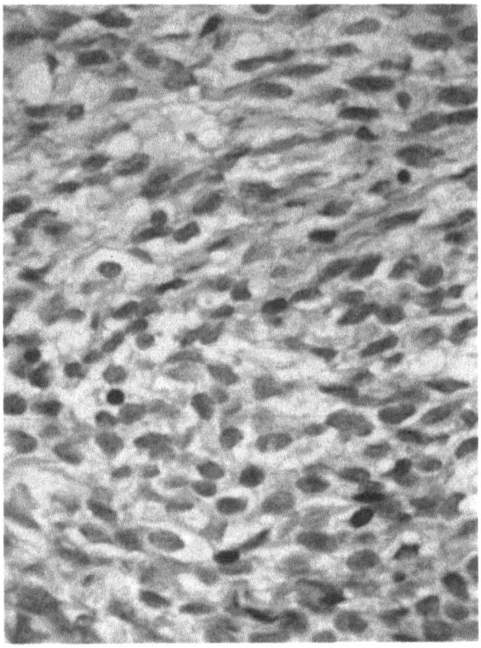

Fig. 1 The *syncytial meningeoma* contains numerous whorls and a few psammoma bodies, Hematoxylin-Eosin, X 130.

Fig. 2 In the *fibrous meningeoma*, neoplastic cells are elongated and spindle-shaped, Hematoxylin-Eosin, X 325.

Meningeomas outnumber any other tumor of the craniospinal region. For the diagnostic histopathologist these meningiomas fall into three groups. The most frequent one is the endotheliomatous or syncytial meningioma which is composed of regularly appearing almost epithelial-like cells (fig. 1), very much resembling nests of arachnoidal cells which are frequent serendipitous finding to the careful post mortem pathologist. Whorl formation about tumor cells or small vessels and theirs subsequent hyalinisation and mineralisation (fig. 1) may result in well known psammoma bodies which, particularly in older meningiomas, may be sometimes so frequent that they seem to have eliminated viable syncytial tumor cells but that they owing to their morphological characteristics not only allow the correct diagnosis of a meningioma but actually warrant sub-classification of such a mass as a psammomatous meningioma.

Usually less conspicuous, small areas of syncytial growth and psammoma bodies may be encountered in the fibrous meningioma, another subvariety of this mesenchymal tumor. Here, slender, often spindle-shaped tumor cells (fig. 2) grow in parallel trains interrupted by various amounts of collagen.

Rich vascular supply to the meningioma delineates the angioblastic type of meningeoma which, according to recent, largely electron microscopic studies, must not be confused with the meningeal haemangiopericytoma (fig. 3 a, b) which unfortunately often offers a more guarded prognosis.

a b

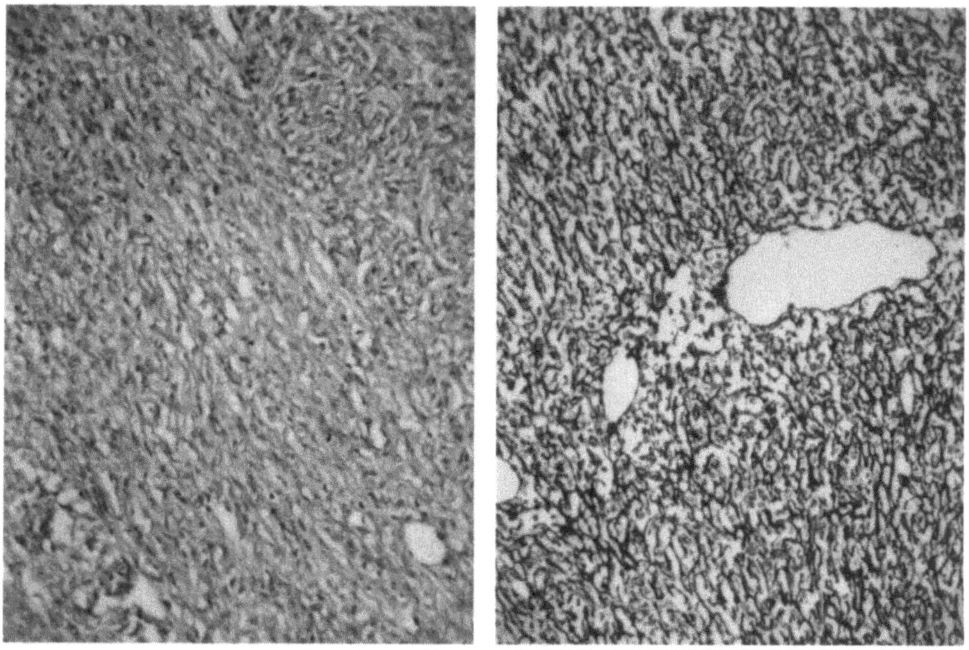

Fig. 3 The *haemangiopericytoma* of the meninges contains numerous small vascular channels, a: Hematoxylin-Eosin, X 130, which are conspicuously outlined by the teticulin network, b: Gömöri's reticulin stain, X 130.

Referring to recent more sophisticated morphological techniques beyond the purely descriptive level it is worthy of note that meningiomas of all sorts are marked by vimentin, the intermediate filament of many mesenchymal cell types [10] which may also be encountered with the electron microscope (fig. 4) in the perinuclear cytoplasmic extensions which, largely in the syncytial type, form an elaborate network often connected to each other by desmosome-like thickness of the cellular membrane.

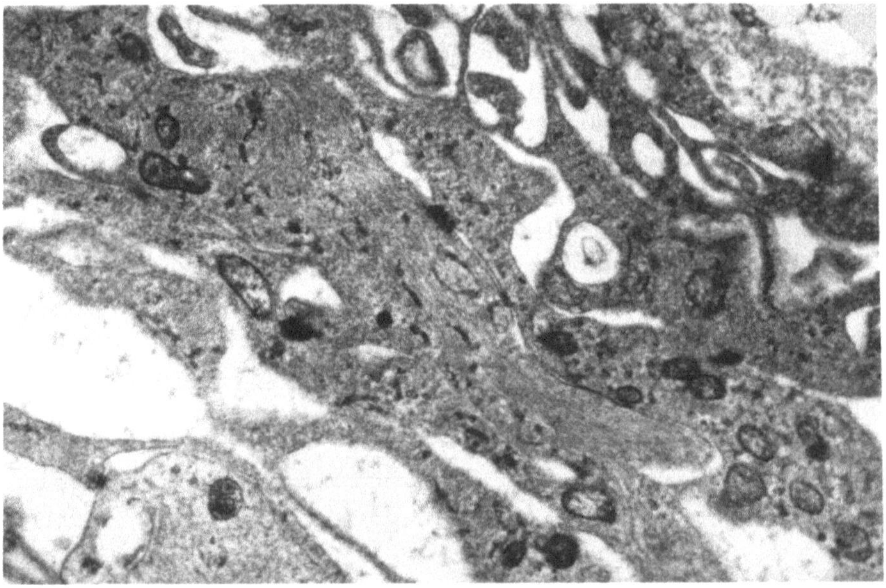

Fig. 4 Seen in electron microscopy, the *meningeoma* is composed of numerous processes attached to each other by junctional complexes and often replete with bundles of filaments, X 27,200.

The ultrastructure of the meningeal haemangiopericytoma, quite like that of extracranial and extraspinal haemangiopericytomas [5] reflects the possible origin of this tumor from vascular pericytes [9].

When located in the subarachoid space of the craniospinal region the Schwann cell may give rise to the *neurinoma* (fig. 5 a) or *neurofibroma*, the second most frequent tumor in this area. Developing from preexisting cranial or spinal roots, the neurinoma (fig. 5 b) displaces the parent nerve to its periphery while the neurofibroma, being composed of Schwann cells and fibroblasts, expands the nerve by intrinsic separation of preexisting nerve fibers further enhanced by the accumulation of a basophilic matrix rich in mucopolysaccharides; but both types of Schwann cell tumors contain neoplastic Schwann cells marked by S-100 protein and invested by a basal lamina (fig. 5 c).

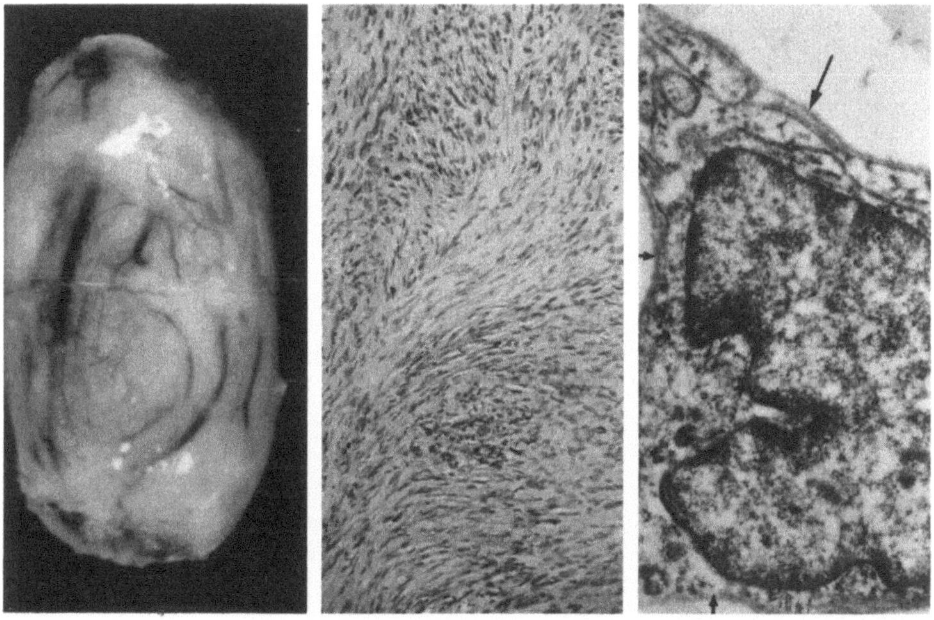

a b c

Fig. 5 The *neurinoma* represents a well demarcated, easily removable mass (a), which is composed of densely packed bundles of spindle-shaped Schwann cells, b: Hematoxylin-Eosin, X 100. The Schwann cell, by electron microscopy, is marked by a continuous basal lamina (arrows), c: X 27.000.

Both, the meningioma and the neurinoma/neurofibroma are commonly benign tumors although the meningeal haemangiopericytoma has a higher rate of recurrence and a malignant Schwannoma may occasionally be encountered in von Recklinghausen's neurofibromatosis.

Among the *neuroectodermal* tumors, i. e. those of the medulla and cervical cord, *astrocytomas* (figs. 6 a, b) both of the pilocytic and fibrillary types prevail. They grow by diffuse infiltration and along preexisting tracts of the neuroaxis, i. e. rostro-caudally and vice versa. Typical histologic features, and glial fibrillary acidic protein of intermediate filaments (figs. 6 c, d) mark this most frequent of all neuroectodermal neoplasms.

Diffuse tumefaction over several segments are another characteristic of such primary intrinsic neuroectodermal tumors, among which oligodendrogliomas and glioblastomas are extremely rare while ependymomas (figs. 7 a – c) are more frequently found in more caudal areas of the spinal cord and in ventricular and periventricular regions of the adjacent medulla oblongata.

a b

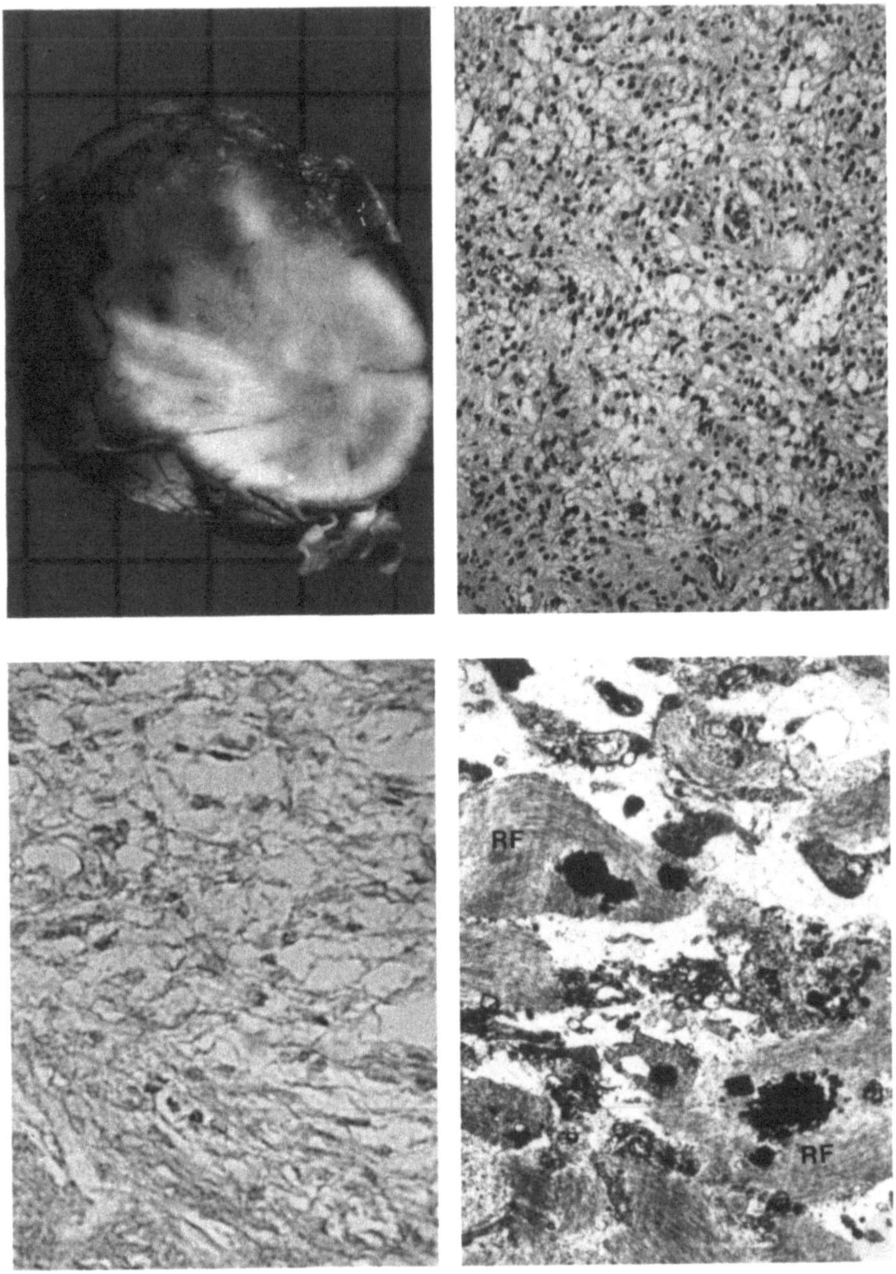

c d

Fig. 6 An *astrocytoma* grows diffusely within the medullo-cervical region (a). A fine fibrillary network among small round astrocytes is conspicuous, b: Hematoxylin-Eosin, X 130. The astrocytic processes become faintly apparent in immunohistological preparations for glial fibrillary acidic protein (GFAP), c: X 180. By electron microscopy, such astrocytomas contain processes filled with dense bundles of filaments, here also marked by central electron dense material, Rosenthal fibers (RF), d: X 30.000.

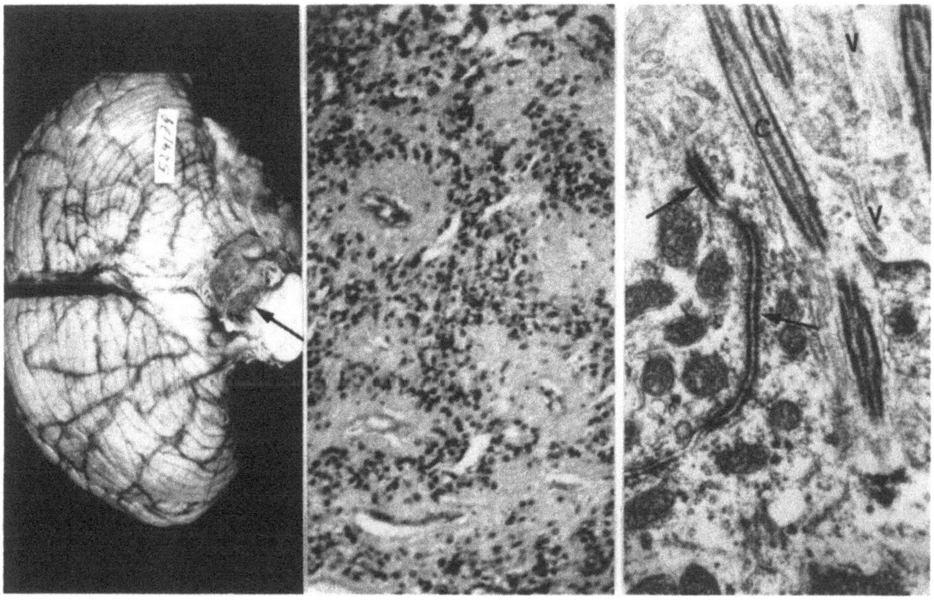

a b c

Fig. 7 An *ependymoma* grows over the dorsal surface of the medullo-cervical region (arrow), [a]. Histology emphasizes the perivascular nuclear-free arrangement of neoplastic ependymal cells, b: Hematoxylin-Eosin, X 100. By electron microscopy, ependymomas may be marked by cilia (C), villi (V) and lengthy junctional processes (arrows), c: X 50.000.

As the *haemangioblastoma*, not to be confused with the angioblastic meningeoma or the meningeal haemangiopericytoma, though overall rare, is seen most frequently among all sites of the neuraxis in the area of the infratentorial-cervical cavities including the cerebellum, it is thus not surprising to encounter such a mesenchymal intraspinal-medullary haemangioblastoma (fig. 8 a) extending over numerous segments, which fine structurally is composed of numerous vessels (figs. 8 b, c) and fat laden foamy stromal cells.

The third category of FOM tumors is derived from extradural structures largely the bone, comprising angiomas [7], osteomas, occasionally myelomas, histiocytosis X or chordomas [2]. The latter type of neoplasm may take origin from the clivus (fig. 9 a) or less frequently from the dens [1], competing with the sacrococcygeal area for the most frequent site along the neuraxis. Their vacuolar or physaliphorous cells may aggregate or form rows often surrounded by and not infrequently vanishing into a mucopolysaccharide-rich ground substance (fig. 9 b).

This basophilic matrix and single tumor cells therein may simulate or even represent islands of chondroid tissue thus evoking the differential diagnosis of a slow growing well differentiated chondrosarcoma which may sometimes finally

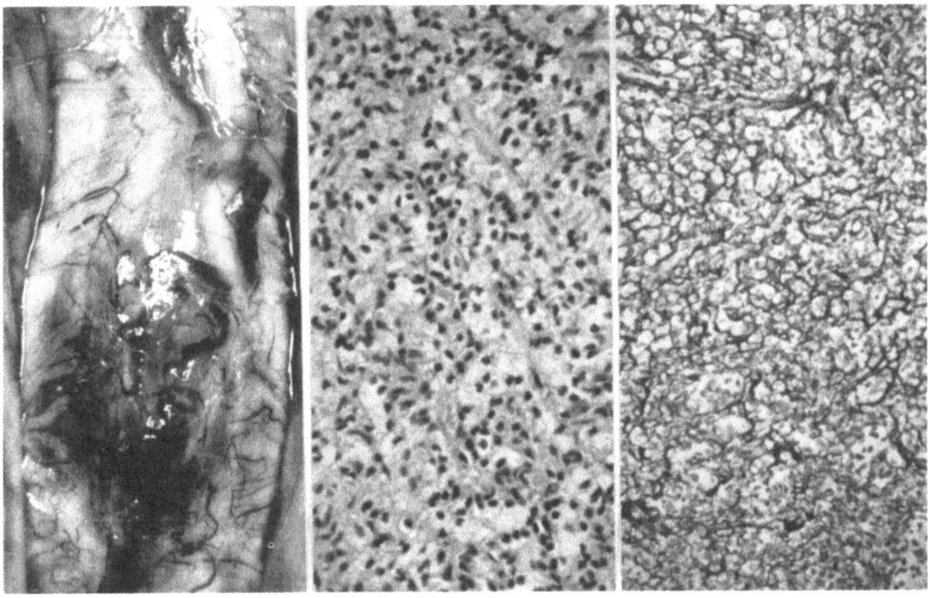

a b c

Fig. 8 A *haemangioblastoma* discolors an expanded upper cervical cord (a). In such a haemangioblastoma, vascular channels and stromal cells alternate, b: Hematoxylin-Eosin, X 200, while the reticular network further delineates the net of small vessels, c: Gömöri's reticulum stain, X 100.

only be resolved by employing electron microscopy (figs. 9 c, d) and immunohistological techniques that demonstrate cytokeratin in the chordoma but vimentin in the chondrosarcoma [8].

Other neoplasms of the FOM seem to be extremely rare [6], among them the extramedullary cavernous haemangioma [7] the lipoma, or the teratoma [3], usually reported in single case studies.

Though carcinomas may metastasize to every remote location of the body and thus also to the bony, meningeal and neuroectodermal compartments of the craniospinal region (fig. 10), isolated metastatic nodules in these tissue seem to be very rare but if present may be more often evidence of other metastatic nodules or even a meningeal carcinosis within the craniospinal cavity, thus alerting the physician to additional neurological deficits originating from functional impairment distant to the craniospinal region.

Similarly, neoplasms may present themselves in the craniospinal region because of expansion from neighboring compartments, largely the infratentorial cavity and its contents. Such tumors may also extend rostrally and/or compromise CSF flow, thus engendering a heterogeneous complex of clinical symptoms.

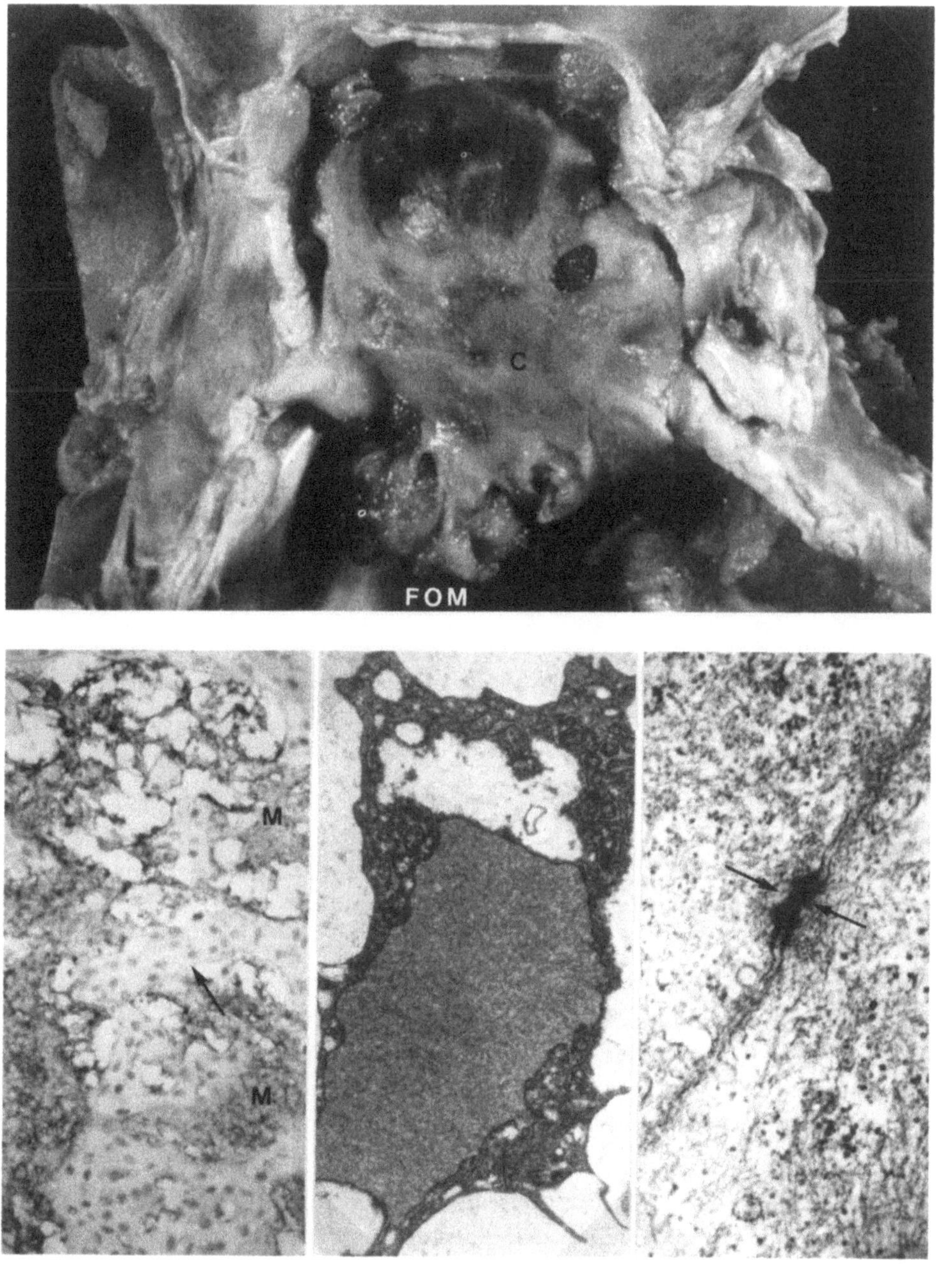

a

b c d

Fig. 9 A *chordoma* (C) of the clivus bulges into the foramen occipitale magnum (FOM) [a], being composed of epithelial-like cells (arrow) embedded in a cell-free matrix (M), rich in mucopolysaccharides, b: Alcian-blue, X 300. The vacuolar bubble-like appearance of the physaliphorous cells is conspicuous in this electron micrograph, c: X 1.968. Typically, chordoma cells may be attached to each other by junctional complexes (arrows), d: X 60.800.

Fig. 10

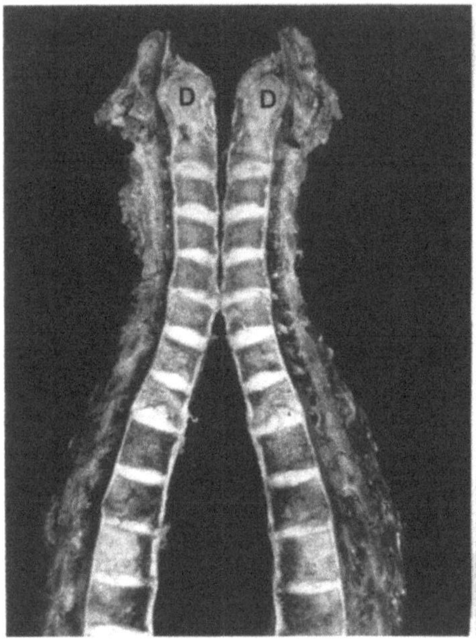

Fig. 11

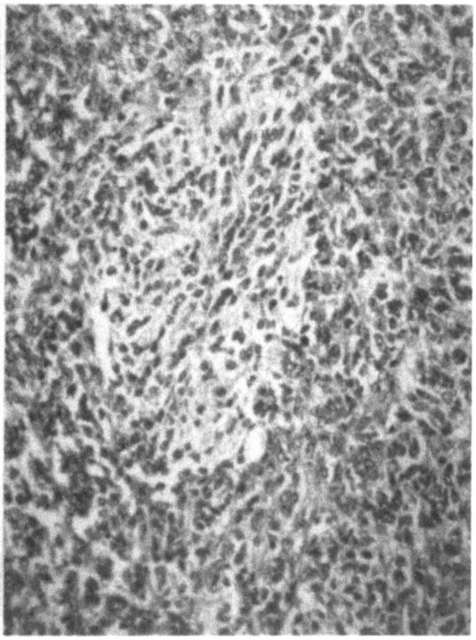

Fig. 10 Numerous vertebral bodies and the dens (D) are infested with *metastatic carcinoma*.

Fig. 11 Within a *medulloblastoma*, a light central island of loosely arranged tumor cells is surrounded by more densely packed neoplastic elements, Hematoxylin-Eosin, X 300.

In addition to those tumors just described above such as meningioma, neurinoma/neurofibroma, haemangioblastoma, and astrocytoma, however, excluding extradural tumors, neoplasms of a different histogenetic pattern, because of their different site of origin, have briefly to be enumerated.

Development of the childhood medulloblastoma (fig. 11) from the vermis or its adult type from a cerebellar hemisphere, when at the caudal region of the cerebellum may grow toward the spinal cavity both in the subarachnoid space as well as within the neuroaxis. Likewise, the subependymoma and the plexuspapilloma (figs. 12 a, b) extend downwards into the FOM from the fourth ventricle.

Large cystic growths of mal-developmental character containing tissue elements of the skin, so-called epidermoids and dermoids may occupy or extend into the cranio-cervical region.

Due to their aggressive behaviour glomus tumors or paragangliomas derived from glomus cells which aggregate in the extradural cranio-cervical region, and which are attached to the cranial nerves may give rise to tumors, histologically marked by islands of well developed round cells. Compression of the tumor and

a b

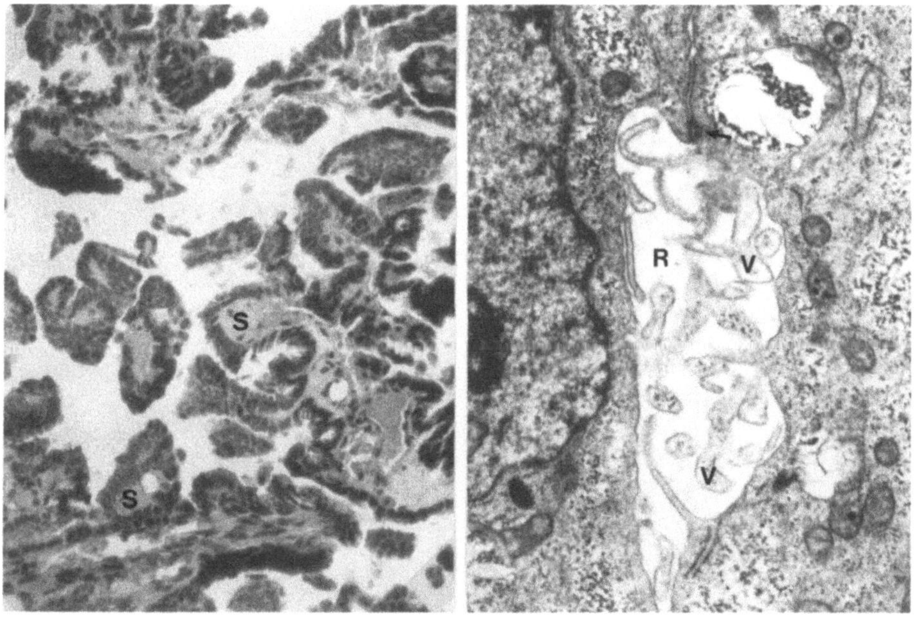

Fig. 12 A ventricular *plexus papilloma* is marked by a thick layer of cylindrical neoplastic cells situated upon the slender plexus stroma (S), a: Hematoxylin-Eosin, X 300, while such neoplastic choroid plexus epithelial cells sometimes form small rosettes (R), similar to ependymal rosettes because of apical junctional complexes (arrow) and villi (V) but different from ependymal rosettes because cilia are lacking, b: X 32.000.

other effects inimical to morphological preservation occasionally demand an electron microscopic investigation where the so-called "dense core" vesicles (fig. 13) usually turn up.

Miscellaneous cysts of mal-developmental or acquired origin such as neuroepithelial or arachnoidal cysts, respectively may act as space occupying lesions although they extend from above or below rather than originate from the craniospinal junction proper. They usually concern more the pediatrician and the neurologist than the neurosurgeon.

Similarly, other tumefactions, though not necessarily of neoplastic origin, encompass chronic inflammatory processes, granulomas of infectious type like gummas, tuberculomas, or infectious granulomas infested by fungi or parasites.

Fortunately, however, such lesions, for historical and geographical reasons, are not only extremely infrequent, but almost unheard of in our today's practice, while space-occupying arterial berry aneurysms which happen to be located in the FOM represent an extreme rarity in view of the comparably abundant number of saccular aneurysms located farther rostrally in the circle of Willis. Situated in

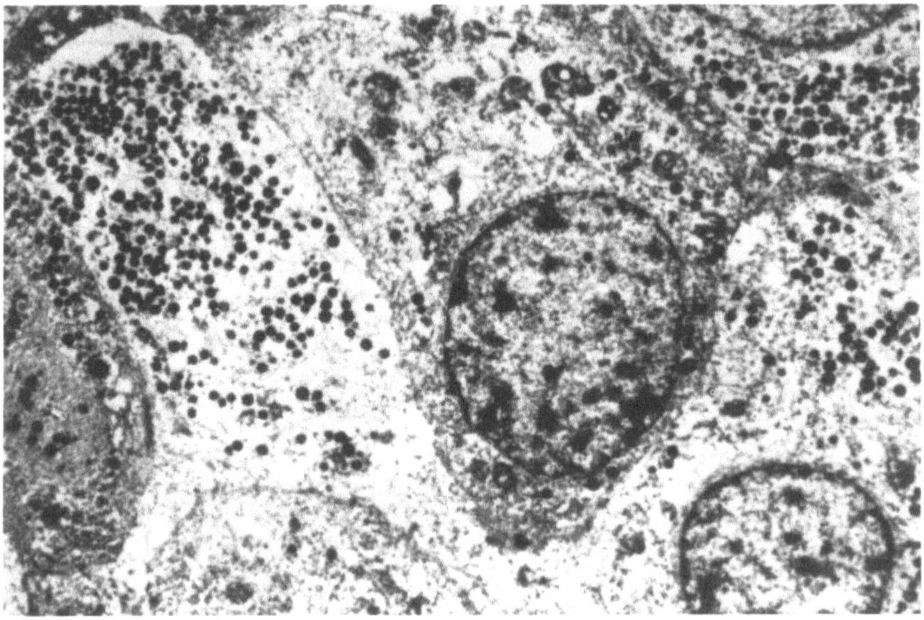

Fig. 13 Typical dense core vesicles of a *glomus tumor (paraganglioma)* are still present after reembedding for electron microscopy from a paraffin block, X 11.520.

the FOM, rupture of such an aneurysm may kill the patient instantaneously, before the examining physician may be able to record any neurological symptoms.

Conclusion

Untoward morphological sequelae to the cord because of intraspinal medullary neoplastic growth or external neoplastic compression of the spinal-medullary region may not always be distinguishable from consequences of surgical intervention at or after operation and thus should not concern us here but rather those reporting on complications of admittedly difficult surgery of such tumors.

As FOM tumors are infrequent, largely because of the spatial smallness of the craniospinal region, precise statistics of these tumors in the FOM area and their statistical subtyping based on morphological patterns are hard to come by and of questionable connotation to the clinician and neuropathologist because such numerical data have to be viewed against different, i. e. post-mortem, epidemiologic, clinical, or surgical backgrounds. The fallibility of statistics also include change in nomenclature and the frequent problem of retrospective diagnosis based on published reports rather than personal reinspection, emphasized for instance when reading about a high frequency of "arachnoidal fibroblastoma (meningeoma)" suggesting fibrous meningioma encountered as the most frequent FOM tumor – although in an admittedly small series – [11]. This would refute the common experience that the endotheliomatous or syncytial meningioma represents the most frequent subtype of all meningeomas including those of the FOM region. Furthermore, statistics are only remotely beneficial to the patient for whom his disease represents 100 percent. He is more concerned with clinical symptoms produced by such tumors, their location as regards surgical removal and prognostication, factors that inspite of the numerical infrequency of such tumors when matched with those from other areas of neurosurgical intervention constitute the significance of neoplasms in this area and the necessity for the physician to familiarize himself with such factors, an honourable reason that united us in this conference.

Summary

Though rare in number the spectrum of neoplasms in the craniospinal region appears rather diversefied. Intra-medullary tumors may be separated from those of the meninges and from extradural mesenchymal tumors. By far, the most frequent tumor encountered in the craniospinal region is the meningeoma followed by the Schwann cell tumor. Other tumors appear of extreme rarity and some only fall into the category of foramen occipitale magnum tumors because they extend into this area from vicinal more spacious cavities such as the medulloblastoma or the plexus papilloma.

Although the neuroanatomic aspect of the FOM may give rise to specific clinical symptoms, such symptoms may be associated with other neurological findings when tumors not only occupy the FOM region but reach it by expansion from districts of different function.

References

[1] Boemke, F., W. Joest: Chordome im Bereich des Schädels. Virchows Arch. **297** (1936) 352–367.

[2] Cervós-Navarro, J.: Die Morphologie der hinteren Schädelgrube. Radiologe **12** (1969) 458–463.

[3] Cohen, L.: Tumors in the region of the foramen magnum. In: P. J. Vinken, G. W. Bruyn (eds.): Handbook of Clinical Neurology, Vol. **17**, pp. 719–729. North Holland Publishing Co. Amsterdam – American Elsevier Publishing Co., Inc., New York 1974.

[4] Cohen, L., D. MacRae: Tumors in the region of the foramen magnum. J. Neurosurg. **19** (1962) 462–469.

[5] Horten, B. C., H. Urich, L. J. Rubinstein, et al.: The angioblastic meningeoma: a reappraisal of a nosological problem. J. Neurol. Sci. **31** (1977) 387–410.

[6] Hughes, J. T.: Pathology of the spinal cord. J. B. Lippincott Company, Philadelphia – Toronto 1966.

[7] MacCarty, C. S., L. E. Lougheed, J. R. Brown: Unusual benign tumor at the foramen magnum. Report of a case. J. Neuro-Surg. **16** (1959) 463–467.
[8] Miettinen, M., V.-P. Lehto, D. Dahl, et al.: Differential diagnosis of chordoma, chondroid, and ependymal tumors as aided by anti-intermediate filament antibodies. Am. J. Pathol. **112** (1983) 160–169.
[9] Peña, C. E.: Meningioma and intracranial hemangiopericytoma. A comparative electron microscopic study. Acta Neuropath. (Berl.) **39** (1977) 69–74.
[10] Schwechheimer, K., J. Kartenbeck, R. Moll, et al.: Vimentin filament-desmosome cytoskeleton of diverse types of human meningeomas. Lab. Invest. **51** (1984) 584–591.
[11] Smolik, E. A., E. Sachs: Tumors of the foramen magnum of spinal origin. J. Neurosurg. **11** (1954) 161–172.

Meningiomas and neurinomas of the cranio-cervical region – Diagnosis and operative treatment

W.-P. Sollmann, V. Seifert, D. Stolke, H. Dietz

Introduction

Because of their rare existence, localisation and multiform symptoms meningiomas and neurinomas of the cranio-cervical region often escape early diagnosis. The following mechanisms have been considered to create neurological deficits: The compression of spinal cord or medulla oblongata, the irritation of upper cervical nerve roots or cranial nerves, the blockage of the cerebrospinal fluid and the obstruction of the vertebral artery and the epidural veins.

Epidemiology

Between 1972 and 1985, 18 patients aged 12 to 69 years were operated on benign cranio-cervical tumours in our clinic. This is less than 1% of all CNS-tumours and 4% of the spinal tumours treated in our clinic. There were 9 patients with meningiomas and 9 with neurinomas (tab. 1). The male to female ratio was 2 : 7 in the meningiomas and 8 : 1 in the neurinomas. The median age was higher in the meningioma group (54.3 years) and less in the neurinoma group (33.1 years).

Clinical and neurological findings

The time interval from appearance of initial symptoms to diagnosis ranged from 3 months to 10 years. Meningiomas had the longer history with an average of 3 years, neurinomas ware recognized after a mean time of 2 years.

Table 1 Age and sex distribution (n = 18)

	All patients	Meningioma	Neurinoma
n	18	9	9
Male/female ratio	10 : 8	2 : 7	8 : 1
Average age (years)	43.7	54.3	33.1
Duration of symptoms (years)	2.5	3	2

13 of 18 patients complained of pain in the occiput, neck and shoulder as initial symptoms (tab. 2). 11 patients noted dysaesthesia, mostly beginning in the hand. The neck pain and dysaesthesia were frequently considered to be caused by cervical spondylosis. These patients often had been treated previously with analgesics, physical therapy, acupuncture or chiropractic manipulation. Months or years after the initial symptoms, gait disturbance and weakness of arms or legs developed slowly. Sometimes the course of the symptoms runs intermitted and/or painless, leading to the diagnosis of encephalomyelitis disseminata. Bladder dysfunction was found in 6 patients.

The neurological examination showed severe paresis, like a spastic hemi- or tetraparesis in 17 of 18 patients (tab. 3). Sensory disturbances usually were irregular and not associated with a certain spinal cord level. 3 patients had a typical Brown-Séquard's syndrome. The signs of Babinski were noted in 16 patients, spastic gait in 14. A restricted movement and deviation of the cervical spine was found in 12 patients. Atrophy of the hand, arm or pectoralis muscles occured in 4 cases, cranial nerve disturbances only in 3 patients. A big dumbbell-shaped neurinoma was palpable at the neck in 1 patient.

Table 2 Symptomatology (n = 18)

	n
Head and/or neck pain	13
Dysaesthesia	11
Gait disturbance	11
Weakness	10
Bladder dysfunction	6

Table 3 Clinical findings (n = 18)

	n
Paresis	17
Sensory loss	16
Babinski's sign	16
Ataxia/incoordination	14
Restricted neck movement	12
Atrophy	4
Brown-Séquard's syndrome	3
Cranial nerve palsy	3
Palpable tumour	1

Radiographic evaluation

In 6 cases the diagnosis was already confirmed by plain X-rays (tab. 4). The myelography detected the tumour in 15 out of 18 patients. Mostly there is a complete or incomplete stop of the contrast media column. Tumours situated cranially or laterally can sometimes escape the myelographic detection. In dumbbell or very large tumours a vertebral angiography is performed in order to detect an extensive tumour vascularisation, an unilateral obstruction or displacement of the vertebral artery (fig. 1). Nuclear magnetic resonance and CT scanning are more informative than the myelography, especially concerning recurrences of tumours and operative results. Figure 2 shows multiple recurring neurofibromas at the level of C 1 – 3 with dorsal displacement of the spinal cord.

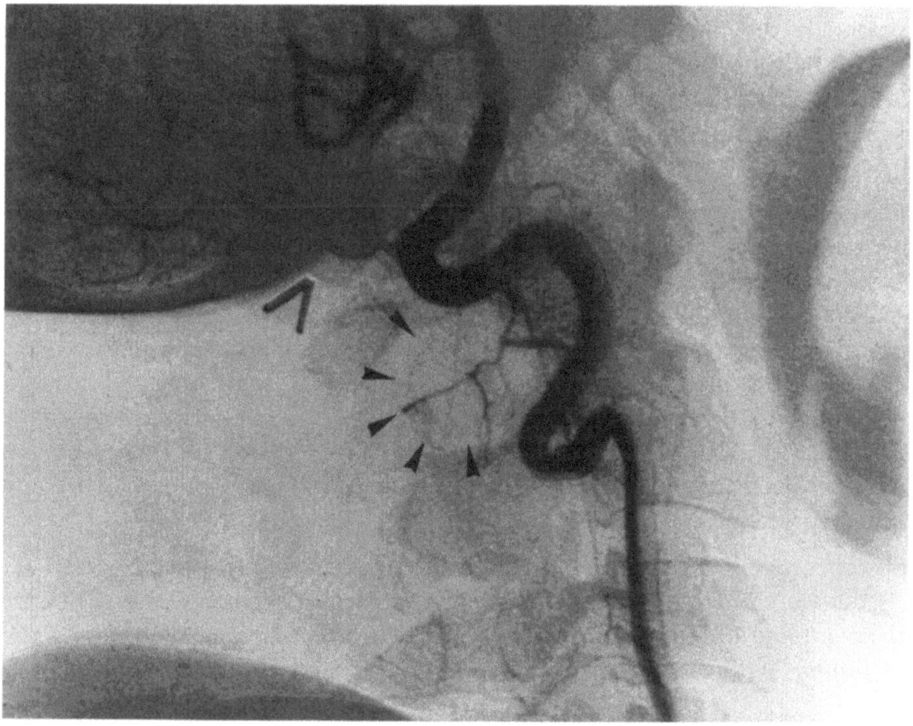

Fig. 1 Vertebral angiography showing tumor vascularisation in the enlarged foramen intervertebrale C 1/2 (arrows). Lateral neurinoma of the left C 2-root.

Operative therapy and results

In all 18 cases the tumour could be approached from dorsal with the patient in the sitting position. 15 of these tumours were situated ventral or ventrolateral

Table 4 Radiological findings (n = 18)

	n
Bony erosion and/or enlarged intervertebral foramen	6
Myelographic evaluation	15
complete stop	5
incomplete stop	9
root compression	1
Tumour stain or vessel displacement in vertebral angiography	4

to the spinal cord (fig. 3). Anteflexion of the patients head should be avoided even if the operative approach is restricted in order to prevent spinal cord compression by the hypomochlion of the premedullar tumour. It may be necessary to sacrifice the roots of C 1 and C 2. A total removal of the tumour was possible in 13 of 18 patients. In one case the remaining extravertebral part of the tumour was removed in a second operation by an anterolateral approach.

Within the first two postoperative weeks there is a high risk of pulmonary complications (tab. 5): two patients died of pulmonary embolism, one of a massive pneumonia. In most of the patients some of the following risk factors were evident: multiple tumours of the CNS, advanced pulmonary and/or cardiac dysfunction, accompanying diseases like myotonic dystrophy and metastazising malignoma. Therefore, early posteroperative mobilisation and heparinisation are indispensible. Postoperative instability of the cervical spine occured in two patients. Following laminectomy one patient developed a kyphotic scoliosis with irritation of the C 3 and C 4 roots. After temporary extension in a halo-cast we performed a dorsal spondylodesis C 1 – C 4. In the second patient physical therapy was sufficient.

The postoperative results are better in neurinomas than in meningiomas (tab. 6). This is due to the lower age distribution, the earlier diagnosis and the more lateral favourable tumour-localisation in the neurinoma group. Concerning the overall results 3 out of 18 patients were symptom- and painfree. In another 11

Table 5 Complications (n = 18)

	n
Pulmonary embolism	2
Pneumonia	1
Cardiovascular disturbance	1
Instability of cervical spine	2
Wound infection	0

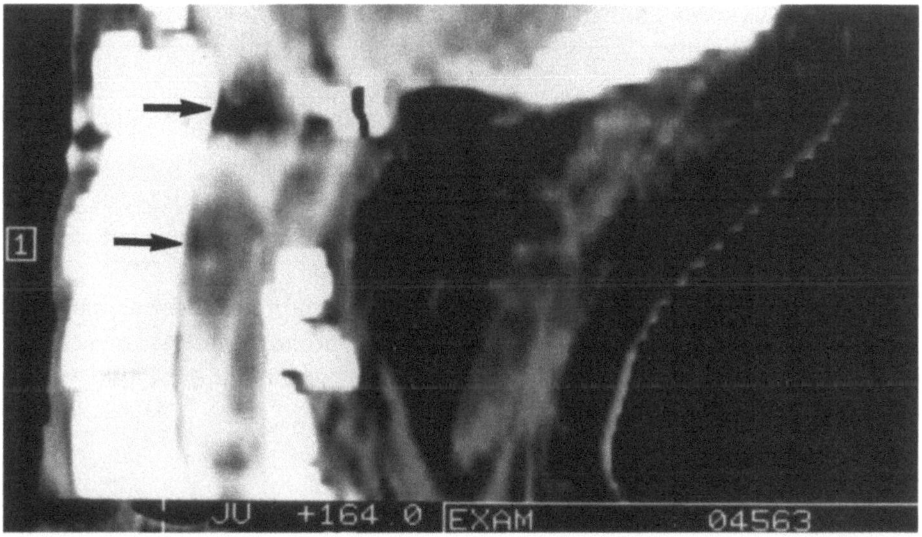

Fig. 2 Sagittal CT-reformation. Multiple recurring neurofibromas C 1 to C 33 with dorsal displacement of the spinal cord (arrows).

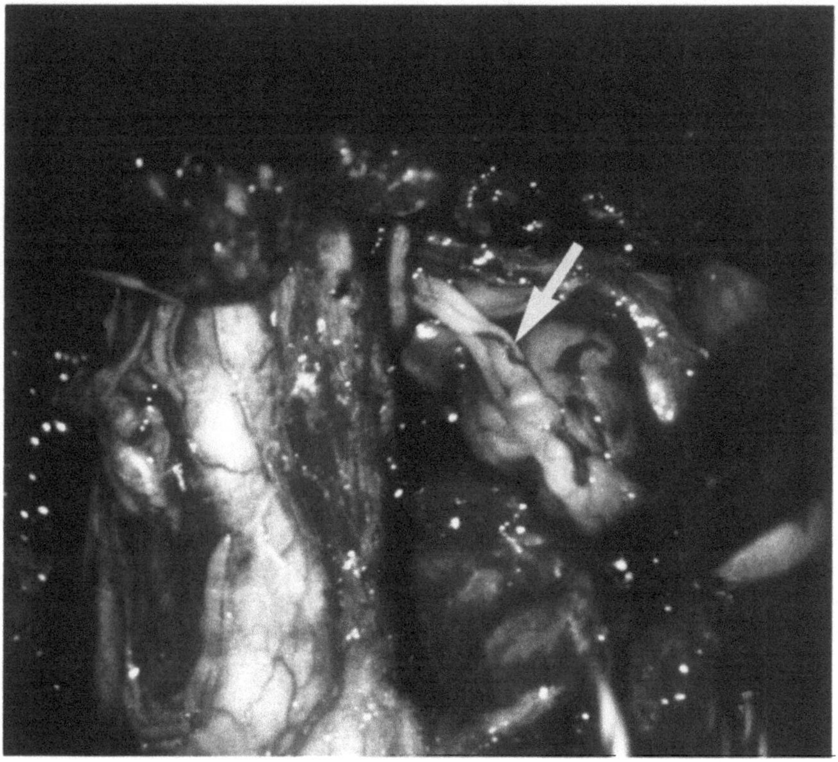

Fig. 3 Neurofibroma situated ventral to the nerve root C 2 (arrow). Introperative photo.

Table 6 Surgical results (n = 18)

	All patients	Meningioma	Neurinoma
Full recovery	3	0	3
Improvement	11	6	5
Deterioration	1	1	0
Dead	3	2	1

patients the neurological deficits were considerably improved. In one case the preoperative bladder dysfunction showed further progression. As mentioned above 3 patients died of pulmonary complications within the first two weeks postoperatively.

Discussion and Summary

Benign tumours of the cranio-cervical region are rare. According to different authors [2, 5, 6] they comprise of approximately 2.4 to 9.4% of all spinal tumours. Sophisticated neuroradiological methods like myelographic computerized tomography and nuclear magnetic resonance imaging [3] ameliorate diagnosis of this tumour group. Vertebral angiography is still necessary to show the vascular supply of the tumour and compression or displacement of the vertebral artery. Using a dorsal approach and microsurgical techniques a total removal of the tumour is possible in most of the cases [1, 4, 5]. Postoperative instability may need additional dorsal or ventral stabilisation. In spite of the considerable risk factors and advanced neurological deficits prior to operation the surgical results with satisfying functional recovery in most of the patients are encouraging.

References

[1] Eggert, H. R., et al.: Unilateral microsurgical approaches to extramedullary spinal tumours. Operative technique and results. Acta Neurochir. (Wien) **67** (1983) 245–253.
[2] Fortuna, A., et al.: Spinal neurinomas and meningiomas in children. Acta Neurochir. (Wien) **55** (1981) 329–341.
[3] Galanski, M.: Röntgen-diagnosis of the posterior part of the base of the skull. Röntgenblätter **37** (1984) 178–186.
[4] Hakuba, A., et al.: Transuncodiscal approach to dumbbell tumours of the cervical spinal cord. J. Neurosurg. **61** (1984) 1100–1106.
[5] Meyer, F. B., et al.: Benign tumours of the foramen magnum. J. Neurosurg. **61** (1984) 49–52.
[6] Yasouka, S., H. Okazaki, J. R. Daube, et al.: Foramen magnum tumours. Analysis of 57 cases of benign extramedullary tumours. J. Neurosurg. **49** (1978) 828–838.

Craniospinal lipoma in infancy

R. Kalff, V. Reinhardt, K. Roosen, W. Kocks, W. Castro

Introduction

Intradural spinal lipomas are rare and account for 1% of all intraspinal tumours [1, 3, 5, 13, 24, 25–27, 29]. They are mostly localized in the cervico-thoracal region [13].

They are considered malformation tumours [30] often combined with other deformations [2, 17, 28] or, in rare cases, with other kinds of tumours [6].

Obré [22] was the first to mention an intradural lipoma in 1851. In 1857 Johnson [21] described an intraspinal lipoma combined with spina bifida. A survey of published cases was given by Ehni and Love [13] in 1945, as well as by Caram [7] in 1957 and in 1966 by Giuffre [15] and Bischof [5]. Further publications followed [1, 3, 4, 8, 9, 10–12, 14, 16, 18–20, 23, 25].

Case report

We report the case of a 6 month-old-boy with an intraspinal lipoma extending from the posterior fossa to the upper thoracic region. Because of the lack of control of his head and reduced movement of his arms and legs, he was admitted to a neuropediatric department.

The *neurological examination* showed a paralysis of the accessory nerves on both sides. The infant was not able to lift its head. There were no other deficiencies of cranial nerves. A completely flaccid paralysis of the muscles of the upper extremities and shoulders was present with a deformed contraction in a bent position of the hands and fingers and muscular atrophy. At the lower extremities a spastic paralysis was dominant. The muscle tone of the anal sphincter was flaccid and there was no anal reflex.

Neuro-radiological examinations

X-ray of cervical spine

A widening of the spinal canal in the cervical region was visible, but no indication of a dysraphic malformation (fig. 1).

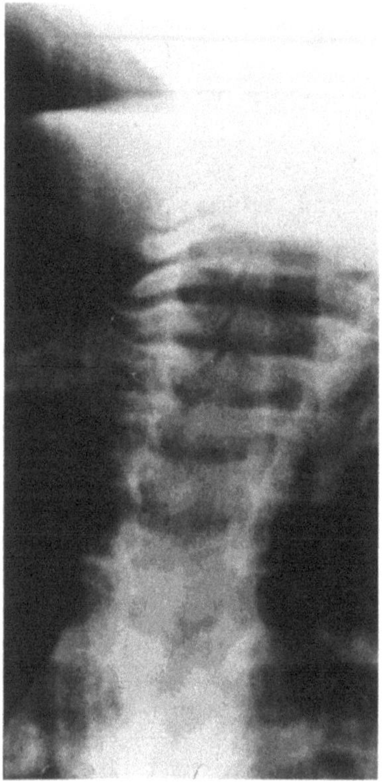

Fig. 1

Cranial and spinal computerized tomography

A hypodense space occupying lesion of 111 HE in the posterior fossa in the region of the fourth ventricle and cisterna cerebello-medullaris extending continuously into the spinal canal down to the level of Th 3 was present mainly in the right posterior area (fig. 2 a, b). Besides this another hypodense region in the soft tissue extraspinally could be seen.

NMR

At the level of T 1 a tumour is visible with a sharp demarcation in the region of the floor of the fourth ventricle extending into the spinal canal down to the upper thoracic region (fig. 3). The brainstem is evidently lifted ventrally and in a sagittal view a lipomatous tumour in the neck without any relationship to the spinal canal is apparent.

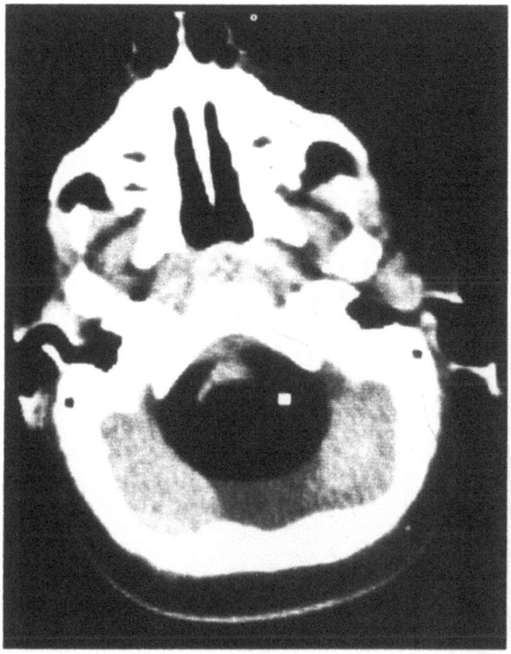

Fig. 2 a

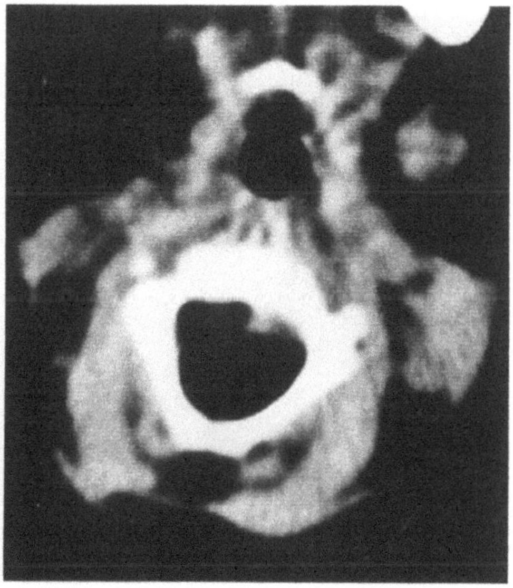

Fig. 2 b

Myelography

After application of Solutrast intradurally into the lumbar region and visualising the cervico-thoracic region, a complete and relatively sharp demarcated arrest of the dye occurs at the level of Th 4 (fig. 4).

Therapy and clinical course

On account of the typical neuro-radiological findings, the diagnosis of an intradural lipoma and another small one in the soft tissue of the neck could already be ascertained before the operation.

After osteoclastic trepanation of the posterior fossa and laminectomy from C 1 – C 4 the dura mater, which showed clear evidence of tension, was opened. A tumour of white-yellow colour filling the cisterna cerebello-medullaris was found. This mass extended through the foramen magnum into the spinal canal. Cranially it was blown up like a balloon and extended to the pons. In this area it was easy to dissect the tumour. Furthermore it was tried to mobilize the

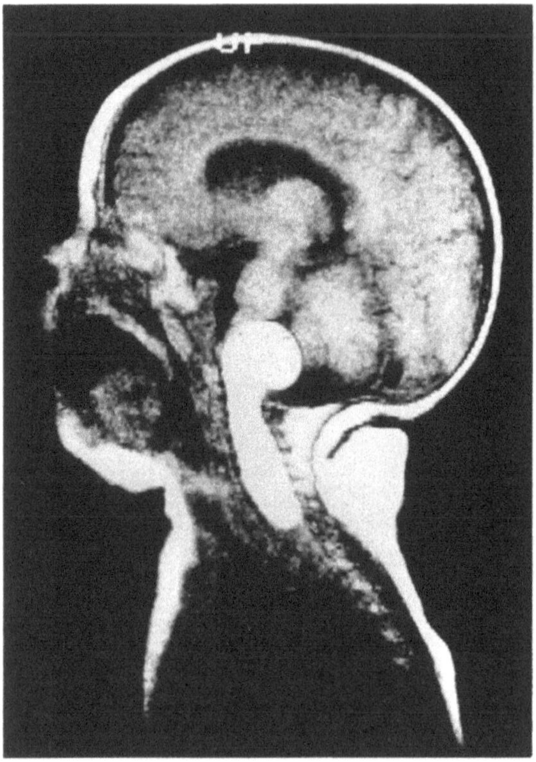

Fig. 3

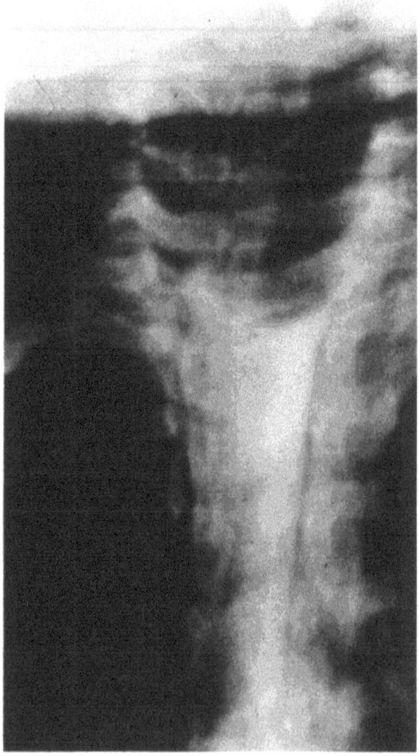

Fig. 4

tumour downwards into the spinal canal. We could soon recognize that the tumour seemed to infiltrate the spinal canal at the level of C 3. No demarcation between tumour and nervous tissue was evident. Since a complete exstirpation was impossible, only the cranial part of the tumour in the posterior fossa and upper cervical region was resected. The lipoma in the soft tissue of the neck showed no relationship to the intraspinal tumour.

One day after the operation the infant could be detubated because pCO_2 and pO_2 levels in the blood were good and spontaneous breathing was sufficient. The neurological examination showed no deterioration in comparison with the preoperative state. During the day paradox respiration occurred. One day later the infant died of central disregulation.

Autopsy

During autopsy in the area of the operation-defect, the upper cervical cord appeared flattened like a strip (fig. 5). From the caudal side of the operation

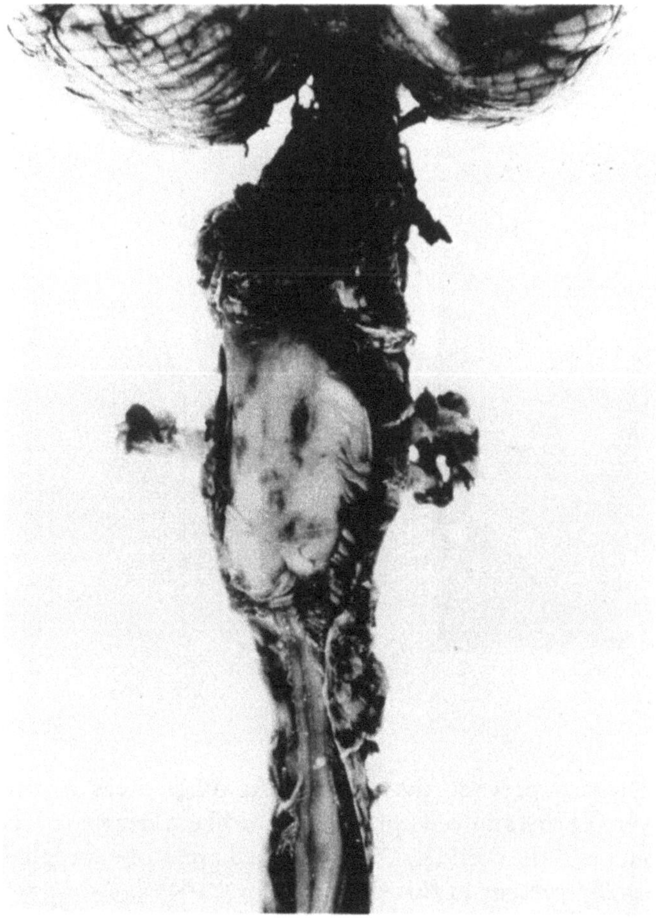

Fig. 5

defect to the beginning of the thoracic cord an intradural sharply-demarcated orange-yellow tumour was present at the dorsal side, which had flattened the cord ventrally (fig. 6). It also seems that intradural nerve roots are enclosed in the tumour. The cord caudally to the tumour showed a normal coinfiguration. Malformations, expecially a dysraphic disformation, were not demonstrable.

Histology

Microscopically the tumour, that looks like a lipoma consisting of mature cells, is demarcated from the compressed cord by a divergent, broad partly scarlike cover consisting of collagenous connective tissue with a rich mixture of elastic fibres (fig. 7 K). Vessels embedded in fibre strips of this cover radiate into the

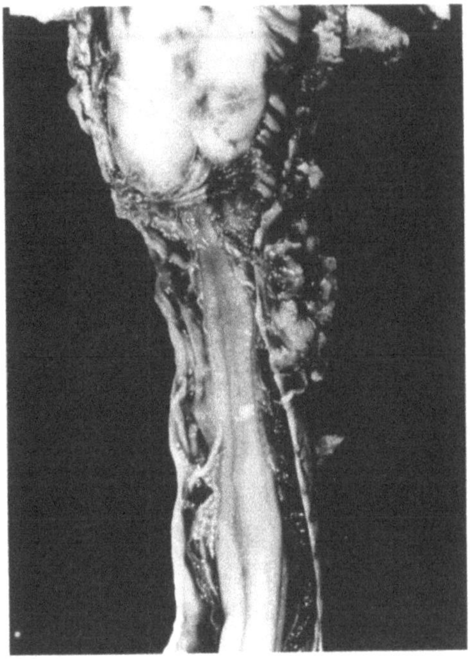

Fig. 6

cord (fig. 7 →). Nerve roots also pervade the tumour. At other areas a disc consisting of concentric layered Schwann-cells proliferations like a neuroma has developed between the lipoma and the cord (fig. 7 N). Isolated areas of neuroglial tissue (fig. 7 G), are occasionally present in this disc.

Discussion and Summary

Intradural spinal lipomas are histologically well differentiated lipomatous tumours which although demarcated from the cord by a tissue layer, radiate into the myelum from the outer side of the membrane with connective tissue-strips, which contain vessels.

In our case too, the same observation could be made. Besides, the neuroma-like tissue disc had no clear boundary to the myelum and there were within these tissue parts glious centers that were probably connected to the cord. This partially narrowed connection from the tumour with the nervous tissue accounts for the operative impression that the tumour had infiltrated the cord. A radical extirpation proved impossible without worsening the neurological status.

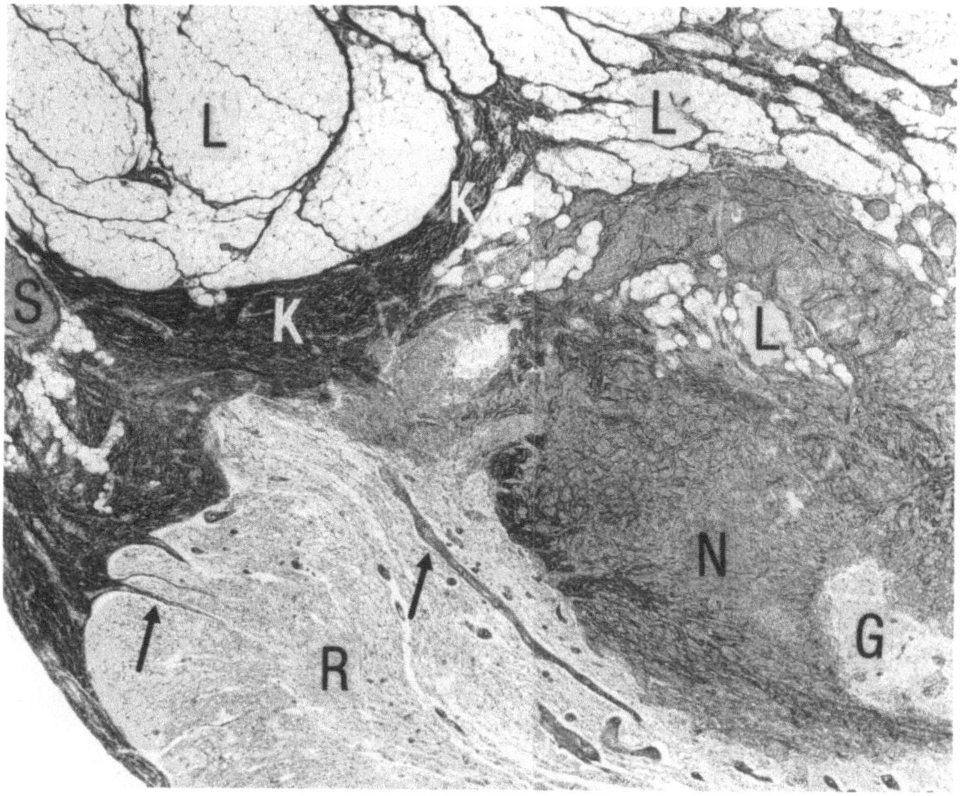

Fig. 7 L = lipoma; K = connective tissue with elastic fibres; → = vessels embedded in fibres radiate into the myelum; N = Schwann-cell proliferations like neuroma; G = neuroglial tissue; S = spinal root.

Retrospectively, the question arises whether a lipoma which – on the basis of neuro-radiological examinations – could be preoperatively diagnosed as such, should be operated upon at all, considering its wide dispersion and the poor separation from the cord.

References

[1] Ammermann, B. J., J. M. Henry, U. De Girolani, et al.: Intradural lipomas of the spinal cord. A clinicopathological correlation. J. Neurosurg. **44** (1976) 331–336.

[2] Ashley, D. J. B.: Evans histological appearence of tumours. 3rd ed., pp. 54–65. Churchill Livengstone, Edinburgh–London–New York 1978.

[3] Barson, A. J.: Symptomless intradural spinal lipomas in infancy. J. Path. **104** (1971) 141–144.

[4] Beaudoing, A., M. Dieterlen, M. Bost, et al.: Les lipomes sous-duraux rachichiens chez l'enfant. Arch. Franc. Pédiat. **29** (1972) 431–432.

[5] Bischof, W., W. Müller: Beitrag zur Biologie der intramedullären Lipome. Dtsch. Z. Nervenheilk. **189** (1966) 1 – 10.
[6] Budka, H.: Intracranial lipomatous hamartomas (intracranial "lipomas"). A study of 13 cases including combinations with medulloblastoma, colloid and epidermoid cysts, angiomatosis and other malformations. Acta Neuropathol. (Berl.) **28** (1974) 205 – 222.
[7] Caram, P. C., G. Scarcella, C. A. Carton: Intradural lipomas of the spinal cord with particular emphasis on the "intramedullary" lipomas. J. Neurosurg. **12** (1957) 28 – 42.
[8] Caram, P. C.: Intradural lipomas of the spinal cord. A clinicopathological correlation. J. Neurosurg. **44** (1976) 331.
[9] Chapman, P. H.: Congenital intraspinal lipomas. Child's Brain **9** (1982) 37 – 47.
[10] De Sousa, A. L., J. E. Kalsbeck, J. Mealey, et al.: Intraspinal tumors in children. A review of 81 cases. J. Neurosurg. **51** (1979) 437 – 445.
[11] Di Lorenzo, N., R. Giuffre, A. Fortuna: Primary spinal neoplasms in childhood: analysis of 1234 published cases (including 56 personal cases) by pathology, sex, age and site. Differences from the situation in adults. Neurochirurgia **25** (1982) 153 – 164.
[12] Drapkin, A. J.: High cervical intradural lipoma. J. Neurosurg. **41** (1974) 699 – 704.
[13] Ehni, G., J. G. Love: Intraspinal lipomas: report of cases; review of the literature, and clinical and pathologic study. Arch. Neurol. Psychiatry **53** (1945) 1 – 28.
[14] Geindre, M., G. Crouzet, M. Coulomb, et al.: Un cas de lipome intrarachidien chez l'enfant. Evolution radio-clinique. Ann Radiol. **12** (1969) 571 – 576.
[15] Giuffre, R.: Intradural spinal lipomas. Review of the literature (99 cases) and report of an additional case. Acta Neurochir. **14** (1966) 69 – 95.
[16] Giuffre, R., D. Gambacorta: Lipoma of the spinal cord. Case report. J. Neurosurg. **35** (1971) 335 – 337.
[17] Giuffre, R.: Spinal lipomas. In: P. J. Vinken, G. W. Bruyn (eds.): Handbook of clinical neurology, vol. 20, pp. 435 – 480. North-Holland Publishing Company, Amsterdam – Oxford 1976.
[18] Giuffre, R., N. Di Lorenzo, A. Fortuna: Primary spinal tumors in infancy and childhood. Zbl. Neurochirurgie **42** (1981) 87 – 98.
[19] Grote, W., F. Römer, W. Bock, et al.: Langzeitergebnisse in der Behandlung spinaler Tumoren des Kindes- und Jugendalters. Mschr. Kinderheilk. **123** (1975) 112 – 119.
[20] Hubert, J. P., G. Monseu, N. Stoupel, et al.: Lipome spinal. Observation anatomiclinique. Acta Neurol. Belg. **72** (1972) 338 – 346.
[21] Johnson, A.: Fatty tumour connected with the interior of the spinal canal of sacrum. Tr. Path. Soc. Lond. **8** (1957) 28.
[22] Obré: Transactions of the London Patholog. Society: 1851 – 1852, Vol. III p. 248. Ref. Virchow's Geschwülste Bd. I, p. 387.
[23] Pani, K. C., J. S. Chopra, V. K. Kak: Intramedullary lipoma of the spinal cord. Neurochirurgia **15** (1972) 33 – 35.
[24] Rand, R. W., C. W. Rand: Intraspinal tumours of childhood. Charles C. Thomas, Springfield 1960.
[25] Rogers, H. M., D. M. Long, S. N. Chou, et al.: Lipomas of the spinal cord and cauda equina. J. Neurosurg. **34** (1971) 349 – 354.
[26] Rubinstein, L. J.: Tumors of the central nervous system. In: Atlas of Tumor Pathology. Institute of Pathology, Washington, DC, Armed Forces (1972) 56 – 74.
[27] Russel, D. S., L. J. Rubinstein: Pathology of tumours of the nervous system, pp. 38 – 39. 4th edition. E. Arnold, Ltd., London 1977.
[28] Shuman, R., W. A. D. Anderson: Mesenchymal tumors of soft tissues. In: W. A. D. Anderson, J. M. Kissane (eds.): Pathology, vol. 2, pp. 1874 – 1904, 7th edition. Mosby Company, St. Louis 1977.
[29] Taniguchi, T., J. A. Mufson: Intradural lipoma of the spinal cord. Report of a case. J. Neurosurg. 7 (1950) 584 – 586.
[30] Zülch, K. J.: Histological typing of tumours of the central nervous system. WHO, Geneva 1979.

The clinical importance of a delayed diagnosis in cases of craniospinal tumors

K. E. Richard, P. Sanker, R. A. Frowein

Introduction

Clinical experience shows that craniospinal tumors are very difficult to diagnose. They are rare and have an ambiguous symptomatology [1 – 4]. In the following we would like first to discuss the typical false primary diagnoses, by which craniospinal tumors were treated until true recognition of the space-occupying process.

Brief histories of patients

In the period 1952 to 1984, 51 patients – 24 female, 27 male – were operated on for tumors of the craniospinal junction in the Neurosurgical Hospital of Cologne. At operation the youngest patient was 1 year old, the oldest was 70 years old. Histologically the tumors were ependymomas (n: 30), meningiomas (n: 8) and rare types (n: 13) (tab. 1).

Table 1 Tumors of the craniocervical junction – patients' material 1952 – 1985

	n
Ependymoma	30
Meningeoma	8
Spongioblastoma	3
Chordoma	1
Chondrosarcoma	1
Plexuspapilloma	1
Neuroblastoma	1
Hemangiopericytoma	1
Dermoid	1
Unclassified	4
Total	51

Results

Symptomatology (fig. 1)

Ependymomas

In general, ependymomas can grow from the floor of the 4th ventricle through the foramen occipitale magnum into the upper cervical canal.

The patient's age at operation is 17 years on the average. In nearly 90% of the patients nausea and vomiting were the first symptoms and in 5 patients as long as 1 year before admission.

During the further course more than half of the patients complained of headache and neck pain. Later on gait disturbances were noticed and in the initial examination such disorders, as ataxic gait, dysdiadochokinesia, and papilloedema dominated.

ANAMNESIS	TOTAL %	EPENDYMOMAS % N	MENINGEOMAS % N	RARE TUMORS % N	N
Nausea/Vomiting	65	26	0	7	33
Headache	63	18	5	9	32
Gait disturbance	63	17	6	9	32
Neck pain	51	14	5	7	26
Dizziness	29	11	0	4	15
Visual disturbance	28	8	0	6	14
Loss of weight	14	5	0	2	7
Bladder disturbance	14	0	4	3	7

Fig. 1 *Anamnestic symptomatology* in tumors of the craniocervical junction 1952 – 1985.

Meningiomas

The meningiomas always originated in the upper cervical canal. Only secondarily did they invade through the occipital foramen into the posterior cranial fossa.

The patients' average age at operation is considerably higher, i.e. 48 years. Prominent initial complaints were neck pain and headache and increasing spastic gait. These patients never complained of nausea and vomiting unlike the patients with craniospinal ependymomas. On examination spastic hemi- and tetrapareses and perception disorders were found.

Rare tumors

The rare tumors of the craniospinal junction do not constitute a uniform syndrome group. The most important complaints were headache, neck pain and gait disturbances.

Typically wrong primary diagnoses

Craniospinal ependymomas (fig. 2)

16 out of 31 patients with ependymomas, i. e. 50%, were treated in view of wrong diagnoses over a period of up to 11 years. The median period until the definitive diagnosis was up to 12 months. Only patients with a maximum length of anamnesis of 2 years survived.

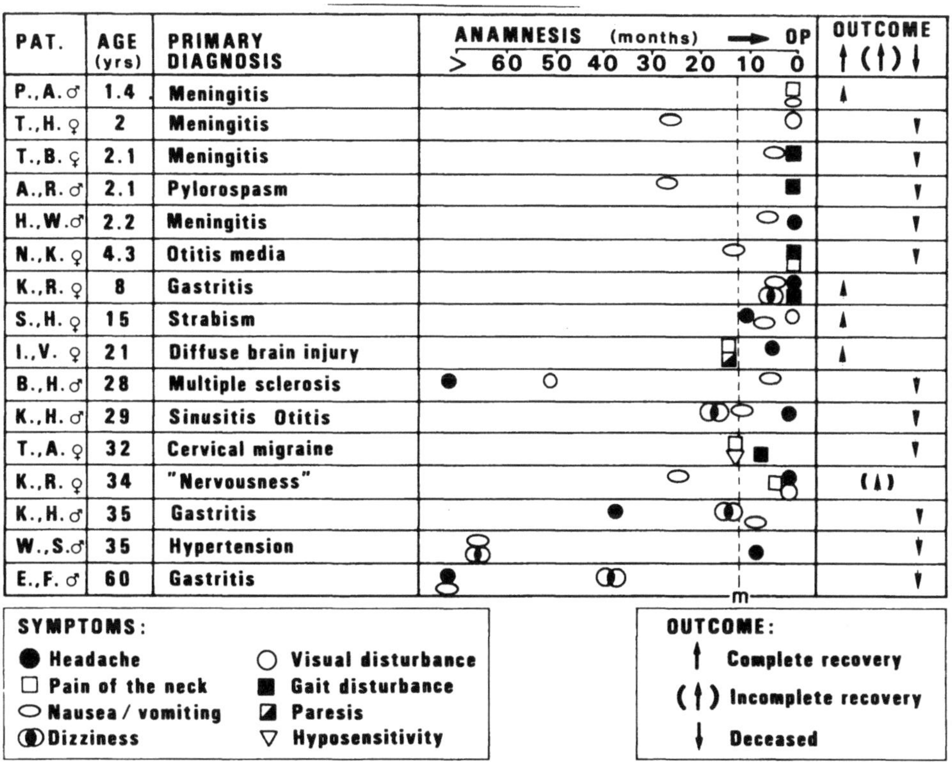

Fig. 2 Craniocervical *ependymomas*: Typical primary diagnoses, length and mean duration of anamneses, type of symptoms and patient's outcome (1952–1985).

We refer here to a typical case a 60-years-old missionary who had been suffering from paroxysmal headaches during his studies. For 11 years he suffered from frequent gastric disorders. In the last 5 years he complained of intermittent nausea, finally with unabated vomiting for days. After fruitless conservative attempts directed at gastralgia, a tropical disease was finally assumed in view of his work in New Guinea. During the last months before admission, increasing imbalance and gait disturbance with continuous headaches were present. Computed tomography, carried out externally, revealed an expanding lesion in the fossa cranii posterior together with hydrocephalus occlusus. On examination dysdiadochokinesia, ataxic gait were present. In the positive ventriculogramm considerable dilatation of the ventricles and a large filling defect in the 4th ventricle were visible. During operation a tumor was found which started from the floor of the 4th ventricle, filling it and extending caudally through the foramen occipitale magnum into the upper cervical canal down to C 2. Histologically the tumor was an epèndymoma.

The patient died 2 months after operation as a result of an acute renal failure.

Spinocranial meningiomas (fig. 3)

In cases of spinocranial meningiomas headache and neck pain combined with hemiparesis were the cause of wrong primary diagnoses such as a cervical syndrome or a cerebral circulatory disturbance. Lack of papilledema was responsible for the late diagnosis. On average 14 months passed until the diagnosis of the expanding craniospinal lesion was made.

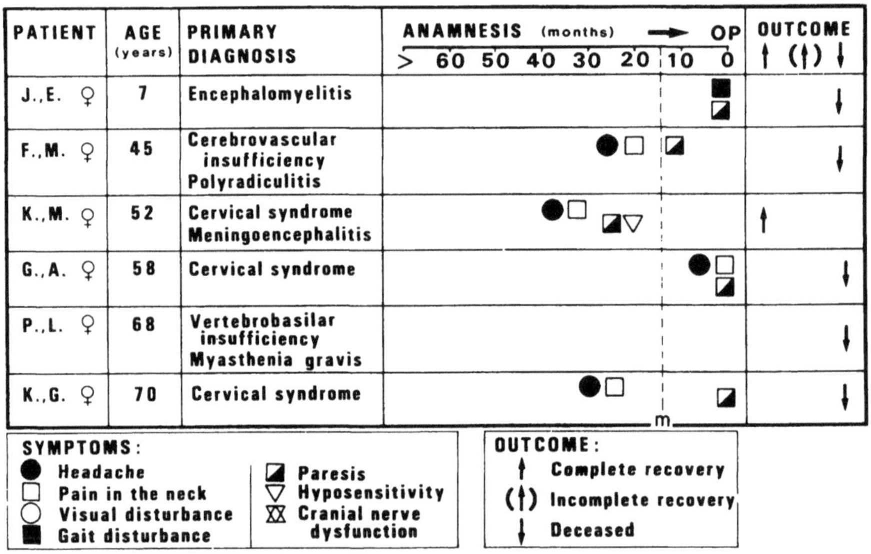

Fig. 3 Craniocervical *meningiomas*: Typical primary diagnoses, length and mean duration of anamneses, type of symptoms and patient's outcome (1982 – 1985).

In contrast to the ependymomas a 53-year-old female survived, having suffered from headache and neck pain for 3 years.

In a 45-year-old female, increasing neck pains for the last 2 years were noticable. Gradual weakness of the right arm with numbness and tingling sensations was reported. A neurological examination could not clarify these complaints. 2

months before operation, when admitted by another hospital, a right-sided spastic hemiparesis had developed. There was discrete left glossoplegia and bilateral dysdiadochokinesia. In the computed tomography ischemic necrosis within the left cerebral hemisphere was suspected. Treatment with drugs stimulating the cerebral blood flow and with psychopharmacological agents was complemented with additional physiotherapy and occupational therapy. During this treatment development of a tetraparesis with bladder disturbances and striking dyspnoea occured. In the suboccipital CSF 15/3 cells with 85 mg% protein were present and in the lumbar CSF 1/3 cells with 224 mg% protein. Suspecting a Barré-Guillain syndrome we started an induction of a cortisone therapy.

To exclude an expanding lesion in the upper cervical region the patient was transferred to the neurological hospital. The cervical myelogram revealed a distinct expanding lesion at the level of the foramen occipitale magnum ventral to the cord. In the CT of the craniospinal junction, a distinct space-occupying mass surrounded by a soft contrast border was observed. At operation a meningioma was found, which had surrounded the cervical cord down to the level of C 2. A part of the tumor extended into the posterior fossa, anterior to the medulla oblongata. The tumor could be removed only subtotally. Postoperatively, an initial good recovery and involution of the tetraparesis was observed. Nine days after operation the patient died following an acute cardiac and respiratory arrest.

Rare tumors of craniospinal junction (fig. 4)

Patients with rarer craniospinal tumors had already undergone either an operation for removal of a meniscus, a protracted conservative treatment of an amyotrophic lateral sclerosis, a treatment for encephalitis, for rheumatism or for an endogenous psychosis. In these patients the mean duration until the final diagnosis of the expanding lesion was made, lasted up to 24 months.

Mortality

The mortality of our patients was 77% within the period 1952 to 1977, after 1978, 33%. However, since the introduction of the computed tomography in 1978 the number of delayed diagnoses did not decrease to any substantial extent (fig. 5).

Discussion

Ependymomas of the craniospinal junction lead to nausea and vomiting in the early stages and after the development of an obstructive hydrocephalus also to headaches. In about 75% of these patients at the date of admission a papilledema

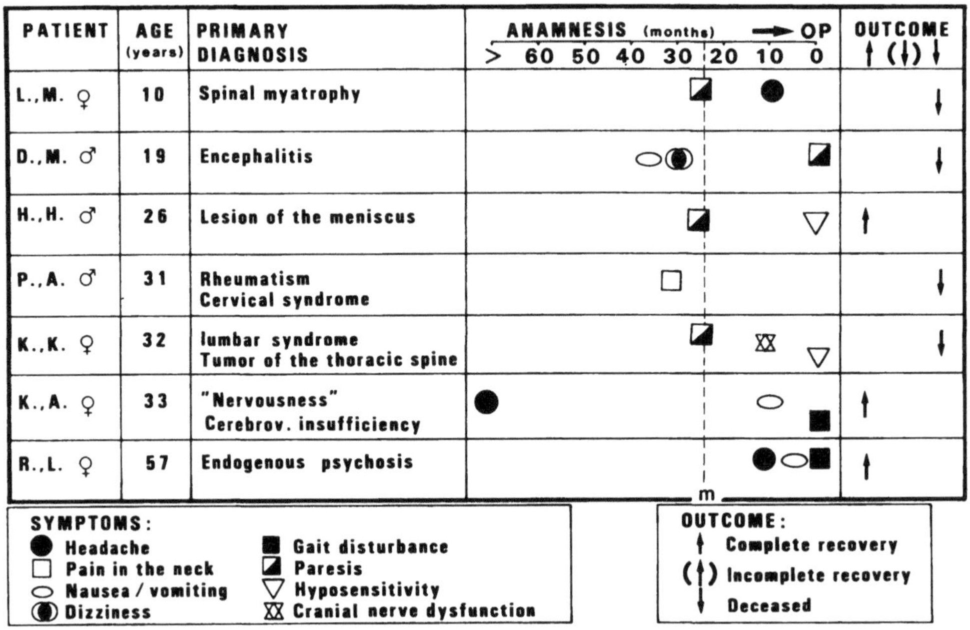

Fig. 4 *Rare* craniocervical *tumors*: Typical primary diagnoses, length and mean duration of anamneses, type of symptoms and patient's outcome (1982 – 1985).

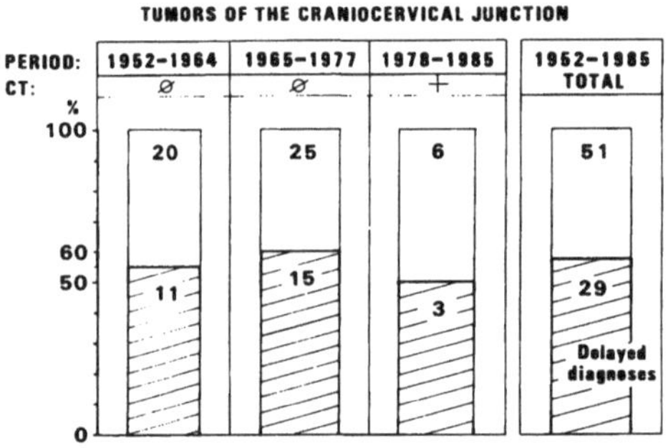

Fig. 5 Number of *delayed diagnoses* at different time periods: in the period after introduction of *computed tomography* the number of delayed diagnoses were approximately the same (50%) as in the two earlier periods (55/60%).

existed. In contrast to the cervicocranial *meningiomas* headaches and neck pain dominated and were followed by pareses. No patient had signs of increased intracranial pressure. Similar observations were also reported by Smolik and Sachs [4] and Fried [2].

Cushing and Eisenhardt had already taken the different syndromes into account by differentiating supra-foraminal and sub-foraminal tumors. Krenkel and Friedmann [3] had drawn attention to the different symptomatology of the supraforaminal, i. e. the craniospinal, and the subforaminal, i. e. the spinocranial, space-occupying lesions.

In spite of this classification valuable for localisation, the clinical analysis of our patients reveals how difficult it is to achieve an early diagnosis of these lesions even nowadays. The time spent on a long treatment after more obvious diagnoses has not diminished noticeably.

However we express the hope that further developments of imaging methods, for example nuclear magnetic resonance tomography, will detect the cervicocranial disease process earlier and improve the results.

Conclusion

- Most frequent expanding lesions in the craniocervical region are ependymomas and meningiomas, in our material 30 and 8 patients respectively, i. e. 75%.
- Patients with craniocervical ependymomas were as a rule not admitted before development of an increase in intracranial pressure.
- The spinocranial meningiomas were diagnosed as a rule not before development of severe spastic pareses. These patients had no papilloedema.
- Computed tomography had not perceptibly improved the early diagnosis of craniocervical expanding lesions, as until now this investigation has been performed only late.
- Prerequisites for an early diagnosis of craniospinal tumors which are difficult to recognize are the analysis of anamnesis, neurological state and early application of the modern diagnostic methods: computed tomography, NMR, evoked potentials.

References

[1] Cushing, H., L. Eisenhardt: Notes on first reasonably successful removal of intracranial tumor. Bull. Los Angeles Neurol. Soc. 3 (1938) 95 – 98.

[2] Fried, H.: Zur Klinik und Behandlung hoher Halsmarktumoren. Zbl. Neurochir. 27 (1966) 95 – 107.

[3] Krenkel, W., G. Friedmann: Diagnose und Therapie der kraniospinalen Tumoren. Fortschr. Neurol. Psychiat. 35 (1967) 237 – 262.

[4] Smolik, E. A., E. Sachs: Tumors of the foramen magnum of spinal origin. J. Neurosurg. 11 (1954) 161 – 172.

Pathological spontaneous activity in the EMG of a patient with a foramen magnum meningioma

H. Beck-Mannagetta, E. Kazner

Introduction

Clinicians as well as electrophysiologists usually decide to investigate a patient by needle electromyography if a lesion of the lower motor neuron can be expected. If evidence of a lesion of the peripheral motor neuron such as pathological spontaneous activity is present in a case of a central lesion it can lead to diagnostic misinterpretation. This disregards the findings of Goldkamp [3] who described fibrillation potentials (FP) in 57% and positive sharp waves (PSW) in 70% of 116 hemiplegic patients as early as 1967.

Cases of "denervation-activity" due to central lesions so far reported had been diagnosed mainly in clinical investigation. They were based on lesions, especially cerebral insults, but also spinal cord injuries, which could not be operated on [5]. Our case of pathological spontaneous activity after a foramen magnum meningioma is special, due to the fact that the lesion could be localized exactly by the nuclear magnetic resonance tomography (NMR) and neurosurgical findings. Moreover the post-operative recovery and disappearance of the electromyographical abnormality after removal of the tumour can be definitly related to the removal of the lesion.

Clinical history and diagnostic approach

The 61 year old patient recognized five years before diagnosis a numbness and heaviness of the left arm and left leg and clumsiness of the tongue. Clinical investigation failed to find evidence for a distinct disorder. Three years later aching of the head and the neck and a weakness with burning dysasthesias in both arms and legs developed. The clinical finding was a slight spastic tetra paresis. In the cerebro-spinal fluid albumin was raised above normal but myelography up to the cervical region discovered no pathological process nor did cranial computed tomography.

The third clinical investigation was carried out already one year later because of progressive pareses and heavy burning dysasthesias. Significantly the small hand muscles were atrophic and deep tendon reflexes were hyperactive with a stress of the left side where Babinski' sign was demonstrable. No disturbance of sensibility could be found.

Considering amyotrophic lateral sclerosis, electromyography and electroneurography were performed. However nerve conduction velocities were normal in all investigated muscles of the hands and lower leg (left M. gastrocnemius, right M. tibialis anterior, left M. tibialis anterior, right M. abductor pollicis brevis, right M. abductor digiti V, left M. abductor pollicis brevis) but sustained PSW and FP could be demonstrated (fig. 1).

Albumin in CSF was raised to 64 mg% and lack of bulbar involvement gave way to another investigation of the upper cervical region, this time by NMR (fig. 2).

Having evidence of a process in the atlanto-occipital region the meanwhile almost completely tetraplegic patient now could be rendered to neurosurgery.

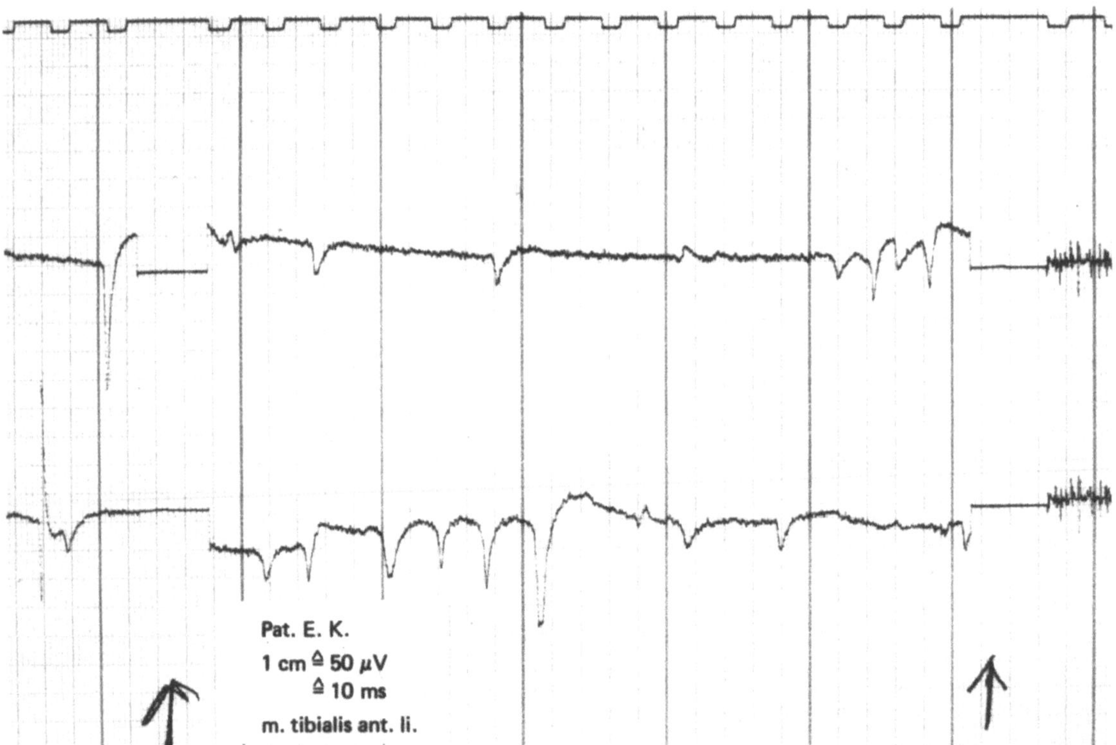

Fig. 1 Example of positive sharp waves and fibrillation potentials.

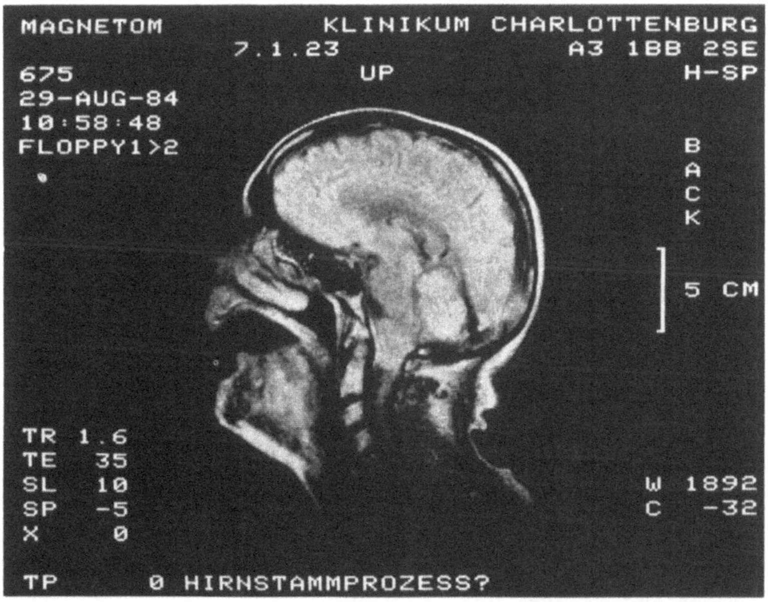

Fig. 2 Medio-sagittal nuclear magnetic resonance tomogram showing an extramedullary situated spinal tumour in the cranial cervical region pressing the medulla oblongata resp. the upper cervical cord to the dorsal circumference of the foramen occipitale magnum. (NMR illustration were kindly supplied by the Radiological University Clinic Charlottenburg, Free University Berlin.)

Using a dorsal approach and after opening the stretched dura mater the medulla oblongata was found to be displaced to the right and dorsally by a solid well encapsuled tumor situated left and ventrally. Using microsurgical technique the protuberant meningioma reaching from the cervical roots C_2 to the fusion of the Aa. vertebrales and being fixed to the anterior circumference of the foramen occipitale magnum, was completely removed saving all nerve roots, cranial nerves and vessels. The spinal cord showed an impression even after removal of the tumor at the level of the foramen magnum.

Already at the night of operation the patient could move hands and feet and after seven days startet to walk completely recovering after ten weeks. Eight weeks after operation the electromyographical controls of the previously investigated muscles showed no pathological spontaneous activity.

Discussion

Spontaneous pathological muscle activity caused by foramen magnum meningiomas has been reported by several American authors [6, 7]. The transgress of a disturbance from the upper to the lower neuron, however, needs further explanation. An ischaemia or oedemae due to compression of vessels especially the A. spinalis anterior, hydromyelia secondary to compression of the central canal, tractions of the roots by torsion due to the tumor have been held responsible for anterior horn cell damage caudal to the lesion. No evidence of such a direct injury, however, could be found by autopsy and the functional importance of the A. spinalis anterior for the lower regions of the spinal cord is uncertain. Models of transsynaptic degeneration appear to be more suitable to explain anterior horn cell damage so far distant from the lesion. According to the concept of Benecke et al. [1, 2] the motor neurons will undergo degeneration owing to lack of trophic inputs, which they normally receive from descending motor pathways. The distal arm and hand muscles which are especially under cortical control showed most striking changes in their studies as it did in our case. We have to assume that descending fibres have not completely degenerated but have been functionally impaired by neuropractic mechanisms at suprasegmental level by the tumor. After operation the structurally undamaged α-motoneurons regained their activity quickly and PSW and FP disappeared after recovery of muscular strength and retrogression of atrophy.

Gutjahr, et al. [4] put more emphasis on the functional significance of the γ_1-motoneurons interrupting their innervation of the muscle spindle cells due to a deficiency of afferent impulses of nigrospinal and pontoretinospinal tracts. By this means sensory spindle impulses reaching the α-motoneurons are reduced, which could produce functional denervation, development of atrophies and pathological spontaneous activity. As soon as the lesion is being removed – by recovery from stroke or through operation as shown before – the α-motoneurons regains its activity very quickly due to its structural integrity with the re-activation of the gamma-system.

Conclusion

The prompt recovery of muscle cell activity needs the preservation of structural integrity of nerve fibres as re-innervation cannot be expected within this short period of time. We assume that a partial transsynaptic degeneration must have taken place which could be repaired relatively quickly.

References

[1] Benecke, R., A. Berthold, B. Conrad, et al.: Pathologische Spontanaktivität im EMG bei zentralmotorischen Störungen. In: A. Struppler (ed.): Elektrophysiologische Diagnostik in der Neurologie. Arbeitstagung der Deutschen Gesellschaft für Neurologie München 1981. Georg Thieme, Stuttgart – New York 1982.

[2] Benecke, R., A. Berthold, B. Conrad: Denervation activity in the EMG of patients with upper motor neuron lesions: time course, local distribution and pathogenetic aspects. J. Neurol. **230** (1983) 143–151.

[3] Goldkamp, O.: Electromyography and nerve conduction studies in 116 patients with hemiplegia. Arch. Phys. Med. Rehabil. **48** (1967) 59–63.

[4] Gutjahr, F., H. Müller-Wahl, H. Schliack, et al.: Elektromyographische Zeichen der peripher neurogenen Schädigung bei Läsionen des ersten motorischen Neurons. In: P. Vogel, D. Seitz (eds.): Hämoblastosen, zentrale Motorik, iatrogene Schäden, Myositiden, Springer, Berlin–Heidelberg 1983.

[5] Johnson, E., S. Henny, J. Kelly: Sequence of electromyographic abnormalities in stroke syndrome. Arch. Phys. Med. Rehabil. **56** (1975) 468–473.

[6] Liveson, J. A., J. Ransohoff, J. Goodgold: Electromyographic studies in a case of foramen magnum meningioma. J. Neurol. Neurosurg. Psychiatry **36** (1973) 561–564.

[7] Yasuoka, S., H. Okazaki, J. Daube, et al.: Foramen magnum tumors. J. Neurosurg. **49** (1978) 828–838.

NMR and the surgery of tumours at the craniocervical junction

A. Ahyai, A. Matsumura, K. Rittmeyer

Introduction

The diagnosis of tumours in the posterior fossa and at the craniocervical junction has always been problematic. Even CT does not always provide satisfactory results, particularly with lesions near the base of the skull. In this problematic region of the brain a clear visualization of the exact extent and relations of a space-occupying lesion is indispensable in assessing whether it is operable. Even though a tumour with its perifocal oedema can be detected by CT, NMR opens new perspectives ot the neurosurgeon; NMR has the primary advantage that it allows the borders of a lesion to be visualized clearly at various levels of section, permitting the lesion's exact topography to be defined in relation to the vital centres of the brainstem [2, 3, 4, 7, 8, 10, 12]. Since 1984 NMR examination was performed in addition to conventional diagnostic procedures in all cases of suspected space-occupying lesion, with the primary aim of obtaining additional information about the advisability of an operation in this critical region.

These cases are presented in 3 groups. *Group I* comprises patients for whom NMR results contra-indicated operation. *Group II* consists of patients who would probably not have been operated on prior to the use of NMR. *Group III* includes patients who would probably have been operated on prior to the use of NMR (e.g. arachnoid cysts, Dandy-Walker malformations, etc); the excellent multi-dimensional imaging by NMR rendered the advisability of operation questionable, so that improved diagnostics may have spared the patients unnecessary operations.

Case reports

Group I. Patients show neurological symptoms due to lesions of the pons, the medulla oblongata or the cerebellum. Computed tomographs (CT scans) show confirmatory signs of a space-occupying lesion, but in no case could the extent of the tumour be determined with sufficient accuracy. The operability of these tumours cannot be assessed unambiguously on the basis of clinical and CT findings. The impressive clarity with which NMR reveals the coordinates of such tumours permits a good assessment of operability. In this group, tumours were considered inoperable due to their infiltrative form of growth, shown in NMR by the absence of clearly defined margins (fig. 1).

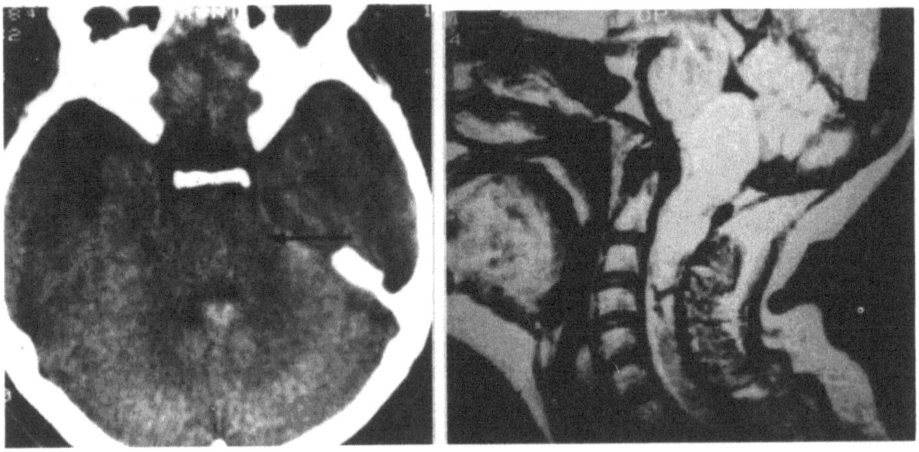

a b

Fig. 1 CT scan shows unspecific signs of a space-occupying lesion in the region of the brainstem with displacement of the ventrobasal cisterns and, possibly, blood in the IVth ventricle (a); in the corresponding NMR, the extent and topographic anatomical relationship of the tumour are clearly seen (b).

Group II. This group comprises cases in which successful operations could be performed: one pilocytic astrocytoma in the region of the pons, two cases of clivus chordoma, and one case of malignant subependymoma of the fourth ventricle.

Case 1: A 4-year old child, whose CT scan showed a circumscribed calcification, presented with signs of a space-occupying lesion ventral to the fourth ventricle (fig. 2 a). Only by means of NMR could the tumour be localized exactly. NMR findings indicated this tumour to be operable: the tumour borders were sharply defined, and the tumour extent was clearly visualized (fig. 2 b). Surgical exploration (performed elsewhere) revealed a pilocytic astrocytoma. Postoperative NMR demonstrated regression of the tumour (fig. 3). Neurological symptoms present at operation (abducens and facial palsy) did not regress, but additional damage did not occur.

Case 2: Both CT and NMR findings show this lesion to be nearly identical with that of case 1 (fig. 4). In view of the good results in case 1, an operative procedure seems likely to succeed here also.

a b

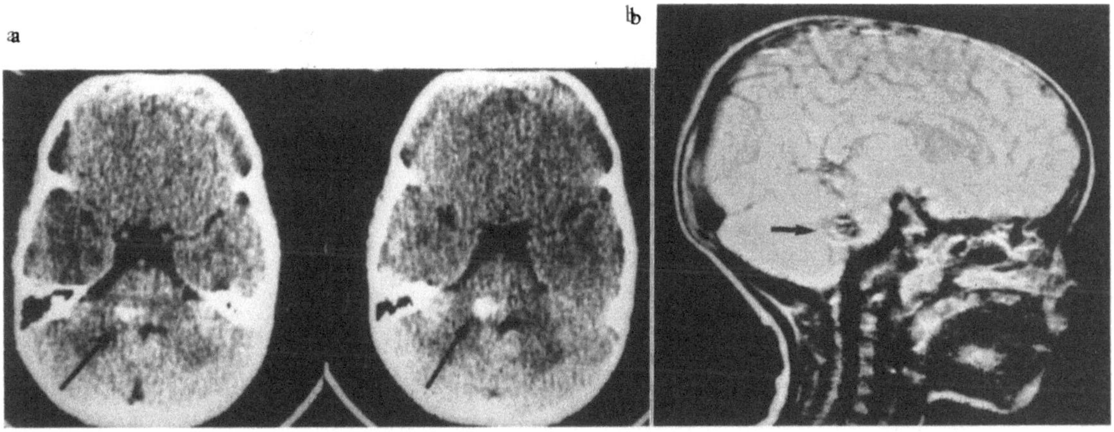

Fig. 2 CT scan shows a circumscribed calcification, with signs of a space-filling lesion, ventral to the IVth ventricle (a); in NMR the extent and sharp borders of the lesion are clearly visualised (b).

a b

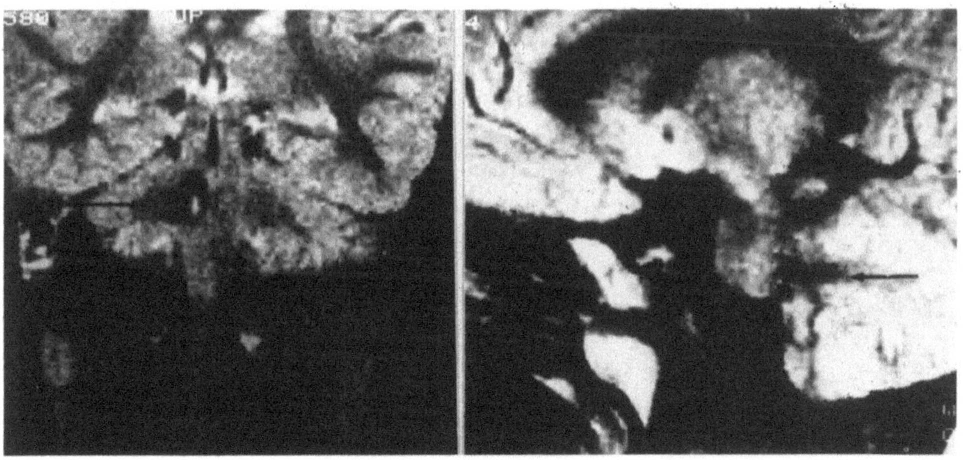

Fig. 3 Postoperative NMR examination proves the regression of the tumour.

Case 3: This patient was admitted because of a hypoglossal palsy, left brachial paresis and cerebellar ataxia of 2 years, standing. CT scan showed a space-occupying lesion at the craniocervical junction (fig. 5 a), and NMR revealed a clearly-delimited tumour extending from the floor of the IVth ventricle to the upper cervical cord (fig. 5 b). This tumour, a malignant subependymoma, could be removed entirely by microsurgery. Unfortunately, the patient died four weeks postoperatively following pulmonary embolism and pneumonia.

a b

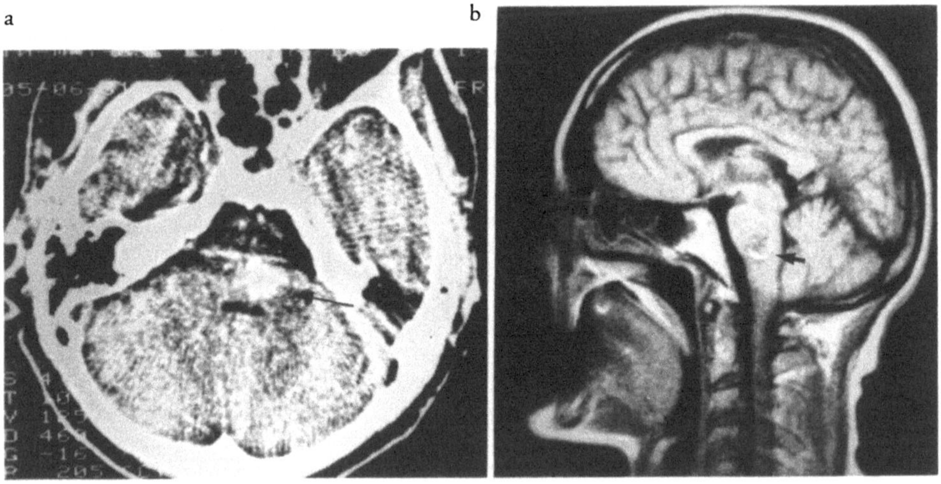

Fig. 4 The tumour localization in CT (a) and the pathological signal behaviour in NMR (b) suggest a tumour of similar type to the previous case.

a

b

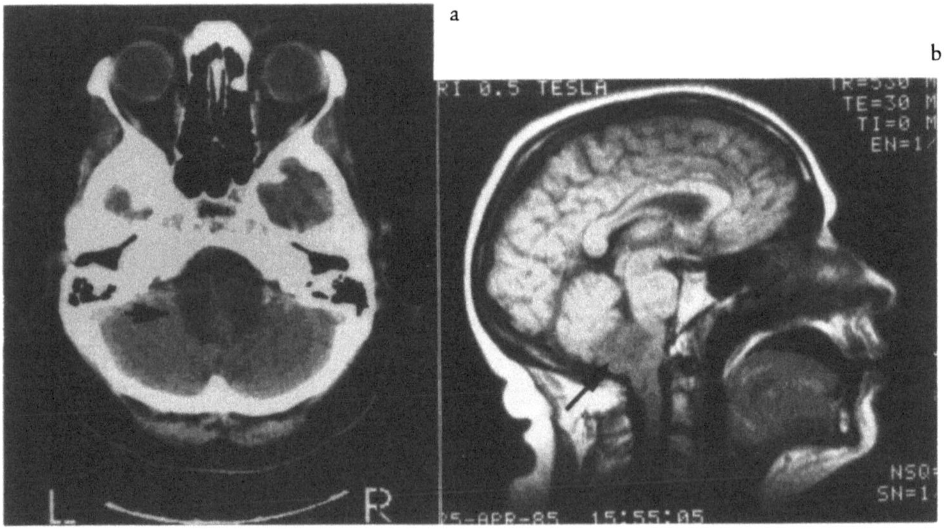

Fig. 5 Signs of space-occupying lesion in the brainstem (a); the tumour and its relationships to the medulla oblongata and cerebellum are clearly seen. It extends from the floor of the IVth ventricle into the upper cervical cord (b).

Cases 4, 5: These comprised two cases of clivus chordoma, both with the radiological symptoms of extensive bone destruction in the region of the middle skull base (fig. 6). The excellent spatial visualization of these lesions provided by NMR suggested operability of the tumour in both patients.

Group III. In this group of patients NMR was especially helpful, due to its excellent visualization of the topographic anatomical relationships in the posterior fossa and at the cranio-cervical junction.

Case 1: CT findings suggested the presence of either a Dandy-Walker malformation or of an arachnoid cyst. However, NMR revealed advanced cerebellar atrophy (fig. 7).

a b

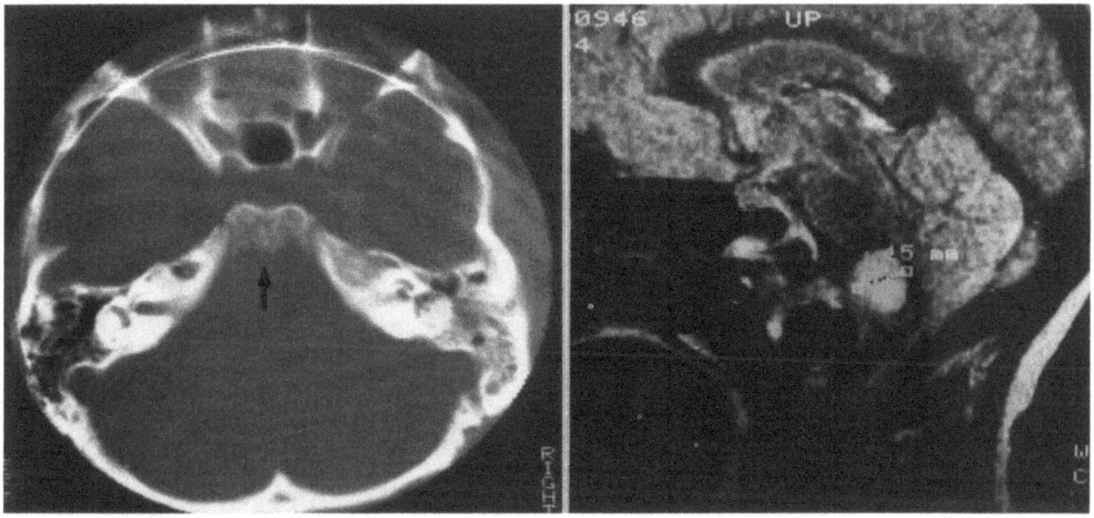

Fig. 6 CT shows extensive bone destruction in the clivus (a); spatial visualisation of a clivus chordoma in NMR (b).

a b

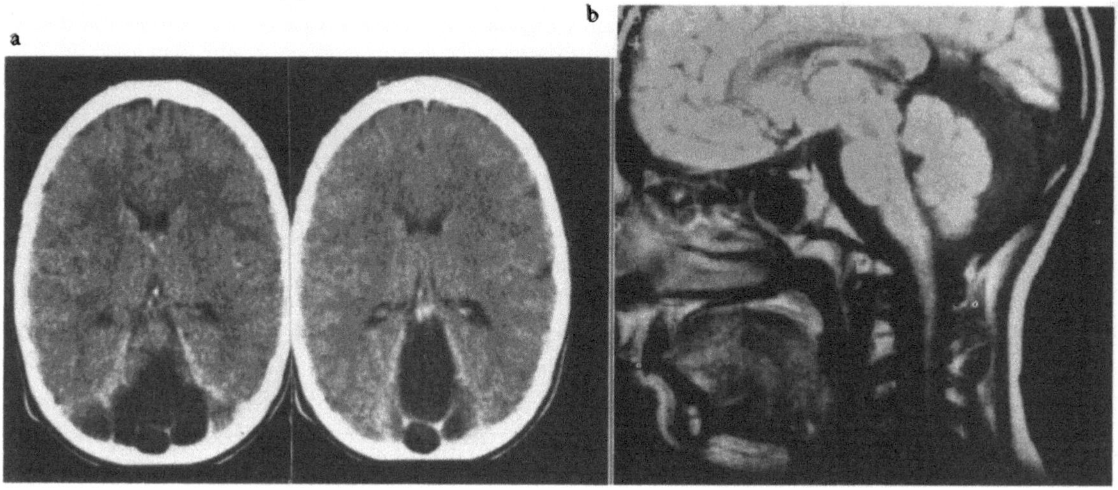

Fig. 7 CT shows multiple arachnoid cysts in the posterior fossa and above the tentorium cerebelli. The images suggest the effect of a possible pressure of a Dandy-Walker malformation (a); NMR reveals an advanced cerebellar atrophy (b).

Case 2: The clinical symptoms of this patient (tetraparesis) suggested a tumour at the cranio-cervical junction or in the upper cervical cord; CT also produced findings suggestive of a tumour (fig. 8a). However, NMR did not confirm this, but produced findings suggesting that the cerebellar tonsils were located relatively deeply (so that the presence of an Arnold-Chiari malformation had to be suspected) (fig. 8b). Because of the discrepancy between the CT and NMR findings a cervical myelography was performed, which showed normal radiological anatomical relationships at the cranio-cervical junction. In the meantime, the typical clinical neurological progression permitted the diagnosis of amyotrophic lateral sclerosis.

a b

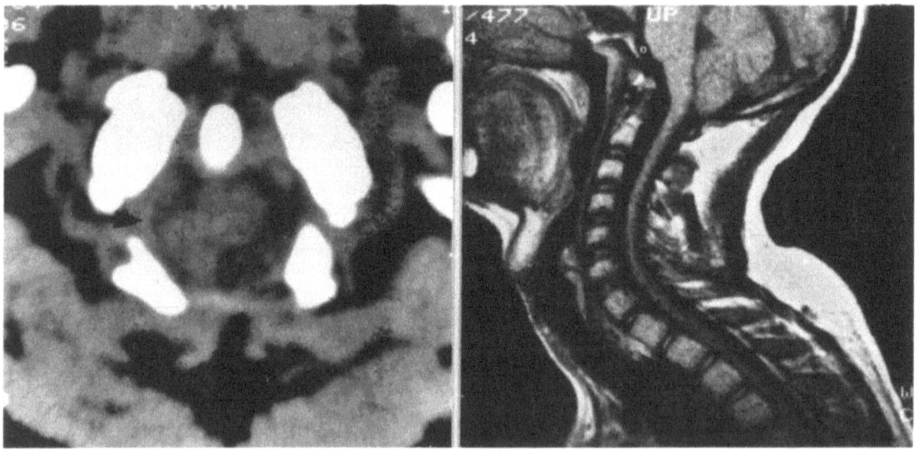

Fig. 8 CT shows signs of space-occupying lesion in the upper cervical cord (a); no signs of tumour in NMR, but the cerebellar tonsils seem to be located more posteriorly than usual (b).

Discussion

With the help of NMR 3-dimensional representation of a tumour has become possible, which was not the case with previously available methods. Although CT revolutionized neuroradiological diagnostics for the cerebral and cerebellar hemispheres, the region of the brainstem, the base of the skull and the craniocervical junction remained a grey area. NMR promises to fill this gap. This diagnostic advance opens new perspectives to the neurosurgeon in assessing the following criteria:

1. The topographic anatomical relationships of a tumour to its neighbouring structures (namely, the pons, medulla oblongata and upper cervical spinal cord) can now be visualized clearly [2, 3, 4, 7, 8, 10, 12].

2. In contrast to CT, NMR is capable of determining whether a neoplasm is sharply bounded or whether it is infiltrating [1, 3, 4, 6, 11].
3. With the exception of meningiomas, NMR offers a clearly improved capacity to define a tumour pre-operatively [3].
4. The resolution of the NMR is now so excellent that fine structures such as cranial nerves and the larger-calibre arteries and veins can be sharply imaged.

It is to be expected that further improvement of the geometric resolution and further development of quantitative tissue analysis will permit yet subtler assessments of the advisability of an operation in any given case than is possible with the present state of the technology. Moreover, it is also to be expected that a pre-operative determination of tumour type will become possible which approaches close to the pathological anatomical diagnosis.

Whether an operation is advisable or not can be decided today significantly better with NMR than with CT. Visualization of tumours by NMR results in a more informed surgical decision, because tumour size and invasiveness can be taken into consideration. We distinguished three groups of patients where NMR findings materially affected the decision to operate. With the cases presented here we have compared the NMR and CT visualization of brain tumours, and discussed how these findings affect the decision to operate.

Summary

Patients suspected of having space-occupying lesions in the brainstem, posterior fossa or foramen magnum were examined by NMR in addition to conventional diagnostic procedures. With the help of NMR the neurosurgeon can now better assess whether or not a tumour in this region is operable.

One group of patients was defined in which the NMR data showed the tumours to be inoperable and consequently, surgery was not attempted. In contrast to CT, NMR permitted exact localisation of tumours in another group of patients. On the basis of the sharply defined tumour borders and the clear visualisation of the extent of the lesions it was possible to consider surgical treatment advisable in these cases. In the final group NMR data, in opposition to CT, made the advisability of operation doubtful; thanks to improved diagnostics the patients could be spared an operation from which they would not have benefited. The cases of tumours diagnosed, and in part operated on, in the region of the pons, medulla oblongata, upper cervical spinal cord and clivus, during 1984 and 1985, are considered here in view of the new diagnostic criteria when using NMR.

References

[1] Bosley, T. M., D. A. Cohen, N. J. Schatz, et al.: Comparison of metrizamide computed tomography and magnetic resonance imaging in the evaluation of lesions at the cervicomedullary junction. Neurology **35** (1985) 485 – 492.

[2] Carr, W. A., R. J. Baumann, R. S. Baker: Nuclear magnetic resonance imaging in the neuro-ophthalmology. Demonstration of a pontine glioma. Surv. Ophthalmol. **29** (1984) 79 – 83.

[3] Di Chiro, G., J. L. Doppman, A. J. Dwyer, et al.: MR imaging of tumors and arteriovenous malformations of the brainstem and spinal cord (Meeting abstract). Radiology **153** (1984) 85.

[4] Han, J. S., C. T. Bonstelle, B. Kaufman, et al.: Magnetic resonance imaging in the evaluation of brainstem. Radiology **150** (1984) 705 – 712.

[5] Hawkes, R. C., G. N. Holland, W. S. Moore, et al.: Craniovertebral junction pathology: Assessment by NMR. A. J. N. R. **4** (1983) 232 – 233.

[6] Holland, B. A., M. Brant-Zawadzki, D. Norman, et al.: Magnetic resonance imaging of the primary intracranial tumors: A review. Int. J. Radiat. Oncol. Biol. Phys. **11** (1985) 315 – 321.

[7] Hueftle, M. G., J. S. Han, B. Kaufman, et al.: MR imaging of brainstem gliomas. J. Comput. Assist. Tomogr. **9** (1985) 263 – 267.

[8] Kaufman, B. A., B. Kaufman, H. L. Rekate: Cervicomedullary junction tumor diagnosed by Nuclear Magnetic Resonance scanning: Case report. Neurosurg. **15** (1984) 878 – 880.

[9] Lee, B. C., J. B. Kneeland, M. D. Deck, et al.: Posterior fossa lesions: Magnetic resonance imaging. Radiology **153** (1984) 137 – 143.

[10] Lee, B. C., J. B. Kneeland, R. W. Walder, et al.: MR imaging of brainstem tumors. A. J. N. R. **6** (1985) 159 – 163.

[11] McGinnis, B. D., T. J. Brady, P. F. New, et al.: Nuclear Magnetic Resonance (NMR) imaging of tumors in the posterior fossa. J. Comput. Assist. Tomogr. 7 (1983) 575 – 584.

[12] Zimmerman, R. A., L. T. Bilaniuk, R. Packer, et al.: Resistive NMR of brainstem gliomas. Neuroradiology **27** (1985) 21 – 25.

Tumors of the cranio-cervical region, diagnostic problems, micro- and laser-surgery

G. Nowak, A. Leppien, H.-D. Herrmann, H. Arnold

Introduction

The first systematic investigations on tumors of the cranio-cervical region were carried out by Elsberg in 1925 and again by Elsberg and Strauss in 1929 [4, 5]. Of a total of 185 extramedullary tumors in the area of the spinal cord, 6 (3.2%) were located at the cranio-cervical region. In 1954, Love and Dodge reported on intra- and extramedullary tumors of the foramen magnum area, and held 40% for operable.

Although there has been marked improvement [2, 3, 6, 8 – 10, 12] in the available diagnostic possibilities (such as myelography, CT – and more recently – NMR) in the meantime there has been a report by Hirano, published in June of 1983 [7], that the average interval between onset of clinical symptoms and surgical intervention still is 37.3 months, which is a little over 3 years.

Material

Between 1968 and August of 1985, 11 patients (tab. 1) with tumors of the cranio-cervical region were operated in the Neurosurgical Department of the University Hospital Eppendorf in Hamburg. Seven of these were extramedullary and four intramedullary. Histology of the extramedullary tumours showed a meningioma in 6 cases and a neurinoma in 1. The intramedullary lesions were one ependymoma, one astrocytoma, one melanoma and one angioblastoma.

Regarding the time between onset of symptoms and surgery the longest interval was 3 years and the shortest 6 months – with the average interval being about 12 months.

Initial clinical symptoms (tab. 2) in half of the patients were pain in the back of the head and neck, which seemed to be uncharacteristic, although it was accompanied by abnormal sensations, and in all patients the correct diagnosis was only made after the onset of motor-weakness or paralysis. The wrong diagnosis most frequently made was that of multiple sclerosis. Two patients were already

Table 1 Tumours of the cranio-cervical region – 1982–1985 (n = 11)

	Age/Sex	Initial symptom	Anamnesis months	Diagnosis
1	47/female	stiffness of the neck	13	meningioma
2	2/female	pain in the neck	6	ependymoma (intramedullary)
3	58/male	dysaesthesia	11	neurinoma
4	28/female	dysaesthesia in the right shoulder	6	meningioma
5	17/male	pain in the neck	12	meningioma
6	63/male	weakness left hand	31	meningioma
7	39/female	pain in the left shoulder	25	meningioma
8	71/female	weakness right leg	36	meningioma
9	50/female	pain in the neck, left side hemidysaesthesia	12	melanoma (intramedullary)
10	47/male	nausea	17	astrocytoma (intramedullary)
11	55/male	left side hemidysaesthesia	6	angioblastoma

Table 2 Tumours of the cranio-cervical region – 1982–1985 (n = 11)
– cranial nerve involvement (n = 6)

	Cranial nerve palsy	Other neurol. findings	Diagnosis
1	$9^{th}-12^{th}$	tetraparesis	ependymoma (intramedullary)
2	11th	tetraplegia	meningioma
3	11th	hemiplegia (right) hemiparesis (left)	meningioma
4	5th	tetraparesis hemidysaesthesia (left)	melanoma (intramedullary)
5	$9^{th}-12^{th}$	astereognosis right hand ataxia right leg	astrocytoma (intramedullary)
6	$9^{th}-12^{th}$	hemidysaesthesia (left) astereognosis left hand	angioblastoma

suffering from complete tetraparesis at the time of correct diagnosis. One female patient even had to be intubated and put on a respirator in the morning of surgery, because she was not able to breath sufficiently on her own. Special note should be made of the fact that a total of six patients presented with cranial nerve problems: in three cases, the accessory nerve was involved, in two there was unilateral involvement of nerves IX–XII, and in one case unilateral dysfunction of the trigeminal nerve.

The obvious problems for early diagnosis are – next to the uncharacteristic primary symptoms – due to the anatomical situation of the area under discussion:

First the general spaciousness of the subarachnoid space in the upper cervical canal and the especially spacious cisterna magna; secondly the fact that more than half of the extramedullary tumours are ventrally located, which facilitated – at least in part – vascular compression and localized ischaemia of the medulla, prior to the filling up of the spinal canal with cord-compression and block of CSF-flow etc. [1, 11, 13–15].

Five patients had an NMR examination prior to surgery and in two patients this modality established to correct diagnosis. In nine patients, the diagnosis was made by myelography and CT or CT-myelography respectively.

Therapy (treatment)

All patients – in a prone position – were operated on with a dorso-medial approach – which means laminectomy of the posterior arch of the atlas and, if necessary, also of the laminae of the second and third vertebrae as well as a small osteoclastic craniotomy of the posterior fossa. In two cases the tumour was resected with help of CO_2-Variopulse-laser technique. Two of the tumours treated with laser technique were intramedullary ones, one a meningioma, which had grown along the upper cervical root into the foramina. Laser manipulation was carried out after hook-up to the surgical microscope via a special adaptor.

Results

In nine patients, total tumour removal was achieved, mainly due to the help of laser. In two patients with an intramedullary astrocytoma and intramedullary ependymoma, only parts of the tumour could be removed (tab. 3).

Surgical mortality was nil. Nine patients were discharged with their symptoms almost completely gone or at least markedly improved; some were transferred to rehabilitation centres. One patient – the one with intramedullary ependymoma – had postoperative radiation therapy. In this patient the symptoms remained unchanged from those prior to surgery. Another patient had improvement of his swallowing problems, but the weakness of his arm became worse. This patient also had a severe gastric hemorrhage on the 6th post-surgical day, and we had to submit him to gastroscopy for definitive treatment. Finally we want to refer to three of our patients.

Case 1: A 17 year-old male patient with a 12 months history of pain in the back of his head and neck. A discrete gait disturbance finally appeared; routine radiographs of the cervical spine show marked widening of the upper portion of the spinal canal. Myelography showed a large mass at the cervico-occipital junction. CT supports this finding by showing a hyperdense tumour in the

Table 3 Tumours of the cranio-cervical region – 1982–1985 (n = 11) – Results

	Histol. diagnosis	Removal	Laser	Clinical result	Complication	Death
1	meningioma I–II	total	–	improved	–	–
2	intramedullary ependymoma II	subtotal (irradiation)	yes	unchanged	aseptic meningitis	–
3	neurinoma	total	–	no complaints	–	–
4	meningioma III	total	yes	improved	–	–
5	meningioma II–III	total	–	improved	aseptic meningitis	–
6	meningioma II–III	total	–	no complaints	–	–
7	meningioma I	total	–	improved	aseptic meningitis	–
8	meningioma	total	–	improved	–	–
9	intramedullary melanoma	total	yes	improved	–	–
10	intramedullary astrocytoma	subtotal	–	improved	gastric bleeding	–
11	angioblastoma	total	–	improved	–	–

foramen magnum and below. In angiography this tumour was hypervascular with a direct supply from the left vertebral artery. The tumour was totally resected by conventional microsurgery. Post-operatively, the patient had transitory worsening of his gait disturbance, and also had an aseptic meningitis. When these symptoms had subsided, he could be discharged.

Case 2: A 50 year-old woman with a 1 year history of complaints of hemihypaesthesia on her left side including the face. Additionally tetraspasticity on the left more than on the right, had developed during the last few months before admission. Routine X-radiography as well as myelography and CT of the cranio-cervical region failed to establish a definite diagnosis of a mass lesion. It required NMR-examination to show the suspected lesion within the medulla. Surgery was done with help of CO_2-laser. After initial incision of the medulla and a biopsy for histological examination, the tumour was removed in layers (which means it was "boiled off" layerwise by laser technique) until normal medullary structures appeared in the area of surgery. Surprisingly, histology showed a malignant melanoma. The search for the potential primary tumour in the skin, the eyes and the intestinal system was without result, and we assume that we were dealing with a primary intramedullary melanoma. The patient was completely mobilized 2 1/2 weeks after surgery; and although her gait was still somewhat instable, she was able to be discharged home without any further measures.

Case 3: A 55 year-old male patient presented with a history of many weeks of complaints about imbalance and altered sensibility on his left side, poor control of his left hand, dysarthria and swallowing problems. CT showed a lesion within the medulla on the right side, without significant mass effect; the fourth ventricle was not encroached upon. NMR proves this finding, however, with much better images and better delineation of topography in regard to neighbourhood structures. Angiography just demonstrated an elongation of the basilar artery without evidence of tumour vessels. The tumour was completely removed by surgery. Histologically, it was diagnosed as an angioblastoma. Postoperatively, there was an initial worsening of the lower cervical nerve symptoms. However, there was improvement of the other symptoms involving the left side of his body and his left hand. There was an incidental complication which we observed for the first time: namely a puncture of the left radial artery for intraoperative blood pressure control resulted in an aneurysm, which required surgical repair.

Summary

Tumours of the cervical-occipital region continue to present a diagnostic problem, especially in view of the remarkably long interval between initial – frequently even serious symptoms until the final diagnosis. Even cervical myelography, CT and angiography frequently remain inconclusive. NMR-imaging, however, proves more and more its value as the main diagnostic tool of choice for this area. In regard to surgery, laser technique certainly provides marked improvement of the surgical possibilities, especially with intramedullary lesions, but also for extramedullary tumours, which grow sheeth-like; they can even be completely removed with optimal avoidance of neighbourhood structures.

References

[1] Abbott, K. H.: Foramen magnum and high cervical cord lesions stimulating degenerative disease of nervous system. Ohio Med. J. **46** (1950) 645–651.

[2] Bortoluzzi, M.: Neoplasms of spinal origin involving the foramen magnum. Neurodiagnostic considerations on 36 cases. J. Neurosurg. Sci. **24** (1980) 71–76.

[3] Dodge, H. W. jr, J. G. Love, C. M. Gottlieb: Benign tumors at the foramen magnum. Surgical considerations. J. Neurosurg. **13** (1956) 603–617.

[4] Elsberg, C. A.: Tumors of the spinal cord and the symptoms of irritation and compression of the spinal cord and nerve roots. Pathology, symptomatology, diagnosis and treatment. Paul B. Haeber, New York 1925.

[5] Elsberg, C. A., J. Strauss: Tumors of the spinal cord which project into the posterior cranial fossa. Arch. Neurol. Psychiatry **21** (1929) 261–273.

[6] Guidetti, B., A. Spallone: Benign extramedullary tumors of the foramen magnum. Surg. Neurol. **13** (1980) 9–17.

[7] Hirano, H., H. Suzuki, et al.: Foramen magnum and upper cervical cord tumors. Clin. Orthop. **176** (1983) 171–177.

[8] Krayenbühl, H.: Special clinical features of tumors of the foramen magnum. Schweiz. Arch. Neurol. Neurochir. Psychiatr. **112** (1973) 205–218.

[9] Meyer, F. B., M. J. Ebersold, D. F. Reese: Benign tumors of the foramen magnum. J. Neurosurg. **61** (1984) 136–142.
[10] Modic, M. T. et al.: Magnetic resonance imaging of the cervical spine. AJR **141** (1983) 1129–1136.
[11] Mullans, S., R. Naunton, J. Hekmat-Ponah, et al.: The use of an anterior approach to ventrally placed tumors in the foramen magnum and vertebral column. J. Neurosurg. **24** (1966) 536–543.
[12] Sartor, K.: Computertomographie bei spinalen Tumoren. Fortschr. Röntgenstr. **132** (1980) 391–398.
[13] Scott, M.: The surgical management of meningiomas of the cerebellar fossa. Surg. Gynecol. Obstet. **135** (1972) 545–550.
[14] Stein, B. M., N. E. Leeds, J. M. Taveras, et al.: Meningiomas of the foramen magnum. J. Neurosurg. **20** (1963) 740–751.
[15] Yasuoka, S., H. Okazaki, J. R. Daube, et al.: Foramen magnum tumors. Analysis of 57 cases of benign extramedullary tumors. J. Neurosurg. **49** (1978) 828–838.

The dorsolateral approach in ventrolateral craniospinal lesions

J. M. Gilsbach, H. R. Eggert, W. Seeger

Introduction

A number of surgical approaches to the craniospinal region are available. The transoral and parapharyngeal paths are well suited for ventral and ventrolateral extradural processes e. g. malformations, tumours, and infections of the vertebrae and the occiput. For intradural pathology, the transoral route is restricted by the deep and narrow operative field and the danger of CSF fistula and infection. For these reasons ventral and ventrolateral intradural lesions are mostly approached via a dorsal standard midline suboccipital trephination and laminectomy of C 1 (and C 2). But in lesions located ventrally to the brainstem and medulla, this approach involves undue manipulation and retraction of these structures. In such cases we prefer a lateral paracondylar approach, which was originally described for operations on aneurysms of the vertebrobasilar junction [14]. It is a combination of a lateral suboccipital approach for acoustic neurinomas [20] and a lateral approach for the vertebral artery in the region of the atlas. It provides enough room without displacement of the brain stem for the preparation in front of the ponto-medullary region.

Approach

All of our patients, with the exception of one, were operated on in a sitting position with a precordial Doppler air bubble detector and positive endexspiratory pressure ventilation. One patient with a severe tetraplegia did not tolerate the upright position and had to be operated on in a prone position. The head was bent, turned, and fixed in a Mayfield clamp. The longitudinal paramedian incision, which was 2 to 3 cm medially from the tip of the mastoid, extended from the level of the transverse sinus to the middle third of the neck (fig. 1). The penetration through the neck musculature (M. splenius capitis, M. longissimus capitis) towards the lateral parts of the arch of C 1 was done bluntly. Due to the distorted position of the craniocervical junction, orientation had to be regained by palpating the lateral parts of the atlas. After having identified the arch of C 1 and the vertebral artery, the neighboring suboccipital region and the medial aspects of the atlantooccipital joint could be dissected free. Then the lateral parts of the arch of C 1, the laterobasal occiput, and the medial parts of the occipital and atlantal condyles were resected (fig. 2). The osteoclastic approach was completed with a more or less extended extradural bone resection towards the jugular tuberculum above the canal of the 12th cranial nerve. In cases of intradural tumours, the dura was opened longitudinally in a cranial direction starting from the entry point of the vertebral artery (fig. 3).

Fig. 1

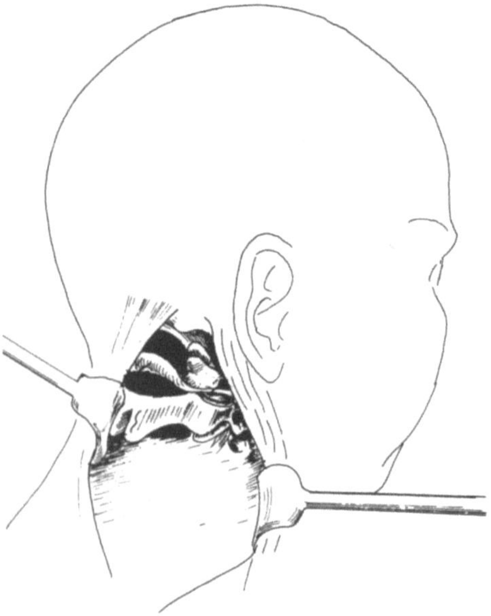

Fig. 2

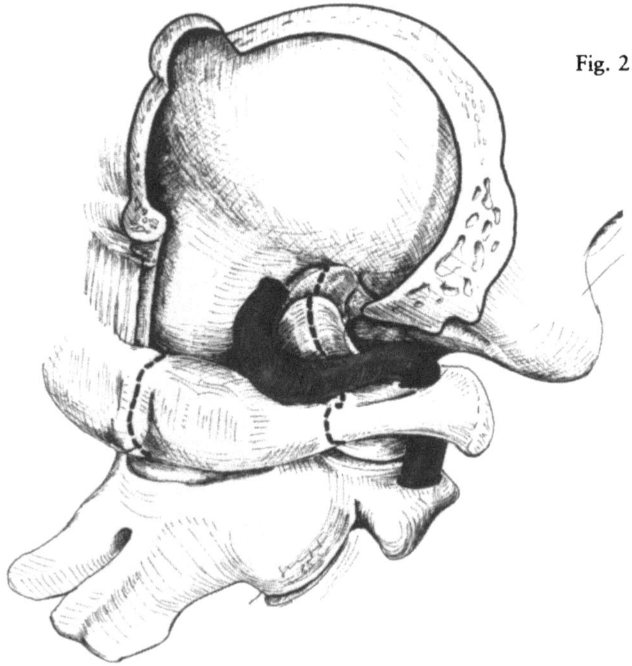

Fig. 1 Position of the head and neck of the sitting patient. Approach to the cranio-vertebral junction with a longitudinal paramedian skin incision and preparation of the musculature centered on the lateral parts of the atlas.

Fig. 2 Small osteoclastic laterobasal trephination of the occiput, including the medial parts of the atlanto-occipital joint and parts of the jugular tuberculum. In cases of spinal extension of the lesion or for a view from below an additional hemilaminectomy of C 1 is necessary.

Patients and results

Eight patients were operated on for tumours. Three had neoplasms originating from the occiput and the region of the atlanto-occipital joint. In the case of an aneurysmal bone cyst, a stabilizing procedure with a metal plate between the

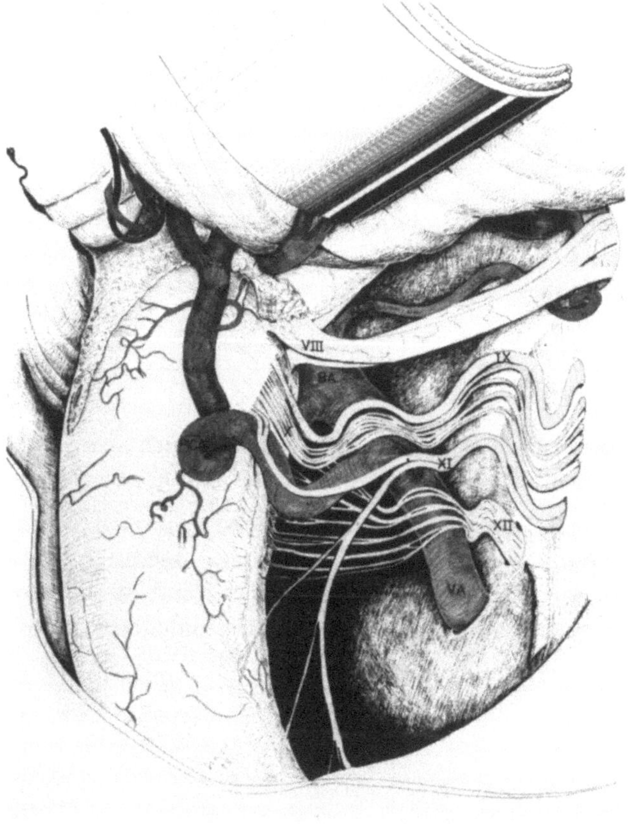

Fig. 3 Intradural view of the lateral aspects of the the pontomedullary region from a right sided paracondylar approach. Note that the vertebral junction, the ipsilateral vertebral artery and the caudal cranial nerves can be viewed totally.

occiput and the lateral mass of the atlas was performed after removal of the destroyed condyles. The other had only (partial) tumour removal without internal stabilization. The pre-operative deficits of the caudal cranial nerves remained constant. New deficits did not occur (tab. 1).

With regard to accessibility, all 5 benign intradural tumours could be removed totally under visual control without compression of the brain stem. In all cases the dentate ligament was incised and, in some cases, the C1 and C2 root as well. In the cases with a marked dorsal and lateral displacement of the medulla, it did not become visible until the end of the operation. In one case, the post. inf. cerebellar artery (PICA) was coagulated inadvertently within a large meningioma which resulted in a lateral medullar oblongata syndrome. Two of

Table 1 Paracondylar approach to craniospinal tumours

Patient	Pathology	Location	Result
F. E. 67 m	meningioma	foramen magnum	fair
W. A. 51 f	meningioma	foramen magnum	fair
S. H. 67 f	meningioma	foramen magnum	good
S. L. 62 f	meningioma	foramen magnum	good
L. G. 28 m	meningioma	foramen magnum	good
M. E. 69 m	carcinoma	condylus occ/C 1	unchanged
W. S. 29 f	chondrosa.	occiput, C 1, C 2	unchanged
K. E. 21 f	bone cyst	condylus occ/C 1	good
M. V. 14 f	aneurysmal bone cyst	condylus occ/C 1	good

the patients presented additional postoperative deficits which were due to the dissection of the tumour from the caudal cranial nerves and not to the approach.

Three aneurysms could be dissected via the paracondylar approach, but only one vertebral junction aneurysm could be clipped without problems. In the case of a large PICA aneurysm, the artery was occluded at the end of the procedure. And in one case of a vertebral junction aneurysm we could only wrap up the aneurysm, as we found no clippable neck.

Discussion

Lateral approaches to the craniocervical region are not new [6, 16, 17, 19]. Although they offered a good view on the ventrolateral aspect of the medulla, these approaches were not widely adapted for intradural processes [7, 11, 15]. Median approaches with enlargement of the foramen magnum and laminectomy of C 1 are usually recommended [4, 5, 9, 11, 21].

Ventrolateral extrapharyngeal approaches [18] and transoral ones [1, 3, 12, 13] were recommended in purely medial lesions in front of the medulla.

Of these approaches the latero-dorsal way seemed to us to be the best suited, because the lesions in our patients were lateralized according to the CT findings. In all cases, the entire area was visible without unnecessary brain retraction. With this approach, we did not have the problems of restricted working space and CSF fistulas, which are inherent with the transoral approach. We were also not restricted by the musculature which hinder a lateral view into the premedullary region when a dorsomedian approach is used.

Orientation during the penetration of the musculature is easily lost and must be reestablished by repeated palpation of the arch of C 1. It is perhaps easier if the head of the patient is not turned, but this position makes it less comfortable for the surgeon to work. Once orientation has been established, the procedure is no longer difficult and can be carried out under microsurgical conditions.

Our approach is relatively dorsal from the course of the caudal cranial nerves and presents no danger to the accessory nerve, which can be cut accidentally if the incision is extended to the sternocleidomastoid muscle. Problems originating from the irritated atlanto-occipital joint could be observed in only one patient who had complained of neck pain.

In cases (not included in this paper) where the lesion lies more laterally in the region of the condyles or in the jugular foramen, we use the same position, but a more lateral curved incision which follows the sternocleidomastoid muscle and which provided a lateral view of the cranio-cervical junction [8, 10].

References

[1] Crockard, H. A., R. Bradford: Transoral transclival removal of a schwannoma anterior to the craniocervical junction. J. Neurosurg. **62** (1985) 293 – 295.

[2] Gilsbach, J., H. R. Eggert: Transoral operations for craniospinal malformations. Neurosurg. Rev. **6** (1983) 199 – 209.

[3] Giroux, J.-C., C. North: Anterior approach for removal of a cervical intradural tumor: Case report and technical note. Neurosurgery **2** (1978) 128 – 130.

[4] Guidetti, B.: Removal of extramedullary benign spinal cord tumours. In: H. Krayenbühl (ed.): Advances and Technical Standards in Neurosurgery, pp. 173 – 197. Springer, Wien – New York 1974.

[5] Guidetti, B., A. Spallone: Benign extramedullary tumors of the foramen magnum. Surg. Neurol. **13** (1980) 9 – 17.

[6] Henry, A. K.: Extensile exposure. 2nd ed., pp. 58 – 66. Churchill Livingstone, Edingburgh 1973.

[7] Koos, W. T., R. F. Spetzler, G. Pendl, et al.: Color Atlas of Microneurosurgery. Thieme, Stuttgart 1985.

[8] Kumar, A., U. Fisch: The infratemporal fossa approach for lesions of the skull base. In: H. Krayenbühl et al. (eds.): Advances and Technical Standards in Neurosurgery. Vol. 10, pp. 187 – 220. Springer, Wien – New York 1983.

[9] Mac Carty, C. S., D. G. Piepgras, M. J. Ebersold: Meningeal tumors of the brain. In: J. R. Youmans (ed.): Neurological Surgery. Vol. 5, pp. 2936 – 2966. Saunders, Philadelphia – London- – Toronto – Mexico City – Sidney – Tokyo 1982.

[10] Mann, W., J. Gilsbach: Die chirurgische Therapie von großen Glomus jugulare Tumoren. HNO **32** (1984) 249 – 251.

[11] Maxwell, R. E., S. N. Chou: Posterior fossa meningiomas. In: H. H. Schmidek, W. H. Sweet (eds.): Operative Neurological Techniques. Vol. 1, pp. 517 – 533. Grune & Stratton, New York – London 1982.

[12] Mullan, S., R. Naunton, J. Hekmat-Panah, et al.: The use of an anterior approach to ventrally placed tumors in the foramen magnum and vertebral column. J. Neurosurg. **24** (1966) 536 – 543.

[13] Pasztor, E., J. Vajda, P. Piffko, et al.: Transoral surgery for craniocervical space-occupying processes. J. Neurosurg. **60** (1984) 276 – 281.

[14] Seeger, W.: Atlas of Topographical Anatomy of the Brain and Surrounding Structures. Springer, Wien – New York 1978.

[15] Shucart, W. A., E. Kleriga: Lateral approach to the upper cervical spine. Neurosurgery **6** (1980) 278–281.
[16] Simmons, E. H., G. jr. du Troit: Lateral atlantoaxial arthrodesis. Orthop. Clin. N. Amer. **9** (1978) 1101–1114.
[17] Southwick, W. O., R. A. Robinson: Surgical approaches to the vertebral bodies in the cervical and lumbar regions. J. Bone J. Surg. A. **39** (1957) 631–643.
[18] Stevenson, G. C., R. J. Stoney, R. K. Perkins, et al.: A transcervical transclival approach to the ventral surface of the brain stem for removal of clivus chordoma. J. Neurosurg. **24** (1966) 544–551.
[19] Whitesides, T. E. jr., R. P. Kelly: Lateral approach to the upper cervical spine for anterior fusion. South Med. J. **59** (1966) 879–883.
[20] Yasargil, M. G., R. D. Smith, J. G. Gasser: Microsurgical approach to acoustic neurinomas. In: H. Krayenbühl (ed.): Advances and Technical Standards in Neurosurgery, Vol. 4, pp. 93–129. Springer, Wien–New York 1977.
[21] Yasuoka, S., H. Okazaki, J. R. Daube, et al.: Foramen magnum tumors. Analysis of 57 cases of benign extramedullary tumors. J. Neurosurg. **49** (1978) 828–838.

Tumors of the cranio-cervical junction

G. Keßel, M. Schwarz, D. Voth, K. Dei-Anang

Introduction

The term cranio-cervical junction used by us embraces the occipital squamous bone, foramen magnum as well as atlas and axis. Space occupying lesions of this region can be divided by histological as well as topico-anatomical criteria.

Within the first group, intramedullar tumors should be mentioned. Usually it concerns brain stem gliomas with a caudal extension into the cranio-vertebral junction area. We have considered them in our statistical analysis only in cases where the plane of the foramen magnum was definitely exceeded and to a large extent.

The second group consists of extramedullar-intradural space occupying lesions. According to the literature, mainly meningeomas, followed by neurinomas of the foramen magnum region are encountered ([2, 4]. However, it is noteworthy that even in great statistics of about 200 meningeomas during an observation period of 15 years we found only 3 of these tumors in the cranio-cervical junction [3]. Meningeomas mainly develop in the anterior dural segments of the superior cervical canal and growing secondarily into the foramen magnum. Tumors in the dorsal region can be simulated by a low tonsillar level or a displacement of cerebellar tissue into the spinal channel. This is the case in the various types of Arnold-Chiari malformations.

The third and last group combines extradural tumors. First of all the metastases in the osseous borders of the cranio-cervical junction have to be mentioned. Less frequently chordomas of the superior cervical canal or the caudal clivus segment are observed.

A number of tumors which, during their growth, can easily reach the cranio-cervical junction, is not listed in our presentation. These are mainly the petroclival tumors as well as the more extensive space occupying lesions of cerebellopontine angle. If one classifies the tumors of the cranio-cervical junction area as described above, only unexpectedly few remain which can definitely be assigned to this area.

Material and results

In the Neurosurgical Department of the University of Mainz we only encountered 22 tumors during the period 1962 – 1985. The pilocytic astrocytomas – 6 – and the neurinomas – a total of 5 – represent the main portion among the neuroepithelial tumors, beside 2 not clearly classified gliomas and 1 ependymoma.

The mesodermal tumors are composed of 3 meningeomas as well as 1 hemangioblastoma and 1 ossified fibroma each. The rest of space occupying lesions represent 2 arteriovenous angiomas, 1 metastasis of an unknown primary tumor, 1 malignant melanoma as well as 1 cystically changed gliosis (tab. 1). A further classification of the mentioned space occupying lesions is shown on table 2. Intramedullary and extramedullary-intradural disease processes represent the most frequent number of cases.

With the small number of cases we cannot make a statistically significant statement regarding age and structure of tumors of the cranio-cervical junction, due to the heterogeneity of this tumor group. However, if one correlates the incidence rate with the various age groups, an increased incidence up to age of 30 and a peak in the age of 40 – 50 can be observed. In the first group the astrocytomas dominate, in the second group meningeomas and neurinomas (fig. 1).

Besides rather short anamneses of 4 – 6 months duration, longer periods occur of 10 – 14 years. Table 3 shows the most frequently mentioned primary symptoms and their percentage distribution. The main and unfortunately non-specific signs are pain in the neck-occipital region in almost 3/4 of all patients. In about 1/4 initially irritative and deficit symptoms were found. Less frequently we have

Table 1 Tumors of the cranio-cervical junction – Histological classification

Neuroepithelial tumors	
Pilocytic astrocytoma	6
Glioma (unclassified)	2
Neurinoma (neuroma)	5
Ependymoma	1
Mesodermal tumors	
Meningioma	3
Hemangioblastoma	1
Ossifying fibroma	1
Others	
Arterio-venous malformation	2
Metastatic tumor	1
Melanotic tumor	1
Cyst (unclassified)	1

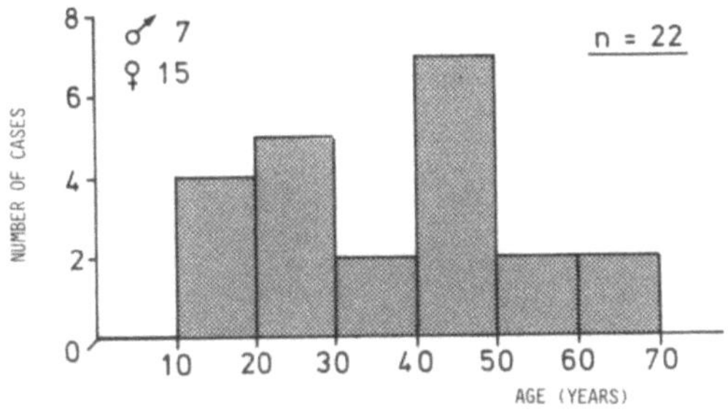

Fig. 1 Age related structure of tumors in the cranio-cervical junction area.

Table 2 Tumors of the cranio-cervical junction. Distribution according to their localization

Intramedullar tumors	
Pilocytic astrocytoma	6
Glioma (unclassified)	2
Ependymoma	1
Arterio-venous malformation	2
Hemangioblastoma	1
Cyst (unclassified)	1
Extramedullar-intradural tumors	
Neurinoma (neuroma)	5
Meningioma	3
Arterio-venous malformation	2
Melanotic tumor	1
Ossifying fibroma	1
Extradural tumors	
Melanotic tumor	1
Metastatic tumor	1

Table 3 Initial symptomatology of tumors of the cranio-cervical junction

Early symptoms	Incidence (Percent)
Pain in the neck-occipital region	70
Sensory disorder	25
Cranial nerve lesion	15
Motor disturbance	15
Posterior cord lesion, ataxia	10

observed cranial nerve deficits, motor disturbances as well as posterior cord lesions with ataxia as a primary symptom.

In the course of the clinico-neurological diagnostics we frequently observed sensory perception disorders among our patients. As can be seen from table 4,

Table 4 Neurological diagnostics in tumors of the cranio-cervical junction

Clinico-neurological examination	Incidence (Percent)
Sensation of pain and temperature	68%
Posture and vibration sense	50%
Pathological reflexes	50%
Severe para/tetraparesis	45%
Cranial nerve deficit	45%
Ataxia	41%
pathological muscle stretch reflexes	36%
Muscle strength (moderate paralysis)	32%
Increase of muscle tone	32%
Disorder of the vegetative system	18%
Dissociated sensory loss	14%
Papilledema	9%
Meningismus	9%

sensation of pain and temperature was affected in 70%, posture- and vibration sense in 50%. In some patients we noted a distribution of disturbances in form of a dissociated sensory lesion, seen in primary centromedullar processes. Severe tetrapareses could be found in almost half of the patients, in parallel with frequently positive pyramidal tract signs and pathological tendon reflexes. Also in almost half of the patients a cranial nerve lesion was present at time of diagnosis. Many patients – more than 40% – showed ataxia, due to the location of the cranio-cervical junction, and based on an involvement of posterior cord or caused by a cerebellar lesion. Less frequently found was a hydrocephalus occlusus, meningeal irritation and congestive symptoms of the fundus of the eye.

Diagnostic approach

The diagnostic fools have received decisive impulses during the last years by the introduction of the computer tomography (CT), and especially by the nuclear magnet resonance (NMR) examination. But the native diagnostics, such as myelography with its great diagnostic accuracy remains in many cases indispensable (tab. 5). Only in 2 out of 22 patients a positive finding could be made in the course of native diagnostics. In one patient a clear dilatation of the upper cervical spinal channel was present with narrowing and flattening of vertebral arch root as indication for a intraspinal space occupying lesion.

Myelography using iodine, hydrosoluble or oily contrast mediums – before air-myelography – is still the most important diagnostic measure. As a rule, the segmental extension of the tumor can be determined so and an operative exposure becomes possible. In 12 myelographies a positive finding was obtained in 11 cases.

Table 5 Reproductive procedure in the diagnostics of cranio-cervical space occupying lesions

	Number of cases	Positive findings
Native diagnostics	22	2
Myelography	12	11
Air-myelography	6	5
CT	6	2
NMR	5	5
Vertebral angiography	9	7

Similarly good results were scored in the pre-CT-era by the application of the air-myelography for demonstrating the cranio-cervical junction. In 6 examinations it was possible to make a diagnosis in 5 cases.

Using CT a tentative diagnosis of an intramedullar tumor originating from a narrowing of the subarachnoid space and the epidural adipose tissue was possible and allows a differential diagnosis between cystic and solid space occupying lesions. Extramedullar tumors which compress spinal cord and medulla oblongata, can be demonstrated well in cases where sufficient CSF is present between the space occupying lesion and the medulla.

The computer tomography after intrathecal application of contrast medium is a supplementary examination [1]. Twice a clear tumor formation was proved in 6 CTs after application of contrast medium. Using nuclear magnet resonance as the latest technique, it is possible to differentiate the dural sheath with its contents from the surrounding structures, and extra- and intramedullar space occupying lesions are well separated. In 5 of our patients the diagnosis of a cranio-spinal tumor was made by NMR-examination.

Case reports

However, a very important examination still is the vertebral angiography. From 9 angiographed patients, 7 clearly showed a pathological finding.

To illustrate the complex signs of the junction we report on a 38-year-old patient suffering for more than 14 months from paresthesias and fine-motor disturbances of the left hand. The same symptoms appeared later on the right side with paresthesias in both legs. Neurologically we found a spastic tetraparesis as well as a posterior cord lesion with spinal ataxia and the presence of a severe atrophy in the right-sided shoulder-girdle-musculature. The Pantopaque-myelography showed an incomplete stop at C 1 (fig. 2). The space occupying lesion was approached in the sitting position through a suboccipital, osteoclastic craniotomy with resection of the atlas arch. A neurinoma was found, proceeding from the right accessory nerve positioned about a 4/5 intracranially and 1/5 extracranially. After this operation the patient worked in his profession again but 10 years later he suffered a relapse. The tumor was clearly outlined in the NMR examination (fig. 3). The second intervention was also well tolerated by the patient and he returned home in a good working condition.

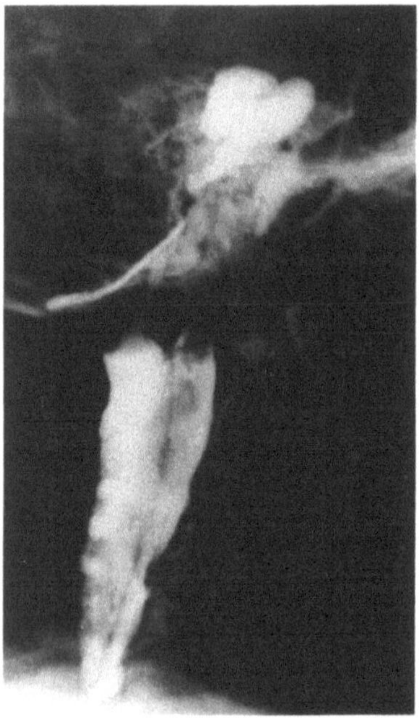

Fig. 2

Fig. 3

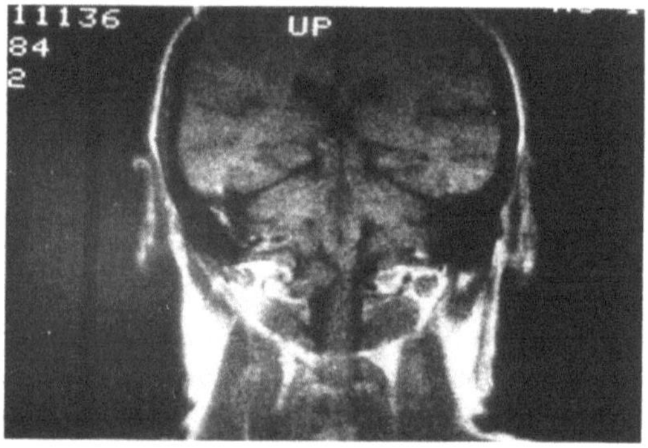

Fig. 2 Neurinoma of the right accessory nerve. Incomplete stop at C 1 in the Pantopaque-myelography.

Fig. 3 Accessory nerve neurinoma right. Same patient as in figure 2. NMR of the tumor recurrence which was diagnosed 10 years after first surgery.

Another illuminating case was a 50-year-old patient. Over 3 years he had suffered from a left-sided cervico-brachialgia. To alleviate his symptoms a ventral fusion by means of a plate had been made as well as a decompressive laminectomy from C4 to C6. The preoperative myelography showed already an incomplete stop in segment C2 as well as a recess of contrast medium as indication for tumor growth. 6 months later a fast progressive paraparesis appeared and the patient was referred to us. Myelography showed the tumor as a large recess of contrast medium (fig. 4). Immediately following the myelography a CT was performed. Figure 5 clearly showes the left-sided dorso-lateral tumor, compressing

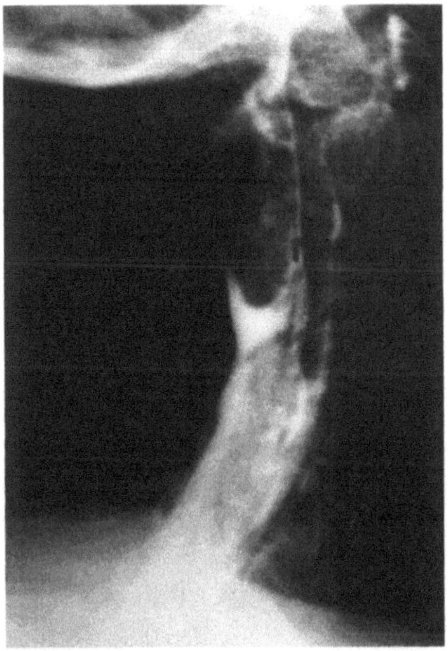

Fig. 4 Fibrillar neurinoma of the cranio-cervical junction. Recess of contrast medium in the myelogram.

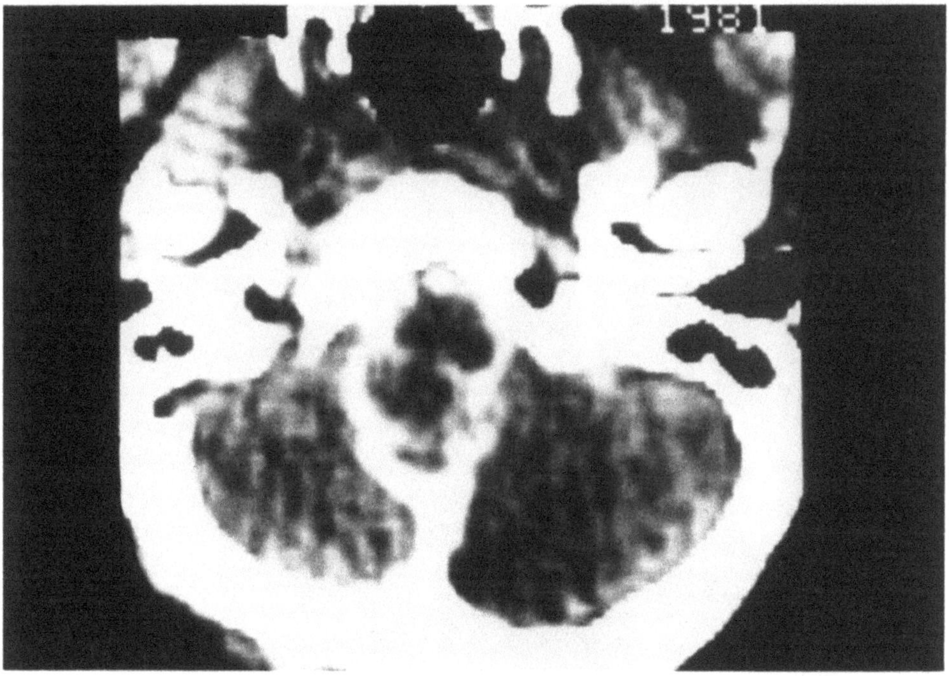

Fig. 5 Same patient as in figure 4. CT immediately after myelography. Compression of the cord by the left-dorsolateral tumor.

and displacing the cord. Total extirpation of a neurinoma was performed after suboccipital craniotomy and laminectomy of C 1/C 2 in the sitting position. But the patient died on the sequelae of a severe meningitis.

The next case, a 29-year-old patient, suffered for many years from perception disorders of the right hand, slowly expanding over shoulder and neck to the right half of the face. Neurologically we found a right-accentuated tetraparesis with right-sided hemihypesthesia and -algesia. The NMR-examination (fig. 6) showed an extensive space occupying lesion in the cranio-cervical junction region, mainly intracranially, with a wide cone growing up to segment C 2. This extension had not be observed in a previously performed CT. In the angiography only discrete signs of a vascular displacement, mainly displacing pontomesencephalic anterior vein towards the clivus. The surgical approach was again done in the sitting position via a suboccipital craniotomy and resection of the arch of the atlas. After incision of the vermis of the cerebellum an ependymoma with the described extension could be totally extirpated. Postoperatively we saw first an increase of the right-sided tetraparesis, but from the third day a clear involution tendency occured and a purulent tracheobronchitis developed with consecutive

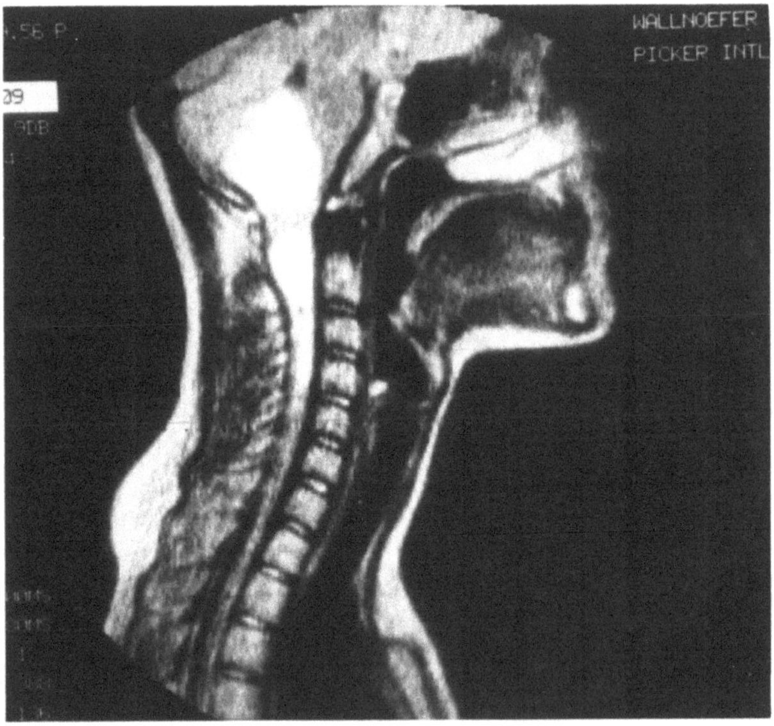

Fig. 6 Ependymoma in the cranio-cervical junction area. NMR picture.

bilateral bronchopneumonia. On the 10th postoperative day a massive infratentorial edema occurred, causing cerebral death.

Finally we still have the rare clinical picture of a pathology of the cranio-cervical junction. A 48-year female patient suffered over a period of more than 6 years from perception disorders of the left hand, in addition a motor weakness proceeding to the left leg. The air encephalography indicated an intramedullar tumor and surgery of the skull base was performed. Intramedullary we found cystic medullary changes. However, the main finding was an arteriovenous angioma of the size of 2 × 3 cm which we considered to be inoperable. In the two following years we observed a progression of the meanwhile severe spastic tetraparesis starting at C 2, a spinal ataxia as well as disturbed micturition with a residual urine of more than 900 ml. The vertebral angiography (fig. 7) shows the more medial and leftsided angioma. Considering the progressive neurological symptomatology, we decided a surgical intervention. The angioma could be totally removed. Its position was mainly intramedullary and it was fed by both Arteriae vertebrales. Fig. 8 shows the postoperative angiography. After surgery patient was able to walk for short distances alone, but a leftsided tetraspasticity of the arm and the disturbed micturition remained, although a marked reduction of residual urine in the bladder had been achieved.

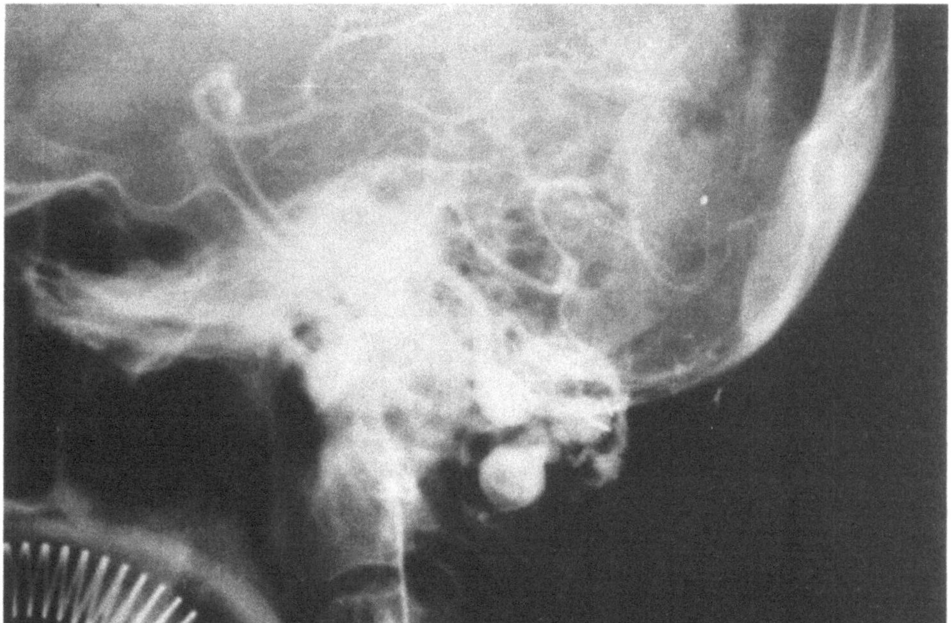

Fig. 7 Vertebral angiography: Angioma of the cranio-cervical junction.

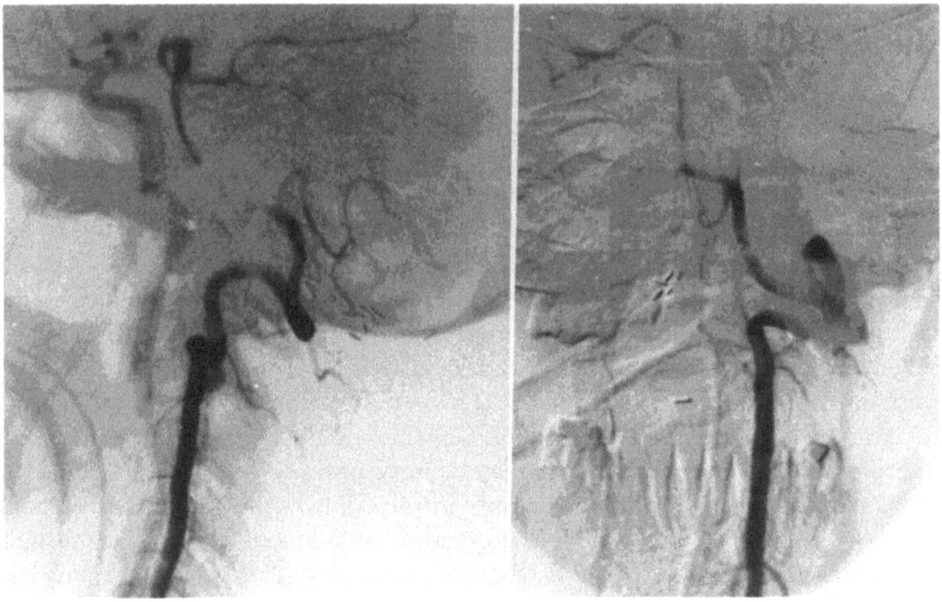

a b

Fig. 8 Vertebral angiography after extirpation of an angioma of the cranio-cervical junction. Same patient as in figure 7.

Table 6 Mortality and long term results after extirpation of tumors of the cranio-cervical junction

Mortality/Results	n = 22
Died, early postop. period	8
Died, late postop. period	3
Long term care patient	2
Able to walk (temporary need of help)	3
Complete independence (also in their professional work)	5
No follow up	1

Finally we want to discuss the mortality rate and the results after tumor extirpations in the cranio-cervical junction area (tab. 6). In 21 out of 22 patients we were able to follow-up the further course. In the early postoperative period 8 patients died. In 2 cases we found meningitis as the cause. In one case pneumonia was the causal factor. A further patient died because of a thrombo-embolism. Four times a central paralysis of the respiratory muscles was the cause for the fatal outcome. Among the patients who died during the later postoperative course, two also showed a primary and central paralysis of the respiratory muscles. Once it came to a coronary circulation failure on the basis of a myocardial failure. 2 patients have to be considered as long term care patients. 3 patients were able to walk with just temporary need of help and 5 patients regained their complete independence, including professional work.

References

[1] La Masters, D. L., T. J. Watanabe, E. F. Chambers, et al.: Multiplanar metrizamide-enhanced CT-imaging of the foramen magnum. AJNR 3 (1982) 485 – 494.
[2] Marc, J. A., M. M. Schechter: Radiological diagnosis of mass lesions within and adjacent to the foramen magnum. Radiology **114** (1976) 351 – 365.
[3] Ojemann, R. G.: Meningiomas: Clinical Features and Surgical Management. In: R. H. Wilkins, S. S. Rengachary: Neurosurgery. Vol. I, pp. 635 – 654. McGraw-Hill, New York 1985.
[4] Tievsky, A. L., D. O. Davis: Radiology of spinal canal neoplasia. In: R. H. Wilkins, S. S. Rengachary: Neurosurgery. Vol. I, pp. 1039 – 1044. McGraw-Hill, New York 1985.

Radiotherapy in metastatic diseases of the cervical spine and the craniospinal region

U. Mende, A. Braun, K. Rieden

Introduction

The results of large autopsy studies indicate that 20 to 30% of all patients with carcinoma will develop sooner or later bone metastases [1, 2]. According to the incidence of the primary tumour itself as well as to its tendency to metastasize into the skeletal system more than 80% of all bone metastases are due to neoplasms of the breast, prostate, bronchus, kidney and thyroid [2]. Most of the metastases are found in the red marrow with an unequivocal preference to the axial skeleton. Galasko reported the results in 50 patients with advanced mammary cancer, where dorsal and lumbar spine, pelvis, ribs and proximal extremities were the preferred sites of metastatic deposits whereas secondaries of the cervical spine and the craniospinal region virtually played a minor role [3]. But the frequency alone does not necessarily reflect the influence on the patient's life or quality of life in case of complications.

Extensive metastatic destructions of the cervical spine and the craniospinal region may cause dysarthria, dysphagia (with consecutive aspiration pneumonia), tetraplegia or death.

Isolated lesions of the cervical spine especially in breast cancer are the very exceptions. In the vast majority of cases a very extended, mostly generalized spread is found which results in a severe worsening of prognosis. A therapeutic concept with curative intention has to be abandoned in favour of palliation with improvement of the quality of life, rarely a prolongation, by relief of pain and prevention of serious complications like pathological fractures and tetraplegia.

Patients and methods

From November 1981 to June 1985, 50 patients under diagnostic and therapeutic care of the Universitäts-Strahlenklinik and the Orthopädische Universitätsklinik Heidelberg underwent radiotherapy of the cervical region with the planned tumour dose because of metastatic lesions of the cervical spine.

The mean age was 57.2 ± 11.5 years (range from 28 to 77 years). The sex distribution was 43 females and 7 males. In all cases the primary tumour site was known. The carcinoma of the breast was the prevailing neoplasm (84%), whereas tumours of the prostate (4%), lung (4%), rectum, bladder, larynx and a non-Hodgkin-lymphoma (2% each) were less frequent occurrences.

All patients had bone scintigrams and radiographs of the cervical spine in two projections. For better evaluation of the metastatic destructions as well as the stability of the affected vertebrae frontal and/or lateral tomograms were done in 38 patients (76%), and only 2 patients (4%) were examined by computerized tomography.

Conservative stabilizing orthopedic treatment alone was done in 47 patients, 14 of which (28%) had external rigid fixation, 7 (14%) a rigid collar and 26 (52%) a soft collar. One patient with fracture dislocation of C 1/C 2, incomplete tetraplegia and beginning paralysis of the respiratory centre received operative treatment with internal fixation followed by a rigid collar (figs. 1, 2). Two patients required no orthopedic devices at all.

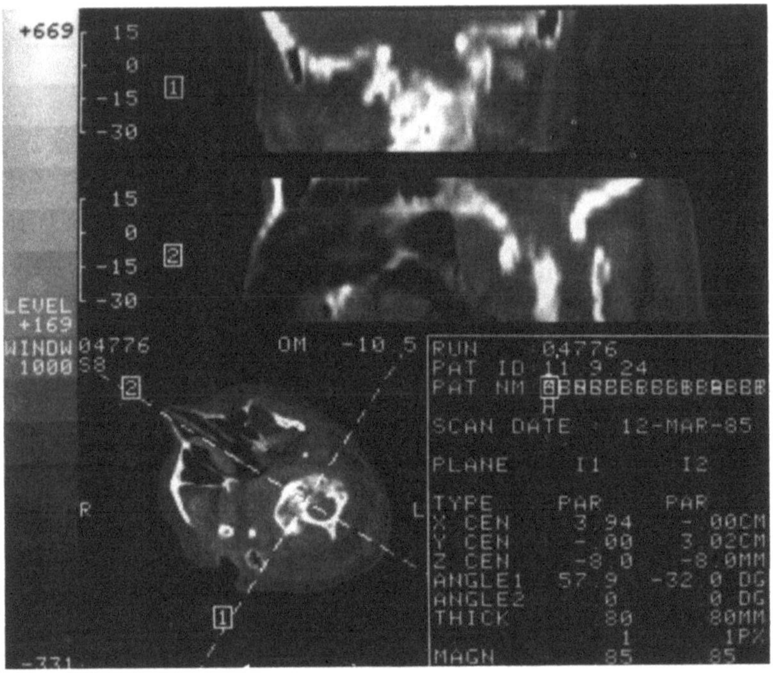

Fig. 1 Diagnosis: Carcinoma of the breast, osteolytic metastases with fracture dislocation C 1/C 2; CT.

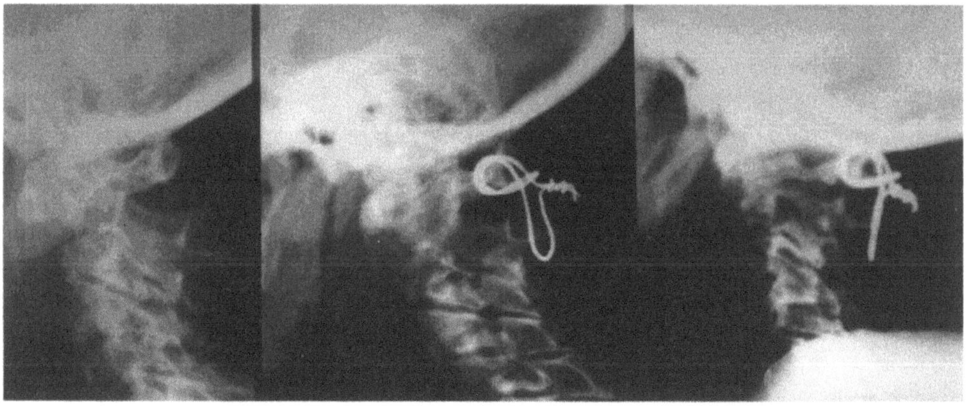

a b c

Fig. 2 Same patient. Before operation; before radiotherapy. Control after radiotherapy (a – c).

After orthopedic cervical fixation radiotherapy was performed with C_0-60-Gamma rays in 49 patients, with 42 MeV photons of a betatron in 1 patient, 43 times over lateral opposing fields, in 7 cases over direct dorsal fields. With single doses of 2 Gy in nearly all cases and weekly doses of no more than 10 Gy the total dose was 42.0 ± 2.9 Gy (range from 34.0 to 50.0 Gy) and NSD-values of 1360 ± 71 rets (from 1188 to 1524 rets). The duration of the radiotherapy course was 38.4 ± 7.4 days (from 26 to 59 days). 4 patients had another radiotherapy series of the cranial cervical spine and the craniospinal region respectively. Two of those patients had undergone radiotherapy of the middle and lower cervical spine only. Because of progression in the previously untreated cranial parts a total dose of 40 Gy was given here. The other two patients had a very rapid generalised progression of the tumorous disease with severe pain in the neck and glossoplegia. They were given another 20 Gy in the second series over the craniospinal region. Two of the cases will be discussed in detail later.

Results

Isolated skeletal lesions of the cervical spine were seen in one patient only. After an interval of 34 months she developed further metastases in other regions of the skeleton. In all other cases the metastatic affections were polytopic if not ubiquitous (fig. 3) [4]. The frequency rates (tab. 1) are in accordance with the results of Galasko [3]. But what is more important is the fact that 40 patients (80%) showed extensive bone destructions resulting in reduced load capacity of the affected skeletal regions.

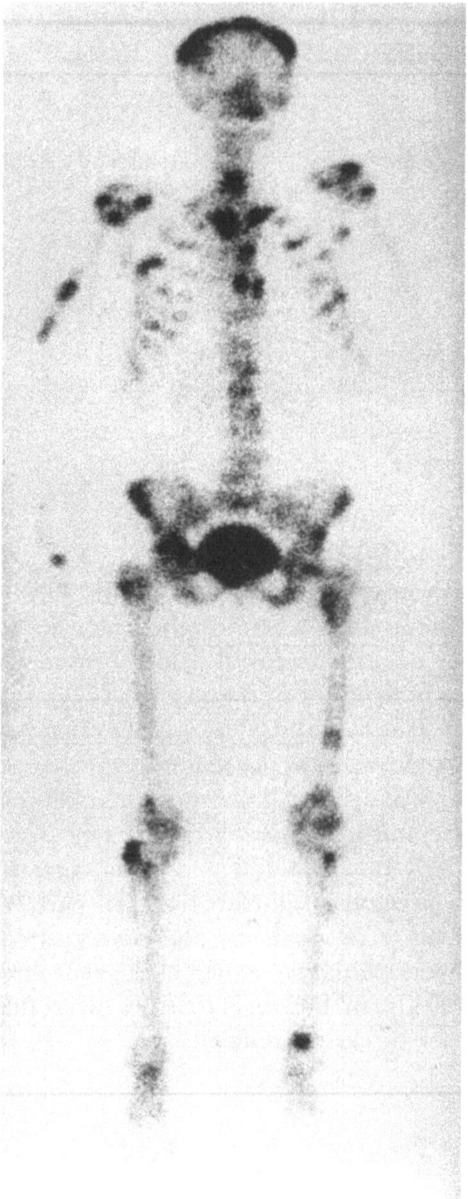

Fig. 3 Diagnosis: Carcinoma of the breast, polytopic metastases; bone scan.

Vertebral deformities like vertebrae planae and wedge vertebrae were seen in 28 and 30% respectively. Whereas in 98% of the cases metastatic lesions of the pedicles were found, the processus spinosi were affected in 70% only. Due to the indication for radiotherapy osteolytic metastases with 74% were over-represented, followed by osteolytic-osteoblastic deposits (26%); the pure os-

Table 1

Metastatic sites except cervical spine		
Spine	48 Pat.	96%
Pelvis	45 Pat.	90%
Ribs	45 Pat.	90%
Extremities	43 Pat.	86%
Skull	34 Pat.	68%
Extensive metastases, reduced load capacity		
Spine	33 Pat.	66%
Extremities	19 Pat.	38%
Pelvis	6 Pat.	12%
None	10 Pat.	20%

teoblastic form was not found. Isolated affection of a single cervical vertebra was not found. In all cases polytopic changes in more than one were seen in the X-ray. Considering the metastatic localisation only there was no statistically significant preference for a certain vertebra. Taking into consideration the extent of metastatic destruction a tendency of decreasing order could be established: From vertebra 6 and 3 over 5, 4, 2, 1 to 7. Very important is the fact that the condylus occipitalis showed changes that were seen in X-ray in 78%, which from phylogenetic reasons is not surprising [7].

In all patients pain in the neck was the principal sign of metastatic bone destructions. By orthopedic treatment, radiotherapy and hormonal and/or chemotherapy a regression of symptoms in all patients was noticed, the vast majority being free from pain in the treated area.

Neurological deficits with paraesthesia, sensory and motor impairment were seen in 8 patients (16%). In 5 cases the symptoms receded. One patient who did not respond to therapy had a tumorous infiltration of the brachial plexus, while the other two died within two months after radiotherapy. The tetraplegic patient with fracture dislocation C1/C2 who had an additional operative cervical fixation could be mobilised without difficulties by the end of the combined treatment.

39 patients (78%) showed signs of recalcification in X-ray (tab. 2); 10 out of the 11 patients without recalcification have died (fig. 4).

45 out of the 50 patients had a restabilisation of the cervical spine. 22 (49%) out of them achieved complete restabilisation without orthotic devices. Partial restabilisation with orthotic devices was seen in another 22 patients (49%) as well as in the one who had been operated. 16 patients out of the latter group have died, 7 are still alive with only one patient showing no signs of recalcification two months after therapy.

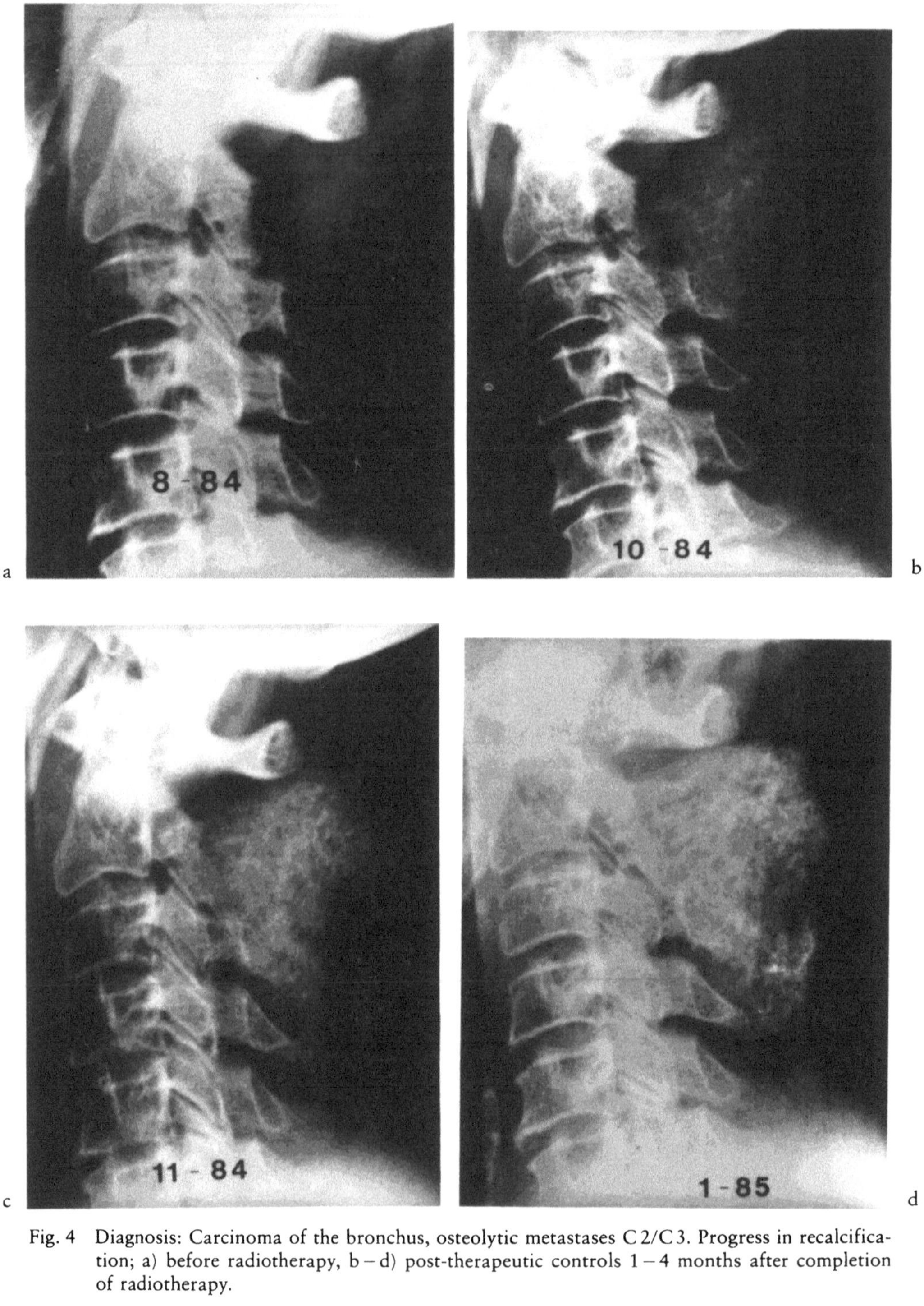

Fig. 4 Diagnosis: Carcinoma of the bronchus, osteolytic metastases C 2/C 3. Progress in recalcification; a) before radiotherapy, b – d) post-therapeutic controls 1 – 4 months after completion of radiotherapy.

Table 2 Degree of recalcification

None	11 Pat.	22%	
Fair to moderate	18 Pat.	36%	78%
Marked	15 Pat.	30%	
Very strong	6 Pat.	12%	

Discussion

Radiotherapy has proved to be very effective in the treatment of bone metastases [5]. In order to ensure optimal results with little side effects a few points should be kept in mind. Pain and neurological deficits do not always coincide with the extent of metastatic destructions. Marked radicular symptoms were noticed in a patient with bone lesions in the segment C6/C7 (fig. 5), whereas in another patients, with extensive tumorous destructions, collapsed vertebrae and narrowing of the spinal canal, a corresponding neurological deficit was missing (fig. 6).

a b

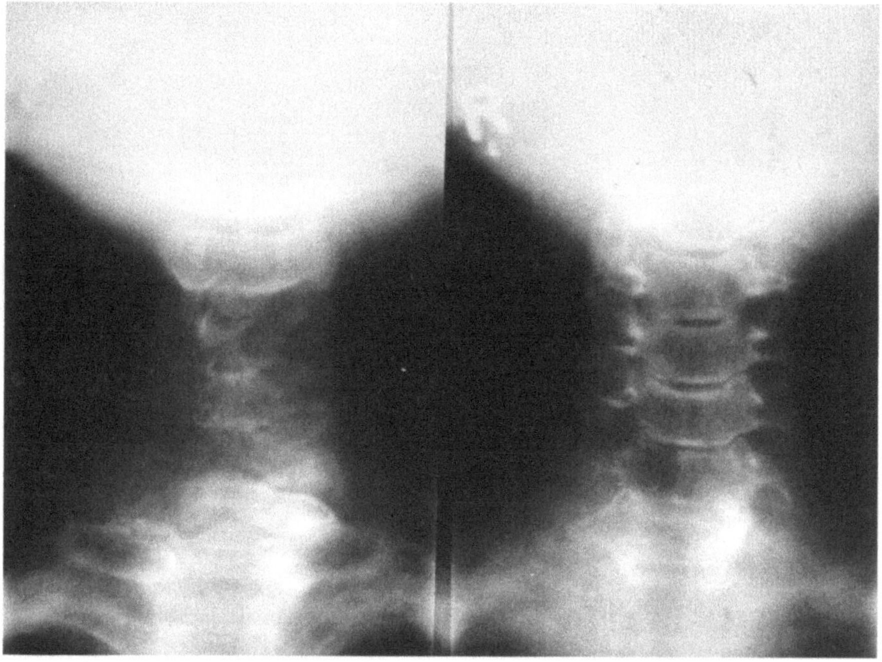

Fig. 5 Diagnosis: Carcinoma of the breast, osteolytic metastases C6/C7 with radicular symptoms on the right side; frontal tomograms.

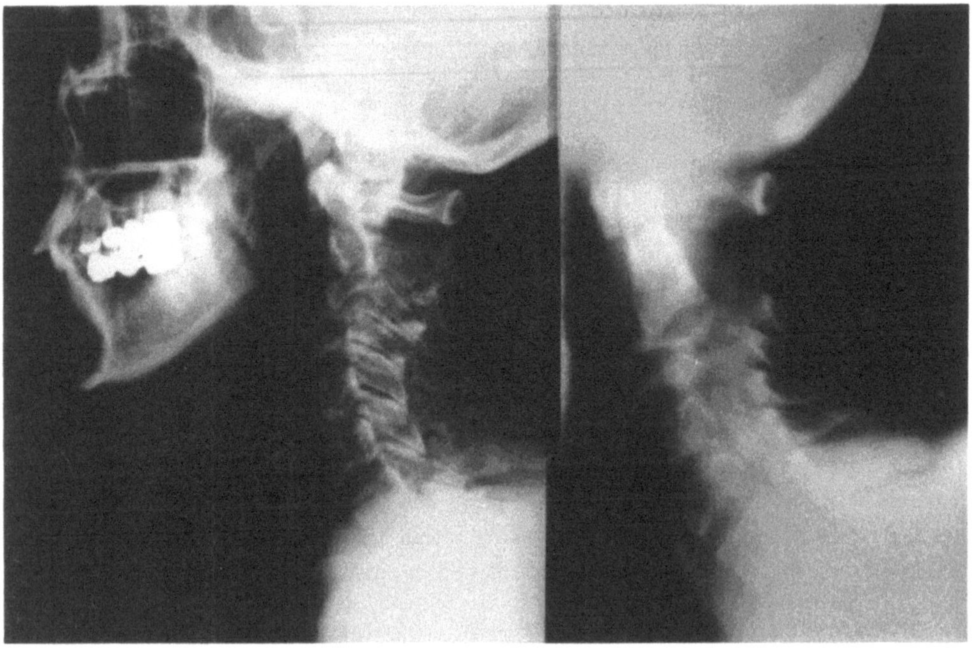

a b

Fig. 6 Diagnosis: Carcinoma of the breast, massive osteolytic destructions, narrowing of the spinal canal, neurological signs absent.

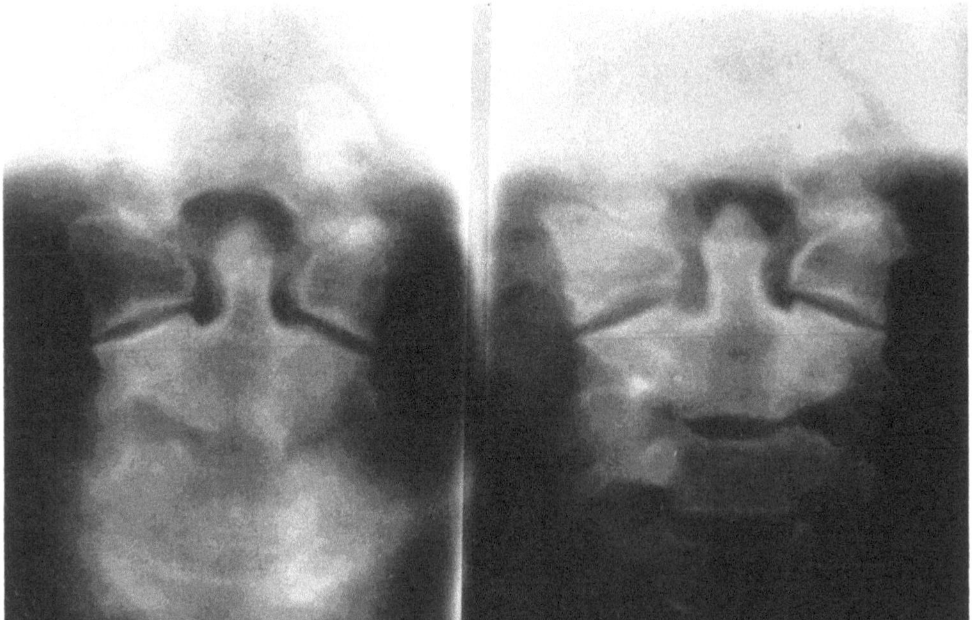

a b

Fig. 7 Diagnosis: Carcinoma of the breast; osteolytic metastases craniospinal region right side; a) before radiotherapy, b) good recalcification after completion.

In case of extensive metastatic lesions radiotherapy may in the beginning cause a transitory increase in porosity of the affected vertebrae, possibly resulting in deformity or collapse with inadequate trauma. The orthotic device has to be adapted before radiotherapy is started. It should be kept until restabilisation has been verified by sufficient recalcification (fig. 7).

Antineoplastic chemotherapy in combination with radiotherapy may result in a massive increase in side effects to risk organs such as skin and mucous membranes. This is especially known for adriamycin, methotrexate and bleomycin [8]. Radiotherapy should therefore be discontinued for the day, when chemotherapy is given.

An effective radiotherapy requires a sufficient dose as well as field size. Especially in case of polytopic metastatic deposits the condylus occipitalis must be included by the field cranially. Apart from special techniques which are the exceptions, irradiation over small fields including parts of the cervical spine only should be avoided. With progression of the tumorous lesions beyond the field margins irradiation over a new adjacent field may result in marginal overdose with the risk of myelopathia [6], or on the other hand of underdose with consequences shown in the following case: A 60-year old patient with carcinoma of the breast and multiple bone metastases had a radiotherapy of the middle and lower cervical spine (with the upper field margin in the caudal third of the axis) (fig. 8). 3 1/2

a b

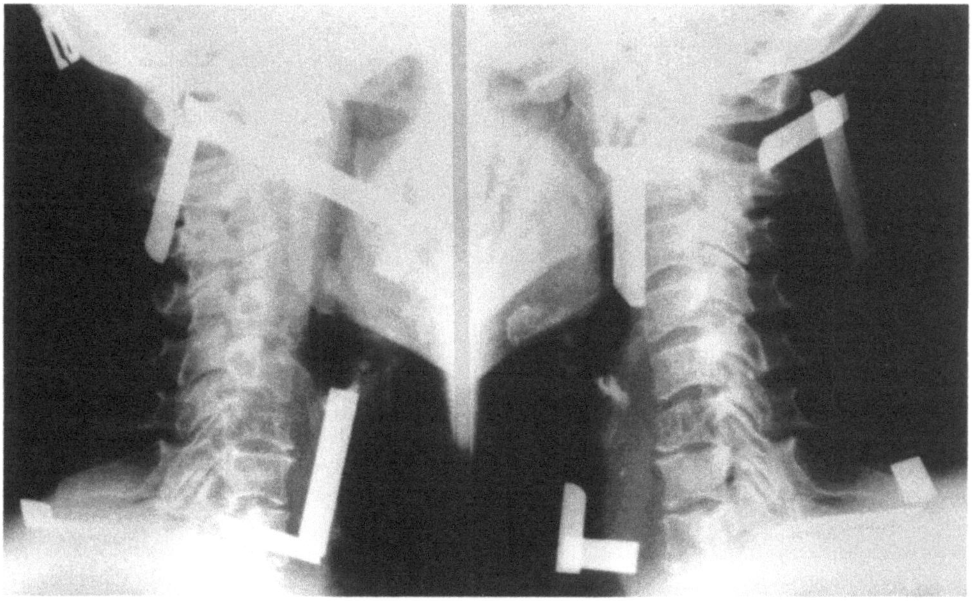

Fig. 8 Diagnosis: Carcinoma of the breast; osteolytic metastases, control X-radiographs of the opposing fields.

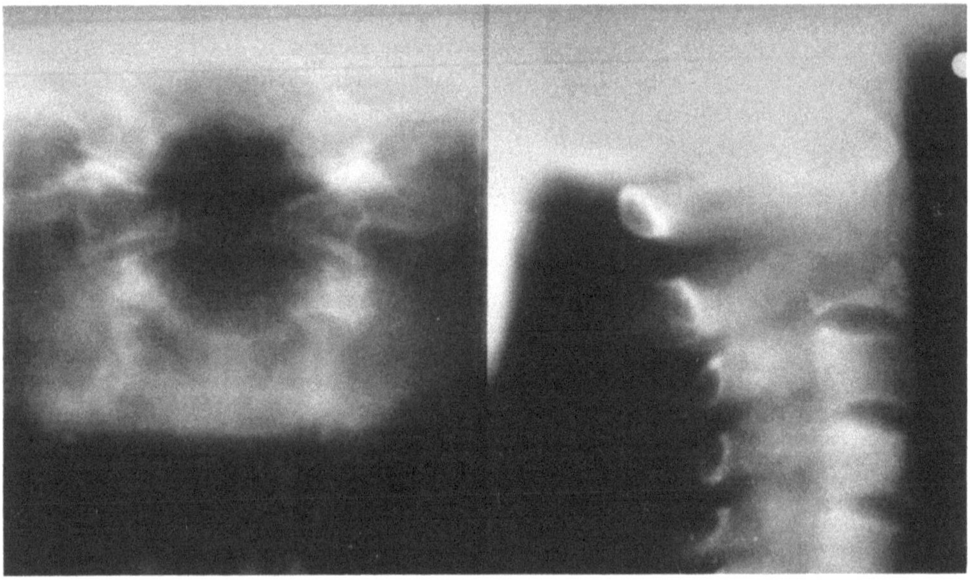

a b

Fig. 9 Same patient; craniospinal region 3 1/2 months after the first radiotherapy series; recalcification caudal, progression in the cranial parts; frontal and lateral tomograms.

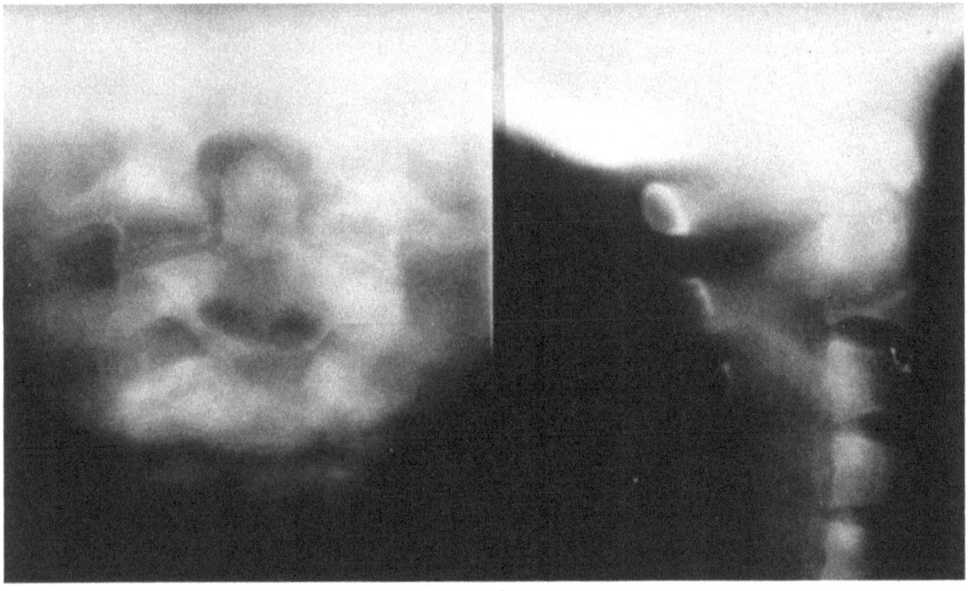

a b

Fig. 10 Same patient; craniospinal region; control 5 weeks after second series of radiotherapy; good recalcification but 3 mm gap between the fields.

months later good recalcification of the irradiated osteolyses was seen, but tumour progression was observed in the more cranial areas, which were now subjected to a total dose of 40 Gy with 42 MeV photons over lateral opposing fields, again with good success (fig. 9). 5 weeks after completion of this course recalcification had occurred, but a 3 mm-gap causing lack of stability was seen, where the fields had apparently not been close enough (fig. 10).

On the other hand in case of massive progression of the malignant disease re-population in the field margins by tumour cells might occur as it is seen in the following case: A 34-year old patient with carcinoma of the breast and ubiquitous skeletal metastases showed recalcification of the osteolytic areas already by the end of the radiation series with 40 Gy (fig. 11). 4 months later she complained of severe pain in the neck, dysarthria and dysphagia indicating an afflication of the left hypoglossal nerve. An additional 20 Gy (amounting to a total dose of 60 Gy) was given to the craniospinal region resulting in regression of the pain and the neurological deficit. The patient died 3 months later from progression of the tumour.

Despite the relative radio-sensitivity of the cranial spinal cord and the medulla oblongata neither here nor in the other cases signs of a myelopathia were noticed.

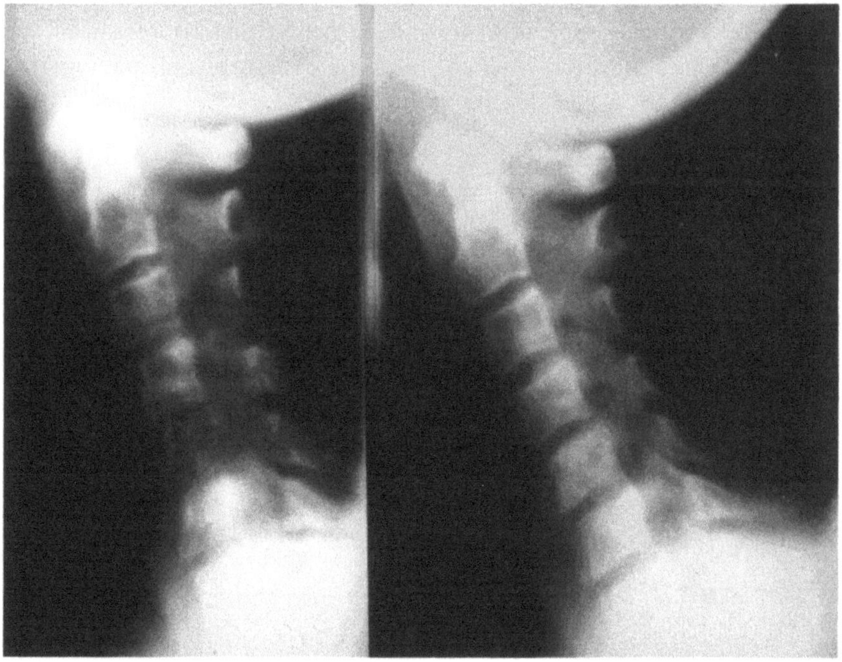

a b

Fig. 11 Diagnosis: Carcinoma of the breast; polytopic osteolytic metastases. a) before radiotherapy, b) good recalcification by the end of radiotherapy. Lateral tomograms.

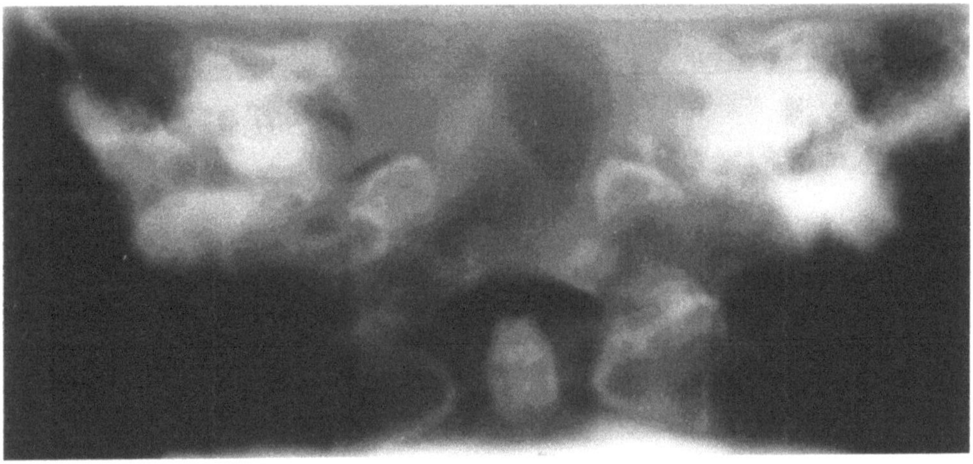

Fig. 12 Same patient, 4 months later. Osteolytic destruction of the left hypoglossal canal.

Conclusion

Combination of conservative orthopaedic treatment, radiotherapy and hormonal and/or chemotherapy offer a therapeutic approach in metastatic disease of the cervical spine with relief of pain, at least partial restabilisation and recalcification in the majority of cases. The indication to operative procedures should be limited to individual cases (in radio-resistent tumours or tetraplegia) paying attention to prognosis, expectation and quality of life.

Acknowledgements

We thank Mr. and Mrs. Bontzol for the photographic reproductions.

References

[1] Abrams, H. L., R. Spiro, N. Goldstein: Metastases in carcinoma. Analysis of 1.000 autopsied cases. Cancer **3** (1950) 74–85.

[2] Freyschmidt, J.: Knochenerkrankungen im Erwachsenenalter, Röntgenologische Diagnose und Differentialdiagnose, pp. 84–88. Springer Verlag, Berlin – Heidelberg – New York 1980.

[3] Galasko, C. S. B.: The Anatomy and Pathways of Skeletal Metastases. In: L. Weiss, H. A. Gilbert (eds.): Bone Metastasis, pp. 49–63. G. K. Hall Medical Publ., Boston, Mass. 1981.

[4] Hermann, H. J., B. Kimmig, B. Kober, et al.: Radiologische Diagnostik von Knochenmetastasen. Röntgenblätter **36** (1983) 203–208.

[5] Kuttig, H.: Die Strahlentherapie von Knochenmetastasen. Röntgenblätter **36** (1983) 209–215.

[6] Rahim, H.: Zur Quantifizierung der biologischen Wirkung von Photonen und Elektronen. Strahlentherapie **159** (1983) 633–641.

[7] Torklus, D. von, W. Gehle: Die obere Halswirbelsäule, pp. 23–24. Thieme Verlag, Stuttgart 1975.

[8] Wannenmacher, M., F. Gauwerky, C. Streffer (eds.): Kombinierte Strahlen- und Chemotherapie. Symposium der Arbeitsgemeinschaften "Strahlentherapie und Onkologie" und "Strahlenbiologie" d. Dt. Röntgenges. 20./21. Oktober 1978 in Bad Krozingen. Urban und Schwarzenberg, München – Wien – Baltimore 1979.

VII Summary and overview

D. Voth

Introduction

The cranio-cervical junction comprises an anatomical region, which harbours within a narrow space vital parts of the nervous system, the upper part of the vertebral column and its connection with the posterior-inferior portion of the skull. Within this skeletal part, long and very short muscles are used to move and steady the skull, while important blood vessels ascend supplying the brain. Diseases of this complex region are manifold but all will affect the functions of spinal cord and medulla. This involvement will lead to severe neural impairment or/and a severe threat to survival. For these reasons surgical intervention is unavoidable but poses a great number of technical and diagnostic problems which will be dealt with by experienced specialists in this field.

Basic research and diagnostics

The embryological, neuroanatomical and topographical morphological aspects have been considered by two internationally known specialists pointing out the complicated development and adult morphology of the region.

Traumatic changes and pathological alterations arising from a number of diseases are treated in relevant chapters refering to malformations such as basilary invagination (impression) and a mobile odontoid process. The congenital abnormalities can cause considerable diagnostic difficulties.

The diagnosis of disease processes in the cranio-cervical junction is normally based on X-rays including computer tomography. Additional information is obtainable by using radio-isotopes which can give clear and significant information in inflammatory lesions.

A completely new period has been opened up by the introduction of nuclear magnetic resonance imaging, NMR. This method proves its great value in tumour diagnosis, in processes causing a narrowing of the spinal canal due to changes of the intervertebral discs and the bony parts of the cervical vertebrae. Further improvement can be expected since the introduction of gadolinium – DTPA.

Contributions from a number of hospitals praise the diagnostic value of the method in space occupying lesions, inflammatory de-myelinated and degenerative conditions. A general advantage of the technique is the reduced stress on the patient and the avoidance of radiation. An addition of the method offers myelography by using computer-assisted myelography (CAM) or a high resolution CT which should be used in selected cases. Furthermore the increasing use of modern electrophysiological methods, such as the use of evoked potentials permits further detailed conclusions in cases where lesions of ascending spinal tracts are suspected, even when distinct clinical signs have not yet developed.

In cases of myelopathy due to spondylosis the evoked potential method allows a differentiated diagnosis and a clear separation from sclerosis multiplex and amyotrophic lateral sclerosis.

Microsurgery and detailed anatomical knowledge supported by modern imaging processes allow careful operational steps to secure maximal conditions for approaching the difficulties when intervention in the cranio-cervical region is necessary. For these reasons standard procedures have been developed, in particular the trans-oral and trans-cervical approach to secure optimal surgical conditions. A lateral access is difficult but often found unavoidable.

Traumatic lesions

In accident surgery fractures of the odontoid process of the atlas or the neighbouring base of skull are in the foreground of surgical intervention. A fusion technique for dens fractures has been communicated to this meeting and the developed tools exhibited. This osteosynthesis using a compression screw appears to be a tissue preserving procedure preventing unnecessary damage, while a direct osseous fusion can be very difficult and to some extent dangerous. However it must be emphasized that 'wiring up' on its own does not achieve rational results and in all cases an apposition with autologous boney material should be attempted to obtain an osseous dorsal fusion.

The occurance of arterio-venous fistulae is rare in the vascular territory of the vertebral artery but distinct flow murmur can be heard, or clinico-neurological signs are present verifiable by angiography. These signs are caused by ischaemia in the brainstem. Intraluminar occlusion or a ligature of the vertebral artery are often unavoidable.

Extensive fractures in the cranio-cervical region combined with condylar damage are very serious injuries and often lethal. These patients are usually unconscious and must undergo a computerised tomography. In case a patient is responsive very severe backpain is the dominant symptom, but no specific signs, apart from occasional failures of cranial nerves.

Patients with high transverse lesions and tetraplegic can now be kept alive by artificial respiration and intensive care units often succeed in keeping them over the worst period after the accident.

Malformations, system diseases and functional disturbances

A neuropathological contribution deals with the complex chapter of malformations demonstrating that malformations of the CNS and of the mesenchymal parts are not independent formations but interdependent needing a complex concept of pathogenesis. Clinicians however maintain that many patients with congenital malformations of the cranio-cervical area show no obvious signs in daily life. A disease connected with congenital disturbances of the cranio-cervical regions is syringomyelia and NMR technique has given considerable insight into its topography and extent, enabling a more secure subarachnoidal drainage.

Functional disturbances were concentrated on the symptoms of spasmodic torticollis. Microsurgery offers a good chance of alleviating symptoms. It is assumed that in the horizontal type of torticollis the primary disturbance is in afferent side of head movements control.

Inflammatory and degenerative lesions

These aspects are of special interest to rheumatologists and neurosurgeons, as morbidity is very high in cases of diseases of the cranio-cervical area and specially so in cases of chronic polyarthritis. Rheumatologists emphasize the well known clinical picture of atlanto-axial dislocation combined with destruction of the odontoid process. In this instance an operational fusion will be necessary in particular when C_2 root irritations and signs of spinal cord compression are present. Rheumatologists have measured the degree of dislocation and the size of the spinal canal in order to establish a firm indication for operation. Surgical methods must correct the dislocation preventing a disease progress. The dorsal fusion by wiring and apposition of antologous bony material is in dislocation of more than 4 mm necessary and usually successful. The Neurosurgical Dept. of Mainz University favours this procedure including a dural resection to relieve compressions of medullary parts. A technical aid offers the compression clamp of Roosen, provided that the atlanto-axial dislocation has a certain degree of mobility.

Definite and urgent surgical intervention is necessary
1. in cases of severe occipital pain,
2. manifest neurological defects and signs of myelopathy,
3. signs of vertebral artery occlusion.

Indicative signs for a preventive surgical intervention are the following factors:
1. Considerable atlanto-occipital dislocation (anterior atlanto-dental distance exceeding 9 mm, posterior distance less than 15 mm (CT), unfavourable conditions of soft tissue components in the region of the clivus, invagination of dens),

2. Clear progression of destructive pathology,
3. Considerable atlanto-axial instability.

In order to be certain whether to operate or not an assessment of the following risk factors of the underlying disease process have to be considered:
1. High systemic activity (laboratory tests);
2. Degree of positivity of rheumatoid factors;
3. Late stage of the disease;
4. The dosage used in cortisone therapy.

The result of fusional operations show for all hospitals the most favourable outcome if the patient had no specific complaints or solely pain. The greater the symptoms, the less satisfactory are postoperative results.

Tumours of the cranio-cervical function

A substantial contribution was made by neuropathologist dealing with meningiomas and neurinomas of the cranio-cervical function. To be certain that diagnosis is correct not only is careful neurological examination necessary but also the whole techniques of imaging including NMR. This technique especially made it possible to visualise the size and extent of gliomas in the medulla and pons and enabled the neurosurgeon to proceed with a microsurgical removal.

Modern techniques certainly have made it possible to reduce the high mortality rate in patients operated on for tumours in the cranio-cervical region. However the high frequency of post-operative complications and the final outcome confirm the high total risks involved in operations of the area under discussion. The problems facing radiotherapy when dealing with metastases in this region were fully discussed by the contributors of the workshop.

List of contributors

Ahyai, A., Dr. med., Med. Einrichtungen der Universität, Neurochirurg. Klinik, Robert-Koch-Str. 40, D-3400 Göttingen
Albrecht, H. J., Dr. med., Rheumaklinik Oberammergau, Hubertusstr. 40, D-8103 Oberammergau
Al-Hami, S., Dr. med., Patholog.-Anatomisches Institut, Abt. Neuropathologie, Langenbeckstr. 1, D-6500 Mainz
Arnold, H., Dr. med., Univ.-Krankenhaus Eppendorf, Abt. Neurochirurgie, Martinistr. 52, D-2000 Hamburg 20
Becker, H., Dr. med., Med. Hochschule Hannover, Neuroradiologische Abteilung, D-3000 Hannover 61
Beck-Mannagetta, A., Dr. med., Neurologische Abt., Karl-Bonhoeffer-Nervenklinik, Oranienburger Str. 285, D-1000 Berlin 26
Besser, R., Dr. med., Neurologische Univ.-Klinik, Langenbeckstr. 1, D-6500 Mainz 1
Bohl, J., Dr. med., Pathologisch-Anatomisches Institut, Abt. Neuropathologie, Langenbeckstr. 1, D-6500 Mainz 1
Brandt, L., Dr. med., Ortopediska kliniken, Lasarettet, S-221 85 Lund
Brattström, H., Doz. Dr. med., Ortopediska kliniken, Lasarettet, S-221 85 Lund
Braun, A., Priv.-Doz. Dr. med., Stiftung Orthop. Univ.-Klinik, Schlierbacher Landstr. 200 a, D-6900 Heidelberg
Brito, N., Dr. med., Neurochirurgische Univ.-Klinik, Langenbeckstr. 1, D-6500 Mainz 1
Castro, W., Dr. med., Neurochirurgische Univ.-Klinik, Hufelandstr. 55, D-4300 Essen 1
Dei-Anang, K., Dr. med., Neurochirurg. Univ.-Klinik, Langenbeckstr. 1, D-6500 Mainz 1
Dietz, H., Prof. Dr. med., Med. Hochschule Hannover, Neurochirurg. Klinik, D-3000 Hannover 61
Eggert, H. R., Dr. med., Neurochirurgische Univ.-Klinik, Hugstetter Straße 55, D-7800 Freiburg
Freckmann, N., Dr. med., Univ.-Krankenhaus Eppendorf, Abt. Neurochirurgie, Martinistr. 52, D-2000 Hamburg 20
Friedburg, H., Dr. med., Abt. Röntgendiagnostik, Sektion Neuroradiologie, Hauptstr. 5, D-7800 Freiburg
Friedrich, H., Prof. Dr. med., Allgem. Krankenhaus Heidberg, Neurochirurg. Klinik, Tangstetter Landstr. 400, D-2000 Hamburg 62
Frowein, R. A., Prof. Dr. med., Neurochirurgische Univ.-Klinik, Josef-Stelzmann-Straße 9, D-5000 Köln 41
Gerner, H. J., Dr. med., Werner-Wicker-Klinik, D-3590 Bad Wildungen-Reinhardshausen
Gilsbach, J., Prof. Dr. med., Neurochirurgische Univ.-Klinik, Hugstetter Str. 55, D-7800 Freiburg
Glees, P., Prof. Dr. med., University of Cambridge, Department of Anatomy, Downing Street, Cambridge CB2 3DY, (U.K.)
Goebel, H. H., Prof. Dr. med., Pathologisch-Anatomisches Institut der Univ.-Klinik, Abt. Neuropathologie, Langenbeckstr. 1, D-6500 Mainz 1
Goebel, K. M., Prof. Dr. med., Zentrum Innere Medizin, Univ.-Klinik, D-3550 Marburg
Grote, W., Prof. Dr. med., Neurochirurg. Univ.-Klinik, Hufelandstr. 55, D-4300 Essen 1
Gschwend, N., Prof. Dr. med., Klinik Wilhelm Schulthess, CH-8032 Zürich
Gutjahr, G., Dr. med., Institut für Klinische Strahlenkunde, Univ.-Klinik, Langenbeckstr. 1, D-6500 Mainz 1
Hahn, K., Prof. Dr. med., Institut für Klinische Strahlenkunde der Univ.-Klinik, Abt. Nuklearmedizin, Langenbeckstr. 1, D-6500 Mainz 1

Harms, J., Prof. Dr. med., Reha-Krankenhaus Langensteinbach, Orthopädie-Traumatologie I, D-7516 Karlsbad

Hasselbach, R., Dr. med., Neurolog. Abt., Landesnervenklinik, Dautenheimer Landstr. 66, D-6508 Alzey

Heckl, R., Dr. med., Reha-Krankenhaus Langensteinbach, Orthopädie-Traumatologie I, D-7516 Karlsbad

Hennig, J., Dr. med., Klinikum Albert-Ludwig-Univ., Abt. Röntgendiagnostik, Sektion Neuroradiologie, Hauptstr. 5, D-7800 Freiburg

Herrmann, H.-D., Prof. Dr. med., Univ.-Krankenhaus Eppendorf, Neurochirurgische Klinik Martinistr. 52, D-2000 Hamburg 20

Hertel, G., Prof. Dr. med., Neurolog. Abt., Rudolf Virchow-Krankenhaus, Augustenburger Platz 1, D-1000 Berlin 65

Hey, O., Dr. med., Neurochirurgische Univ.-Klinik, Langenbeckstr. 1, D-6500 Mainz 1

Hildebrandt, J., Dr. med., Neurochirurg. Univ.-Klinik, Robert-Koch-Str. 40, D-3400 Göttingen

Hilgenstock, J., Dr. med., Landesnervenklinik, Neurologische Abt., Vulkanstr. 58, D-5470 Andernach.

Höllerhage, H.-G., Dr. med., Med. Hochschule Hannover, Neurochirurg. Klinik, Konstanty-Gutschow-Str. 9, D-3000 Hannover 61

Hopf, H. C., Prof. Dr. med., Neurologische Univ.-Klinik, Langenbeckstr. 1, D-6500 Mainz 1

Hüwel, N., Dr. med., Neurochirurg. Univ.-Klinik, Langenbeckstr. 1, D-6500 Mainz 1

Huk, W., Dr. med., Neurologische Klinik, Schwabachanlage 6, D-8520 Erlangen

Hussein, S., Dr. med., Med. Hochschule Hannover, Neurochirurg. Klinik, Konstanty-Gutschow-Str. 9, D-3000 Hannover 61

Jansen, J., Dr. med., Neurochirurg. Univ.-Klinik, Robert-Koch-Str. 40, D-3400 Göttingen

Jensen, H.-P., Prof. Dr. med., Chr.-Albrechts-Universität, Neurochirurgische Klinik, Weimarer Str. 8, D-2300 Kiel

Kalff, P., Dr. med., Neurochirurg. Univ.-Klinik, Hufelandstr. 55, D-4300 Essen 1

Kazner, E., Prof. Dr. med., Univ.-Klinikum Charlottenburg, Abt. für Neurochirurgie, Spandauer Damm 130, D-1000 Berlin 19

Keßel, G., Dr. med., Neurochirurgische Univ.-Klinik, Langenbeckstr. 1, D-6500 Mainz 1

Klawki, P., Dr. med., Neurochirurgische Univ.-Klinik, Langenbeckstr. 1, D-6500 Mainz 1

Kluger, P., Dr. med., Werner-Wicker-Klinik, D-3590 Bad Wildungen-Reinhardshausen

Knöringer, P., Dr. med., Neurochirurg. Abt. der Univ. Ulm, Bezirkskrankenhaus Günzburg, Reisenburgerstr. 2, D-8870 Günzburg

Kocks, W., Dr. med., Univ.-Klinik, Neurochirurg. Abt., Hufelandstr. 55, D-4300 Essen 1

Köhler, D., Dr. med., Neurologische Abt., Rudolf Virchow-Krankenhaus, Augustenburger Platz 1, D-1000 Berlin 65

Koschorek, F., Dr. med., Chr.-Albrechts-Universität, Neurochirurg. Abt., Weimarer Str. 8, D-2300 Kiel 1

Krause, A., Dr. med., Zentrum für Innere Medizin, Univ.-Klinik, D-3550 Marburg

Lang, J., Prof. Dr. med., Anatomisches Institut der Universität, Kollicker Str. 6, D-8700 Würzburg

Leppien, A., Dr. med., Univ.-Krankenhaus Eppendorf, Neurochirurg. Klinik, Martinistr. 52, D-2000 Hamburg 20

Ljunggren, B., Dr. med., Ortopediska kliniken, Lasarettet, S-221 85 Lund

Matsumura, K., Dr. med., Med. Einrichtungen der Univ., Neurochirurg. Klinik, Robert-Koch-Str. 40, D-3400 Göttingen

Meister, B., Dr. med., Werner-Wicker-Klinik, D-3590 Wildungen-Reinhardshausen

Mende, U., Dr. rer. nat., Dr. med., Univ.-Strahlenklinik, Voss-Str. 3, D-6900 Heidelberg

Montazem, A., Dr. med., Zentralklinikum, Neurochirurgie, D-8900 Augsburg

Nowak, G., Dr. med., Univ.-Krankenhaus Eppendorf, Abt. Neurochirurgie, Martinistr. 52, D-2000 Hamburg 20

Nüsslein, B., Dr. med., Neurologische Univ.-Klinik, Schwabachanlage 6, D-8520 Erlangen

Reinhardt, V., Dr. med., Univ.-Klinik, Neurochirurg. Abt., Hufelandstr. 55, D-4300 Essen 1
Renella, R. R., Dr. med., Neurochirurg. Klinik, Med. Hochschule Hannover, Konstanty-Gutschowstr. 9, D-3000 Hannover 61
Richard, K. E., Prof. Dr. med., Neurochirurgische Univ.-Klinik, Josef-Stelzmann-Straße 9, D-5000 Köln 41
Rieden, K., Dr. med., Univ.-Strahlenklinik, Voss-Str. 3, D-6900 Heidelberg
Rittmeyer, K., Prof. Dr. med., Med. Einrichtungen der Univ., Neurochirurgische Klinik, Robert-Koch-Str. 40, D-3400 Göttingen
Roesler, A., Dr. med., Institut für Klinische Strahlenkunde, Univ.-Klinik, Langenbeckstr. 1, D-6500 Mainz 1
Roosen, K., Prof. Dr. med., Neurochirurgische Univ.-Klinik, Hufelandstr. 55, D-4300 Essen 1
Sanker, P., Dr. med., Neurochirurgische Univ.-Klinik, Josef-Stelzmann-Straße 19, D-5000 Köln 41
Schaub, Th., Dr. med., Institut für Klinische Strahlenkunde der Univ.-Klinik, Langenbeckstr. 1, D-6500 Mainz
Schilling, F., Prof. Dr. med., Rheumatologe, (Univ. Mainz), Hebbelstr. 20, D-6500 Mainz-Lerchenberg
Schleich, A., Dr. med., Rheumaklinik Oberammergau, Hubertusstr. 40, D-8103 Oberammergau
Schmitt, H. P., Prof. Dr. med., Institut für Neuropathologie der Universität, Im Neuenheimer Feld 220 – 221, D-6900 Heidelberg 1
Schörner, W., Dr. med., Neurologische Abt., Rudolf-Virchow-Krankenhaus, Augustenburger Platz 1, D-1000 Berlin 65
Schürmann, K., Prof. Dr. Dr. med. h. c., Neurochirurgische Univ.-Klinik, Langenbeckstr. 1, D-6500 Mainz 1
Schumacher, J., cand. med., Neurochirurgische Univ.-Klinik, Langenbeckstr. 1, D-6500 Mainz 1
Schumacher, M., Prof. Dr. med., Abt. Röntgendiagnostik, Sektion Neuroradiologie, Albert-Ludwigs-Univ., Hauptstr. 5, D-7800 Freiburg
Schwarz, M., Dr. med., Neurochirurgische Univ.-Klinik, Langenbeckstr. 1, D-6500 Mainz 1
Seeger, W., Prof. Dr. med., Neurochirurgische Univ.-Klinik, Hugstetter Str. 55, D-7800 Freiburg
Seifert, H., Dr. med., Neurochirurg. Klinik, Allgem. Krankenhaus Heidberg, Tangstetter Landstr. 400, D-2000 Hamburg 62
Seifert, V., Dr. med., Med. Hochschule, Neurochirurgische Klinik, Konstanty-Gutschow-Str. 9, D-3000 Hannover 61
Sollmann, W.-P., Dr. med., Med. Hochschule Hannover, Neurochirurg. Klinik, Konstanty-Gutschow-Str. 9, D-3000 Hannover 61
Steiger, U., Dr. med., Klinik Wilhelm Schulthess, CH-8032 Zürich
Stolke, D., Prof. Dr. med., Med. Hochschule Hannover, Neurochirurg. Klinik, Konstanty-Gutschow-Str. 9, D-3000 Hannover 61
Terwey, B., Dr. med., Chr.-Albrechts-Universität, Abt. Neurochirurgie, Weimarer Str. 8, D-2300 Kiel 1
Thümler, R., Prof. Dr. med., Neurolog. Abt., Landesnervenklinik, Dautenheimer Landstr. 66, D-6508 Alzey
Trauschel, A., Dr. med., Neurochirurg. Univ.-Klinik, Hufelandstr. 55, D-4300 Essen 1
Treig, T., Dr. med., Neurochirurgische Univ.-Klinik, Schwabachanlage 6, D-8520 Erlangen
Trempenau, B., Dr. med., Neurolog. Abt., Rudolf-Virchow-Krankenhaus, Augustenburger Platz 1, D-1000 Berlin 65
Voth, D., Prof. Dr. med., Neurochirurg. Univ.-Klinik, Langenbeckstr. 1, D-6500 Mainz 1
Wackenheim, A., Prof. Dr. med., Service de Radiologie, 1, Place de l'Hôpital, F-67091 Straßbourg Cedex
Wallenfang, Th., Dr. med., Neurochirurg. Univ.-Klinik, Langenbeckstr. 1, D-6500 Mainz 1
Weller, E., Dr. med., Rheumaklinik Oberammergau, Hubertusstr. 40, D-8103 Oberammergau
Westerburg, K. M., Dr. med., Rheumaklinik Oberammergau, Hubertusstr. 40, D-8103 Oberammergau

Author's Index

Subject Index

Bei Fragen zur Produktsicherheit wenden Sie sich bitte an:
If you have any questions regarding product safety,
please contact:

Walter de Gruyter GmbH
Genthiner Straße 13
10785 Berlin
productsafety@degruyterbrill.com